UNINTENDED CONSEQUENCES

A Novel

Copyright © 2007 Alberta L. Mason

ISBN: 978-1-4675-5208-0

Published by:
Mason & Company
321 Englenook Drive
DeBary, Florida 32713
Email: almason@att.net

UNINTENDED CONSEQUENCES is a complete work of fiction. Names, characters, places, and incidents are products of the author's imagination or are used fictitiously. Any resemblance to actual events or locales or persons, living or dead, is entirely coincidental.

Cover Background Art: Shutterstock/Molodec

Cover Design: A.L. Mason

Cover Photograph: A.L. Mason

First Edition Published: 2013

Printed in the United States of America by Lulu.com

Visit Author's Websites: http://albertamason.info/ and http://www.lulu.com/spotlight/albertamason

UNINTENDED CONSEQUENCES

A NOVEL BY

ALBERTA L. MASON

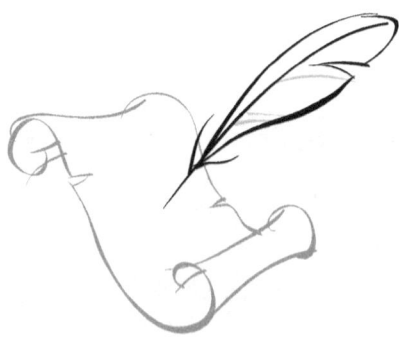

To all the Zingerellas of the world,
carry on.

PROLOGUE
San Francisco ~ 1977

When the private investigator who worked for her father's attorney finally tracked her down, Martina Fiasconi had been hiding out in San Francisco for nearly two years. And although Martina had adopted the use of her uncle's surname after running away, and had taken every possible precaution to conceal her whereabouts she was stunned by how seemingly easy it was for the investigator to locate her. Martina could not even deny she was the daughter of Professor Martino Fiasconi since the determined investigator was armed with a file about two inches thick and an 8x10 glossy of her Millborough High School graduation photo, which he was only too happy to hold up for her inspection. Clutching her eighteen month old son tightly against her chest, she hoped the large framed man did not notice that she was trembling with fear. Even now, more than two years after having fled from her father's stranglehold, the mere mention of his name filled her with a dreadful sense of panic.

"For the record, I must verify that you are indeed Martina Fiasconi, the nineteen year old daughter of Professor Martino Fiasconi," the Private Investigator informed, noticing that the exotically beautiful young woman standing before him had suddenly turned pale and was trembling. "I use the name 'Denault" now," Martina said, with a detectable note of defiance in her soft voice.

The investigator, a results oriented fellow in his mid-forties named Mike Farrell, gave Martina an appraising stare and nodded. He could certainly understand why the trembling young woman would want to change her name, even though she was thousands of miles from her former home. It was entirely possible the bizarre story about her father had made national, if not worldwide, headlines. No one could blame Martina Fiasconi, who now called herself Martina Denault, for disassociating.

Considering the number of times Farrell had seen Martina's photo on the front page of his local newspaper or flashed upon a television screen over the past many months, it felt surreal to actually be in her physical presence. So mythologized had she become by the incredible volume of media coverage, now seeing her in the flesh was like a sighting of the last unicorn. Farrell could not help but be proud of his investigative skills, since it was he who had single handedly traced Martina to the Pacific Heights address, where he was now standing. For the most part, Farrell's mission was impelled by a morbid curiosity. Martina Fiasconi was, after all, a pretty young runaway at the center of a huge scandal, one which did not show any signs of losing the public's interest, and her disappearance was the subject of numerous theories and speculations. Even so, Farrell considered himself a true professional in his field and tried not to unduly stare at the intriguing young woman with the exotic sea-green eyes and flawless caramel skin. Even in the flesh, Farrell noted, Martina Fiasconi looked like the personification of an airbrushed photo from some high-end glamour magazine.

Farrell had traveled all the way from the very traditional New England college town of Millborough, where Martina had once lived with her father, and he was perhaps more familiar than most with the lurid details of the scandal. From the outset of the case, Farrell had the inside advantage of working hand in glove with Vittorio Travante, Esquire, who was Professor Fiasconi's criminal defense attorney. That the people of Millborough were still talking about Martino Fiasconi's fall from grace with shocked disbelief, even these many months after the Professor was sentenced to prison, was no surprise to Farrell. It seemed that the "Fiasconi Fiasco," as Farrell had dubbed the sensational case, was doomed to incite conversation in the parlors, restaurants, and any variety of social gatherings in the town of Millborough, probably until the day the cozy burg ceased to exist.

As it were, Martino Fiasconi had been not only a respected college professor at Wingate University, an Ivy League school established by the purest of the town's blue bloods, and where only the most renowned of scholars were invited to join its faculty, but the man was also an eminent Doctor of Philosophy, having received his letters from the venerable Universita de Roma, in Rome, Italy. The professor's two inch-plus thick Curriculum Vitae that was the veritable A-List of academic and scholarly merit, not the least of which were his long-term postings with the Sorbonne, Cambridge and Harvard, among other hallowed halls of academia. Later, when the sordid speculations of Professor Fiasconi's "unnatural interests" in his young daughter and the attempted murder of the girl's boyfriend had blackened the town's lily white image, the phrase most commonly repeated around town and to the press was, "...*but Doctor Fiasconi came to us with the most impeccable of credentials.*"

Farrell found it difficult to not stare at the little boy Martina was holding, but his investigator's curiosity prodded him to inspect the child's dark curly hair and large green-blue eyes. Farrell was all too familiar with the gossip about Martina's baby and the ugly innuendos as to who its father might be. The most rabid of all the rumors he heard floating around Millborough was the one about some sort of "selective breeding experiment" the Professor had going on. That one really peaked Farrell's interest. He did a lot of poking around to find something – anything – to either confirm or disprove such an outrageous allegation but found nothing to substantiate the hearsay. Facts, not innuendo, were Farrell's guideposts. A good detective, as Farrell was determined to be, could not hang his hat on wagging tongues, so he discounted the numerous rumors he heard about experiments and unconventional relationships as products of either overblown imaginations or very sick minds. Nor could Farrell believe that a man of Fiasconi's background and credentials would be so insane as to impregnate his own daughter, whatever else might have been going on behind the walls of the very private Georgian mansion located on the outskirts of town, where the once respected academic and his teenaged daughter had lived together.

Farrell was not so naïve as to think incest did not occur in polite society, but he had interviewed Professor Fiasconi countless times in preparation for his legal defense and just simply could not believe a man of Fiasconi's dimension, intelligence, and soft temperament would even consider such a thing. The man was so handsome, dignified, and personable, it would seem he could pick and choose from all available women of substance on the entire planet and be assured of captivating any and all of them. Fiasconi was that impressive. But who really knew. Stranger things have happened.

Gut feelings and instincts had a definite place in Farrell's line of work and most often his instincts about people served him well. But the Fiasconi case troubled him immensely. There were too many unanswered questions and unverifiable statements. And while Farrell probably relied on his gut feelings eighty percent of the time, he relied on empirical evidence one hundred percent, which was why he took the time to search through the birth records on file at the Bureau of Vital Records immediately after arriving in San Francisco yesterday morning. Sifting through public records and ferreting out pertinent information were the things Farrell loved most about his job. For Ferrell, it was the meat and potatoes of his investigative work. And yesterday, when he came across the birth record of Martina Fiasconi's son, Roderick McDonough, Jr., it was like a celebratory banquet of

6

prime rib, with a giant baked Idaho potato oozing with butter and sour cream. Farrell nearly jumped out of his chair and did the dance of joy right there in the office of the Bureau of Vital Records.

According to the Certificate of Live Birth he found, Martina's son was born at San Francisco's St. Luke's Hospital on February 28, 1976, about seven months after she ran away, which meant she was indeed pregnant when she left Millborough in July of 1975. The real surprise to Farrell was the name shown on the birth certificate as the baby's father: that of Roderick J. McDonough. But the odd kicker was that McDonough was listed as being "deceased" and the date of his death was recorded as "July 18, 1975", which Farrell knew was the date of McDonough's shooting, and the same date Professor Fiasconi was arrested for having shot McDonough. Farrell wondered if Martina really believed McDonough was dead. Perhaps she had no idea that McDonough had actually survived.

Granted, McDonough was pretty close to death after being shot in the back while riding his motorcycle (in the vicinity of the Fiasconi residence, no less) and subsequently crashing into a tree. The man was laid up in the hospital and then a rehabilitation facility for months afterwards with a head injury and broken bones, but had recovered in time to point a finger at Dr. Fiasconi. In fact, it was McDonough's statement to the police that convinced Dr. Fiasconi that he would be better off to enter a guilty plea and avoid a sensational trial; either way, he knew he was going to jail for attempted murder. In his very brief and only statement to the media about his shooting, Rod McDonough was quoted as saying, "Martino Fiasconi is a sociopath and should be locked up for the rest of his *unnatural* life."

While Farrell waited for the clerk to make him a photocopy of the birth record, he shook his head, truly bewildered. The Fiasconi case had more twists and turns to it than San Francisco's famed Lombard Street.

The entry of Rod McDonough's name on the birth record emphatically answered only one of the several perturbing questions Farrell had about why Martino Fiasconi shot Rod McDonough. Did Fiasconi shoot McDonough because the 22-year old man had impregnated his 17-year old daughter? But what about the revelation that Martina and Rod were secretly married by a justice of the peace and of a nasty juvenile court proceeding that ensued, which basically amounted to a vicious tug of war between Dr. Fiasconi and McDonough? Or was it really a matter of jealous rage borne of incestuous feelings that caused Fiasconi to shoot McDonough? And the

7

fact that McDonough is recorded as the father of Martina's baby is no certain guarantee that he is, in fact, the baby's father. Only a blood test could determine that with any certainty. And therein lay the ongoing problem with the Fiasconi case: It didn't seem that it would ever really be solved. The answer to one question inevitably provoked another question or two. The only thing about the case that was known with any certainty was that Professor Martino Fiasconi shot Rod McDonough, but no one knew for certain why Fiasconi did it. Farrell wished he could forget about the Fiasconi case, but forgetting it was all but impossible. For one thing, Attorney Travante paid him too well to think about it. And the fact of the matter was that he was obsessed with the case. Until every question was answered to his satisfaction and every fact was known he could not walk away from it.

So, it was a bittersweet victory that Farrell located Martina Fiasconi and discovered her baby's birth certificate, and both mother and child were only inches away from him at the moment. The cherub-faced little boy Farrell was now trying not to stare at was obviously the same Roderick McDonough, Jr. whose name appeared on the Certificate of Live Birth, a copy of which Farrell now had in his file. But Farrell doubted the senior Rod McDonough, what little Farrell knew about him, had the slightest idea he had a son. Farrell had to forcibly shake off his meandering thoughts and get back into the moment to respond to her somewhat defiant proclamation that her name was now Denault.

"I understand, Miss...Denault," Farrell said, softening his tone. "But I have to file an Affidavit of Service with the court...so I must ask you for some identification bearing your previous name before I can leave this envelope with you."

Sighing impatiently, Martina quickly glanced at the embossed return address on the envelope and recognized the familiar name of her father's attorney, "Vittorio V. Travante, Esquire."

"What's it about?" She asked, suddenly engulfed with trepidation. "Doctor Fiasconi is in prison...isn't his case closed by now?" She had already been through the emotional ringer with her father, his attorney, the police, the prosecutors, the court system, her court appointed Guardian *ad litem*, the psychologists, and the juvenile case workers. She had no more to give any of them. Why couldn't they just leave her alone?

Farrell noted Martina's annoyed expression and irritated tone, a clear signal that he had better wrap up his mission before she decided to slam the front door in his face. Affecting his most affable don't-shoot-me-I'm-just-the-messenger persona, Farrell sounded sincerely apologetic when he said, "I surely don't know what it's about, Miss Denault. My job is only to find people and deliver envelopes." Then, after a brief pause to flash his most beatific smile, he delivered the line that always seemed to melt the ice crystals for him, "Mr. Travante treats me like the proverbial mushroom, Ma'am... he keeps me in the dark and sprinkles manure on my head." Her expression lightened only slightly. Farrell pressed on. "Do you have any identification with your...uh...other name on it?"

Martina regarded Farrell for a few moments, and he could see she was weighing the merits of his request. He didn't attempt to press her further. Something about Martina's ocean green eyes and caramel complexion triggered Farrell's memory of a knock-out woman he used to see motoring around the streets of Millborough in a bright red Jaguar convertible, her long golden brown hair whipping in the wind like some sort of urban goddess. Back then, Farrell was new in town and not up to speed on the local color, so he had taken to calling the mysterious woman "the Jaguar lady". The woman, who appeared to be in her thirties, stuck in his mind because she, too, had those same strange colored, exotic eyes. Then, one day, Farrell noticed he hadn't seen her around town for a while and wondered what had become of her. The mystery of the Jaguar lady was solved when Farrell took on the investigation of the Fiasconi case. He was astonished to learn the mystical green-eyed woman with the waist length golden brown hair was Professor Fiasconi's wife, Jacqui, the mother of his missing daughter, and the reason she was no longer seen around town was because she had died. Farrell thought it was terribly unfair that someone so beautiful had died so young.

Indeed, according to a news article Farrell had read early on in the case, Jacqui was barely nineteen years old when she made her first sensational debut on a Milan runway and slinked right into the annals of mannequin celebrity. It was the eyes, most all of the photographers who covered her shoots agreed, an amazing sea-green color that was spellbinding, sometimes radiating a strange luminosity that caused people to stare and become entranced. Others, such as the Italian designer to royalty, Alberto D'Oro, opined it was Jacqui's "flawless caramel-hued skin tone" that brought the colors of his signature eveningwear to life. All of that exotic beauty on a five-foot eight-inch frame of lissome elegance immediately captivated the top houses of the fashion and beauty industry throughout Europe. Suddenly, haute couture, from Valentino to Givenchy, were designing their gowns for Jacqui to model, and scrambling to find fabric in the precise shade of green to match her eyes.

Every glossy magazine that catered to the ultra-glamorous feminine lifestyle wanted Jacqui's exotic face on their cover. And she dominated the runways and camera lenses in Europe and New York until her self-imposed exile at the age of twenty-four, when she simply vanished. The article went on to say that months after Jacqui's disappearance it was discovered she was living in Paris with "the eminent philosopher Martino Fiasconi, the guru of the Parisian free-thinking intelligentsia". Her whereabouts came to light when the couple hosted an elaborate dinner party to celebrate their "union of togetherness", and invited the who's who of European academia, the arts and political activism. Apparently, Fiasconi and Jacqui did not believe in traditional marriage ceremonies. Farrell figured it had something to do with their free-thinking lifestyle. The author of the news article, a Thom Yardley-Smith, alleged it was his understanding from sources in the know that Professor Fiasconi had chosen Jacqui for her "exquisite physical features". Farrell had read Yardley-Smith's article months prior to hearing the rumor about Fiasconi's "selective breeding experiment", but even in retrospect he could not give it any credence. What man in his right mind would not be smitten with Jacqui's exquisite physical features? She was an absolute stunner.

And Jacqui's run-away daughter, as Farrell could now see, was every bit as beautiful. "No doubt about it," Farrell would later comment to an interested Vittorio Travante, "Martina Fiasconi could hop right up there on that Milanese runway where her celebrated mother first knocked the fashion world on its ass, pick right up where Jacqui left off, and they probably wouldn't know the difference."

Farrell estimated that Jacqui was only about thirty-nine when she died of cancer. Martina was probably about fifteen at the time. As Farrell studied Martina's face, a bizarre theory began to take shape in his ever probing mind. Perhaps, thought Farrell, that was when all the craziness with the Professor started. After his beautiful, exotic wife died Fiasconi was so bereft he merely latched on to the one person who reminded him the most of Jacqui, her carbon copy daughter, Martina.

Fiasconi was, after all, a free thinker. It was an interesting theory. A sick theory, to be sure, but nonetheless interesting. It might explain why the Professor shot Rod McDonough and why Martina ran away and changed her name. Of course, the theory of an unnatural relationship between the father and daughter was not proven two years ago and it surely could not be proven now. Unless, that is, someone who knew for sure spoke up. The only person who knew for sure was Martina, and her speaking up about it was unlikely at this point. The young woman was obviously trying to move on to a new life, with a new name.

Farrell could have gone on and on with his mental peregrinations but the sound of Martina's voice stopped his mind cold. She had apparently made a decision regarding his request for a Fiasconi identification.

"Just a moment," she said, exhaling a long sigh of resignation. Turning away from Farrell, she walked across the living room and gently placed the little boy in an armchair that just about swallowed him up in its soft cushion. She kissed the top of his head and said something to the boy, but her words were too inaudible for Farrell to make out. Farrell watched her with his obsessed interest as she walked to the other side of the living room. He wished that she was not wearing a floor length skirt.

Farrell snatched another quick look at the little boy, who was now sucking his thumb and eyeing Farrell with suspicion. Even if the rumors of Professor Fiasconi's sexual intimacy with Martina were true, it would be impossible to determine from simply looking at the child whether Fiasconi was the father. Any resemblance the boy may have to his paternal grandfather could be attributable to lineage and not parentage. From the roundness of the child's face, the pale complexion, and dark hair, Farrell wouldn't swear to it in an affidavit but he thought he saw a striking resemblance to Rod McDonough. The only Fiasconi trait he saw in the child was the blue-green eyes, which definitely came from his mother. Professor Fiasconi had dark eyes, an oval face, and a Mediterranean complexion. The child looked nothing like him.

In any event, Doctor Fiasconi was not convicted of the sexual abuse of his daughter. He could not even be charged with such a crime. The police may have had their strong suspicions but they had no hard evidence to support them, and Martina had consistently denied her father ever did anything inappropriate to her. She had even refused to testify against him regarding the solid case the state did have against the disgraced Doctor of Philosophy: that being the attempted murder of Roderick McDonough. And the police did actually have hard and fast evidence of Fiasconi's crime in that regard: they had literally found the smoking gun in the professor's possession.

11

It was always a mystery to Farrell why Martina turned her back on her father if, as she claimed, he had never done anything to deserve her total abandonment. Some speculated she turned on her father because he shot Rod McDonough, but it seemed Martina had also left McDonough in the dust of her rapid departure from Millborough. Of course, if Martina truly believed Rod had been killed by her father, then that would account for her not returning to Millborough to see McDonough during the months he was laid up.

Although Farrell had been privy to a good deal of information by virtue of the investigation he conducted for Attorney Travante, that same investigation actually left many more unanswered questions than those answered, as far as Farrell was concerned. And now, while Farrell watched Martina Fiasconi Denault search for her identification, he consciously clamped his teeth together to keep his mouth shut. There had been a very ugly court battle between two jurisdictions on the subject of Martina's right to privacy, including who could talk to her and about what, and a very strict ruling had been rendered by the presiding judge. Farrell knew he had no standing to speak even one word to Martina about her father's case or why she ran away. If he did, he would undoubtedly lose his investigator's license and maybe even be prosecuted for violating a very strict order of the court, said order having never been challenged or rescinded. As much as he would have liked to find out if she knew Rod McDonough was still alive, Farrell did not dare open his mouth about such a heavily restricted subject. And he had been duly warned by his boss, Travante, not to say or do anything that would instigate the wrath of the court.

As Martina riffled through the compartments of her purse and then her wallet, Farrell's fertile mind was, nonetheless, busy violating the court's order regarding disallowed communication with "MJF (Martina Jacqui Fiasconi), a Minor Child," which was how her original California court case had been titled. Beads of perspiration broke out on Farrell's face and rivulets of sweat ran down his back. If only he could, there were dozens of questions he itched to ask her. At the moment, however, Farrell wished she would hurry up and find the damned ID. It was torture for him to be around her any longer. He had to get out of there. Now! Before he blew it. Unable to take the pressure any more, he blurted, "Have you found the ID?" His voice sounded as strained as he felt.

Nodding affirmatively, Martina slowly removed her Millborough driver's license from a hidden fold in her wallet. When she returned to the front doorway she handed Farrell her original driver's license, which was now expired but bore her photo and the name he needed to see: "Martina Fiasconi."

Farrell eyed the driver's license as a matter of form and nodded his approval. Handing her a typed receipt, he said, "Please sign this receipt, which shows that you did in fact receive Mr. Travante's envelope and I'll be on my way."

After quickly reviewing the receipt, Martina scribbled her signature and handed the paper back to Farrell, wondering why his voice suddenly sounded so strange.

When he handed her the envelope and a copy of the receipt, Farrell said, "Thank you for your time, Miss Denault. Sorry to have bothered you."

Before Martina could make any further comment, Farrell spun around and rushed away.

Closing the front door, Martina stared at the envelope for a long time, too afraid to open it. Since fleeing Millborough, Martina spent countless hours blaming herself for Rod's death. Despite countless hours of therapy and countless reassurances, she could not shake off the feelings of guilt. Guilt was Martina's dogged companion: It shrouded the morning sunrise, shadowed her throughout the day, and lie down with her each night at bedtime. No, she did not pull the trigger on the gun that killed her beloved husband, but what did she do to prevent her father from doing so on July 18, 1975? Instead, she boarded an airplane on that infamous July night and left Rod, the man to whom she had pledged her loyalty, to fend for himself. Now, the specter of her ugly past had stealthily found its way to her front door, bringing with it the old foes she battled so hard to defeat: self-loathing, despair, betrayal. Wasn't it torture enough to be wracked with guilt every time she looked at her fatherless son?

Her atheist father was right about one thing. There is no forgiving God. No all-powerful deity to wipe away the debt of one's ill-conceived actions. Everyone must live with the unintended consequences of their choices.

1.

If it were not for Aunt Catherine and Uncle Jack taking her into their home on that horrific night she fled Millborough, Martina knew her life and the life of her son, Roddy, might have ended tragically. But knowing that fact and accepting it were two different concepts for Martina to make peace with. Each time she suffered a bout of despair and recrimination, her aunt and uncle were quick to remind her that if she had not left Millborough when she did, Martino might have shot her too, and she had her baby to think of. At a rational level, Martina understood that. If it had been a case of simply putting her own life in jeopardy, she should have never left Rod behind to suffer the consequences of her father's insane wrath on July 18, 1975.

But earlier that same day Martina had learned she was pregnant, and her protective, maternal instincts pushed her to flee from the threat of danger. At least that is what she told herself to assuage the guilt she felt about the horrible events that happened that day. If only, Martina told herself over and over, she had handled things differently. She should have never told Martino she was pregnant. Why did she even think he would be happy about such a thing? Her father hated Rod McDonough. But hindsight, as it is so often said, is twenty-twenty.

On that hot, sticky July afternoon when all hell broke loose in the normally peaceful town of Millborough, Martina was only seventeen years old, but her life had already spun seriously out of control. She had gone behind Martino's back and secretly married Rod McDonough months before her high school graduation. Her attempts to appease both a controlling father and a husband who was eager to start their life together ignited a firestorm of hatred between the two men. While Rod battled with Professor Fiasconi in court for Martina's legal custody, the judge trumped them both when he declared Martina a ward of the court, and placed her in a group home for juveniles until either the legality of her marriage could be determined or she turned eighteen, when she would no longer be a minor. No one was happy with that arrangement, least of all Martina, who wanted to be with Rod.

Seething with fury, Martino Fiasconi, however, had other designs for the "experimental child" he raised to be intellectually superior. In his deteriorating mental state he considered Martina more of a legal possession than a person, and it was unthinkable to the Professor that she be placed by the court into what he thought of as a "barracks occupied by the lowest elements of society". He pleaded to the court for Martina to be returned to his custody, despite Rod's photographic proof of horrific physical abuse, and demanded Rod McDonough be jailed for statutory rape. But Professor Fiasconi's usually persuasive arguments and theories had no traction with the presiding judge, who couldn't help but notice that never once did Professor Fiasconi refer to Martina as his daughter or with any expression of heartfelt love.

The proverbial straw that broke Dr. Fiasconi's back, or his tenuous grip on reality, was Martina's elated news on the morning of the shooting that she was expecting Rod McDonough's child. Keeping his cool long enough to trick Martina into his car, her father drove her to a clinic on the outskirts of Millborough and insisted she immediately have an abortion performed. To his rapidly disintegrating mind, there was no way his "genetically perfect" daughter would have the child of "a motorcycle-riding baboon". After leaving Martina at the clinic, Fiasconi then went in search of Rod McDonough to exact his revenge for impregnating Martina. Luckily, Martina was able to escape from the clinic and make her way to a telephone. She attempted to call Rod at his house several times, but he had apparently left to pick her up for their afternoon "date". Panicked, Martina knew she had to get out of Millborough before her father discovered she was on the run and then began looking for her. Millborough was a small town, with few places for her to hide. Terrified and determined to protect her unborn child at all costs, she did the only thing she could think of to do, she placed a collect call to her Aunt Catherine, who lived in San Francisco.

Certainly, Martina could not tell her Aunt over the phone the full story behind her desperate need to leave Millborough. For one thing, it would take far too long. And for another, her Aunt might not want to get into the middle of such a sordid and complex family matter. But just as Martina launched into a tearful, but carefully edited, summary of her straits, her Aunt calmed her down and said she didn't need to hear any reasons for the visit, it was enough that Martina wanted to be with her.

After all, Catherine thought, the poor child was approaching her womanhood without the guidance of a mother, and what little she knew of her deceased sister's husband she could certainly understand her niece's anxiety. So, without question, Catherine immediately arranged for Martina to fly to San Francisco that very day, and she and her husband, Jack Denault, were waiting for Martina at the San Francisco Airport when the girl arrived, bringing only the clothing she was wearing and, of course, her unborn child.

Aunt Catherine was not just the sister of Martina's deceased mother, she was Jacqui's identical twin. Perhaps it was that close connection that made it easier for Martina to relate to her Aunt, even though Catherine was the extreme opposite of her eclectic twin. As maturing young women, Jacqui had been utterly flamboyant about her striking beauty, whereas Catherine was always more understated about her own exotica. Oddly, these incredible looking women came into the world as scrawny, premature babies that no one thought would even survive the first few days of their lives. And their origin seemed the lore from which fairy tales were spun: they were the offspring of a marriage between a red-headed, blue-eyed Merchant Marine sea captain named Duncan MacPherson and a beautiful young native woman he had discovered on a remote, South Seas island, where he had steered his ship for refuge during a bad storm. At first, Captain MacPherson tried bartering with the village elders for the bewitching girl, offering them various foodstuffs, liquor, and even a pig or two, but he was unable to make the trade. So when the storm cleared and it was time for MacPherson's vessel to move on, the Captain and his crew literally kidnapped the beautiful girl, whom MacPherson knew only as Lani, from her village. At the end of his voyage, MacPherson brought Lani back to his home port of San Diego, where she spent her days pining for her people and the lush, tropical island where she was born. San Diego, despite its palm trees and proximity to the ocean, was no substitute for a *Shangri La*.

It was the combination of their parents' opposite coloring that produced Jacqui's and Catherine's perpetually tanned skin, smooth and flawless as it was, and those sea green eyes that always reminded Lani of the color of the ocean surrounding the island where she had once lived. Unfortunately, the twins spent very little time with their mother, because the woman was basically dysfunctional in the modern world, where she thought of electric lights as demons, and the sight of water running from a faucet was beyond her comprehension, so they were raised by their paternal grandparents, who lived in San Francisco. Lani died not too many months after her babies were taken from her. Captain MacPherson went back to his life on the sea, where he eventually disappeared—perhaps the victim of a shipwreck.

When they were only eighteen, Jacqui and Catherine were discovered by Françoise Sandoval, the creative genius behind Les Femmes Mannequin, one of the world's most prestigious modeling agencies, specializing in uniquely stunning women for specialty events

16

and live advertising displays. To get them started, Sandoval first placed them for a Doublemint chewing gum commercial and that one appearance launched them into very successful modeling careers. At nineteen, the twins were the two most highly sought after models on the scene and doing photo shoots all over the world, sometimes working together and at other times they were each in different corners of the globe. They were making a lot of money but had no time to enjoy it.

It was during a photo shoot in front of the Louvre, in Paris, that Jacqui caught the eye of Dr. Martino Fiasconi, a handsome, young philosophy professor who was lecturing at the Sorbonne. Fiasconi made it his business to negotiate an introduction to the exotically beautiful Jacqui and, as it turned out, his timing could not have been better. Suffering from extreme burn-out, Jacqui was more than ready to chuck the frenetic pace of being a top model for the promise of a more languorous life as the trophy companion to a renowned college professor. Soon after her first date with Martino Fiasconi, Jacqui suddenly dropped off the fashion world's radar. The chatter of the literati, the frequent rounds of cocktail parties, and stately three course diners were more to Jacqui's liking. That was how she eventually wound up living in a Georgian mansion in Millborough and driving a red Jaguar convertible.

Catherine, on the other hand, continued with her modeling career until younger, fresher faces emerged to claim her eminent position. By then, however, she had learned all the tricks of the trade from Sandoval and assembled her own agency, setting up shop amidst the upscale dens of interior design on Hotaling Place, directly across the chic alley from the rear entrance to the law office of the redoubtable Elvin Jonas, San Francisco's "King of Courts". Jonas, it seemed, had a keen eye for glamorous women, and after seeing Catherine entering her office on a few occasions, he decided to stop in one afternoon to introduce himself to his beautiful new neighbor. Catherine was too grounded to be taken in by Jonas's mystique and legendary status, but she did find him to be a very endearing man. So, when he invited her to attend one of his famous Solstice parties she heard herself promising to attend even though her good senses told her to steer clear of the gray-haired barrister.

It was at Elvin Jonas's Spring Solstice Party that Catherine met Jack Denault, a wealthy Montgomery Street stock broker, and his friend, Jake ("call me Shotgun") Mitchell. Six months later, Catherine married Jack Denault, and it was really a marriage made in heaven. A pregnant

Jacqui flew out from Boston, where she and Martino were living at the time, to be the Matron of Honor and Shotgun served as Jack's Best Man. It was a small, but wonderful wedding, held under the golden dome of the Palace of Fine Arts, a picture perfect site. Later, there was a sit down banquet at the Mark Hopkins Hotel, on Knob Hill, which had been secretly arranged by Elvin Jonas as a surprise to the newly married couple.

And, so, it was into this sophisticated world of modeling, stock brokers, and larger than life attorneys that Martina landed, literally, via airplane, with only the shirt on her back, scars on her soul, and a baby in her womb. Since Aunt Catherine was also the only living relative Martina had, aside from the man who fathered her, Martina had no other options but to settle into the rather conventional lifestyle of the Denault household. Although, after what Martina had been through since the death of her mother, the unfaltering equilibrium of the Denaults was exactly what she needed in order to begin the healing process. Thus, it didn't take long for Martina and her Aunt to become very close. And she became extremely fond of her Uncle Jack, too. Since Jack and Catherine were never able to have children of their own, for whatever the reason, the arrival of Martina fulfilled their long standing wish for parenthood. And since they were now too old for the diaper scene anyway, a child of Martina's age suited them just fine.

Martina had not as yet told them she was pregnant and worried about how and when to deliver that bit of news. As it turned out, she did not have to.

It seemed the perfect arrangement for Jack, Catherine, and Martina, but the family merger was not without some inherent difficulties. First of all, there were the normal issues of readjustment and realignment that had to be dealt with. While the Denaults restored order and security to Martina's existence, their own lives were turned upside down in the process. But those were only the good, solvable issues. There soon came to light some horribly shocking issues that proved very daunting for the neophyte "parents." Within days of Martina's arrival they found out why the distraught girl was in such a hurry to leave Millborough. Jack and Catherine had just finished eating their usual light breakfast, and Jack was about to leave for his impeccably appointed Montgomery Street brokerage firm, when the telephone rang. Jack answered the call and was astonished when the caller identified himself as an Assistant District Attorney in Millborough, and proceeded to advise Jack of Martino Fiasconi's arrest, for what Jack understood was murder. While the prosecutor refused to elaborate on the details of the ongoing murder investigation, he was more communicative about the status of Martina, advising the Denaults they were harboring an important witness for the state's prosecution of Fiasconi. And if the news about the arrest of their brother-in-law for murder wasn't shocking enough to the conservative Denaults, who never even so much as watched crime dramas on television, the Millborough prosecutor went on to say he was convinced Martina had been sexually abused by her father and the baby she was carrying might possibly be her father's child. (The Prosecutor had not as yet uncovered the fact of Martina's justice of the peace marriage to Rod McDonough, so the Denaults' were spared for the moment that additional shock.) The prosecutor demanded Jack and Catherine to forthwith return Martina to the Millborough jurisdiction, so they could conduct blood tests, depose her, and have her testify against her father. And just to show them he meant business, the Assistant District Attorney crisply advised that he would bring his Subpoena power to bear on the Denaults if they did not comply.

So, that was how the Denaults found out Martina was pregnant, and possibly by her own father, a revelation that sent them reeling in shock. It was a stark introduction to the chaotic world of their niece, which apparently trailed her straight to their front door.

Similarly, Martino Fiasconi's defense attorney, Vittorio Travante, wanted his chance to depose Martina and have her testify on behalf of her father. John and Catherine were appalled by the idea of a seventeen year old, who was still a child in their opinion, being pulled from pillar to post by two warring factions in a serious criminal proceeding, and they decided they would have none of it, neither for Martina nor themselves.

Then along came the civil attorney hired by Roderick McDonough's family to represent the impaired man's interests. That attorney weighed in as also wanting to depose Martina with an eye to establishing that the baby she was expecting was not the progeny of his client, and, further, that Martino Fiasconi shot his client to keep McDonough from interfering in his incestuous affair with his daughter. Since her Uncle and Aunt were themselves confused about the complexities of the numerous legal issues, they decided to keep Martina shielded from any knowledge of this particular litigation, as well as much of the other legal wrangling. It was due to the Denaults' desires to sequester Martina from the Millborough attorneys and

Martino's prosecution that she did not learn that Rod McDonough had survived her father's attempted homicide.

Jack and Catherine viewed the three Millborough attorneys as akin to a pack of rabid wolves circling a wounded fawn, each wolf intent on getting the greater share of the carcass. And the analogy was fairly accurate. In order to protect Martina from a veritable feeding frenzy of lawyers they hired their own top gun attorney, their good friend Jake "Shotgun" Mitchell, who immediately petitioned the court to have John and Catherine appointed as Martina's legal guardians, which was so ordered by the hearing judge. The judge also appointed a Guardian *ad litem* for Martina, to make certain the teenager had her own legal counsel to look out for her interests.

Then taking matters a step further, Shotgun Mitchell motioned the court for psychological counseling for Martina in view of the harrowing experiences she had recently suffered, citing the murder charges against her father, the shooting of her friend, her pregnancy, and the general uprooting of her life as causes necessitating such counseling, as well as a protective order disallowing any and all further communications with Martina by any attorneys or their representatives associated with the criminal charges pending against Martino Fiasconi.

The court granted Shotgun's various motions without reservation. Three oddball attorneys from the Bay Area were hired by the Millborough lawyers to represent their respective interests and appeared at Shotgun's properly noticed hearing to raise objections. The judge sided wholeheartedly with Shotgun's persuasive argument that Martina was in a fragile emotional state, and forthwith issued a comprehensive protective order accordingly. Of course, the Millborough Prosecutor's Office went ballistic over Shotgun's protective order and immediately filed a barrage of motions to get the order rescinded.

2.

Martina had never before met anyone quite like Jake Shotgun Mitchell. He was a far cry from the refined gentry she was used to being around in Millborough. Shotgun was given to loud guffaws and brash behavior, and he frequently appeared wearing stained, wrinkled suits along with his signature snakeskin cowboy boots. He also had a rather obnoxious habit of eyeing people up and down until they withered under his steely-eyed scrutiny. And Mitchell was not above indulging in the most self-serving of braggadocio without the least bit of shame.

The first time Martina met Shotgun she automatically liked and trusted him. She somehow knew that Shotgun was a force to be reckoned with. Of course, she always addressed him as "Sir" or "Mr. Mitchell," which tickled Shotgun to no end. Martina overheard him tell her Uncle Jack that hardly anyone ever called him "sir." "Most everyone calls me a lousy SOB," he announced with great pride one night after a dinner at the Denaults' home. "If my fellow lawyers start calling me 'sir,' I'd better start worrying that I've lost my ability to strike fear into their blackened hearts."

Shotgun was apparently an old friend of her Uncle Jack's, and he came to visit her uncle often. The two men would sit in her uncle's study for hours on end, where the fully stocked liquor cabinet was situated, and proceed to analyze and then solve the problems of the world. Mostly, it was Mitchell pontificating on the follies of the world at large. Martina didn't know whether it was Uncle Jack's patient company or his ample supply of Scotch that routinely brought Shotgun to the house. Whatever the attraction, Martina looked forward to Shotgun's visits. His constant barrage of stories about this sorry-assed lawyer or that tinhorn judge, interspersed with a few raw jokes and cackles, kept her enthralled and amused. She noticed that when Shotgun was within earshot, and he didn't have to be all that close in order to be heard, she completely forgot about all the hurt and anger that usually haunted her thoughts. Her Aunt Catherine did not think it was fitting for Martina to be listening to Shotgun's ribald stories and jokes, so after politely acknowledging Shotgun's presence Martina would excuse herself and sneak off to the dining room (which was only across the hall from the study), and pretend to be busy with some sort of worthwhile project. Luckily, Aunt Catherine would be too enthralled with listening to Shotgun herself to notice that Martina was positioned where she could overhear Shotgun's every off-color word.

Unbeknownst to Martina, it was Shotgun who had insisted that her Aunt and Uncle keep her insulated from all the legal bickering and wrangling going on between him and "those two-bit Millborough bottom feeders," as he liked to call the lawyers back there. He suggested they get Martina back to school and doing the usual things that teenage girls do. "Yep," Shotgun ordered Jack and Catherine, "get some normalcy and routine back in that young girl's life." And so they did.

Then one day Shotgun stopped by the house and to Martina's surprise he announced that he had come by to have a chat with her. Aunt Catherine ushered them into the living room and retreated. Martina felt somewhat nervous because he had refused her Aunt's offer for a glass of Scotch; she figured he was about to deliver some bad news. But Shotgun was not the kind of person who'd let anyone sit wondering for long.

"Just wanted to let you know that I have succeeded in neutralizing that snarling pack of jackals back there in that rinky-dink town…what's its name again? Oh, yeh— Swillborough. They won't be hassling you any more."

Martina wanted to burst out laughing when he called her hometown "Swillborough," but didn't want to appear disrespectful. So, she merely said, "Thank you, sir," and bit her lip.

"Now…," he said, leaning forward as if he were about to advise her of a plea bargain, "In order to get the judge to go along with my motion protecting you from those Ivy League pantywaists, I had to really lay it on thick. I told the judge that you were not able to participate in their three ring circus because you were too traumatized by your father's arrest and such …which I'm sure you are all-in-all…but I took the liberty of advising the judge that you will be needing extensive psychological counseling in order to overcome your traumas, and until we get an all-clear from your counselor it would be injurious to you to have those jackals slobbering all over you in depositions and such. Don't you agree?"

Martina nodded in agreement, even though she was not sure about the counseling business. But she liked the fact that an important lawyer like Shotgun Mitchell would take the time to sit down with her and explain what was going on.

"So…if you wouldn't mind, Miss Martina…I'd appreciate it if you would go along with the program and humor the judge by going to see a good friend of mine who specializes in young women such as yourself…her name is Dr. Chloe Renfrew. And I'm going to tell you right now that there is nothing you can't tell her that she probably hasn't heard before…so don't hold back. She sure as shoot won't be shocked." Shotgun paused in his spiel for a moment to do one of those eye scrutiny things, but this one was quite mild considering what he was capable of. He then added, "And whatever you tell her is confidential, so don't worry that she will be telling anyone else…not even the court can know."

Martina was so flattered by his appeal she could hardly go against his wishes. "Yes, sir. I'll go see her. I wouldn't want the judge to get mad at you because of me."

Shotgun slapped both of his knees so hard Martina could almost feel the pain in her own body. "That's the spirit, girl. Keep me out of trouble with the judges. I ought to get you to come to work for me." With that, he let out a few loud guffaws and then stood up. He placed one of his huge hands on her shoulder. His touch was gentle and his hand was warm and comforting. "You know, Martina— you've got a beautiful, whole new life waiting ahead for you. You go live that life and make the most of it. Just make sure you leave everything that happened back there in old Swillborough behind. Don't take any of that with you. Got it?"

Martina smiled up at Shotgun appreciatively and nodded her understanding. There was the kindest expression she had ever seen in his keen blue eyes. She had just witnessed the softer side of Shotgun that few, if any, knew existed.

In keeping with her promise to Shotgun, but mostly out of reverence for him, Martina immediately began her counseling sessions with Dr. Chloe Renfrew, a child psychologist who specialized in counseling young women who had suffered sexual abuse, although Martina was not aware of Dr. Renfrew's specialty. As far as Martina was concerned, she was only seeing the psychologist to keep Shotgun from getting in trouble with the San Francisco judge handling her case; she had even taken it upon herself to call Dr. Renfrew's office and make her first appointment. Her Aunt Catherine was delighted that Martina took the initiative, but insisted upon accompanying her niece to the first appointment, just to be certain Martina would be in good hands. Martina followed along obediently, but she had already steeled herself for whatever lie ahead in the psychologist's office. Her lines were all scripted and memorized. No one would ever be allowed access to the thick-walled vault she had mentally constructed within herself, in which she had sealed the events of her life after her mother died. But nothing about Chloe Renfrew or her office, an indoor re-creation of a sylvan glade (complete with verdant foliage and a bubbling fountain), was as Martina expected. For all intents and purposes, they found themselves standing in the forest primeval, even though they were actually on the twelfth floor of a downtown San Francisco office building. Even the furniture was made from rough-hewn pieces of wood. All that was missing was the troll under a bridge, but Dr. Renfrew's diminutive hippy receptionist could have easily qualified as the resident troll.

The wary pair was still gawking around in awe of the high-rise forest surrounding them when Dr. Renfrew made her entrance into the arborous outer office through a door that had been incorporated into the trunk of a giant *faux* tree, with leafy branches that obscured the ceiling above it. The woman was short and pudgy, with long, frizzy hair that had been dyed an outlandish color of crimson. Once the shock of the hair color wore off, Martina noticed the Doctor had plump rosy cheeks and sparkling cerulean eyes, which gave her an impish, jovial expression that was at once disarming. She walked toward them with such a light, bouncy gait, it appeared that she might spring upward, above their heads, at any moment like a helium filled balloon. Martina's immediate impression of the Doctor was that she looked like a Hobbit, or at least like what Martina thought a Hobbit would look like in the flesh, albeit wearing a long denim jumper over a tie-dyed jersey.

"Greetings!" Dr. Renfrew called to them, as she bounced across the woven straw rug, wearing multi-colored striped stockings, but no shoes, and thrust her arms outward as though she were welcoming two wayfarers to the Lost Realm of Arnor.

True to her form, Aunt Catherine stood up and extended her hand to the elfin doctor, acting as though the meeting was taking place at the rather posh San Francisco Garden Club, and a tree trunk with a door standing inside of an office suite was an everyday sighting. "I'm Catherine Denault...Martina's aunt.

"It's such a pleasure to meet you after all of the wonderful things Jake Mitchell has told us about you." Martina marveled at her Aunt's ability to maintain her mantle of composure no matter what situation she was thrust into. She knew her ultra conservative Aunt had to be wondering what kind of kook this Dr. Renfrew might actually be.

Chloe Renfrew smiled graciously. "Ah! Yes. Good old Shotgun. We go back a few years…a very good man, he is indeed." The lilt of her Irish brogue seemed to go right along with the bucolic setting and her Hobbit-like appearance. Then turning to Martina, Dr. Renfrew took hold of the young girl's hand and gently squeezed it. The doctor's sparkling eyes radiated a warm, genuine kindness. "And might you be the beautiful and bright Martina that Mr. Mitchell has praised so highly?"

Martina blushed. "A pleasure to meet you, Ma'am."

Suddenly, Martina felt a wonderful energy coming from Dr. Renfrew, and she knew right then she was going to like the strange hobbity woman that stood beaming before her.

After the introductions and the usual exchange of pleasantries, Catherine told Martina she would be back in two hours and excused herself. And wasting no time, Dr. Renfrew then ushered Martina through the door of the faux tree and into her counseling room, which was designed to look as though they were actually inside the trunk of a hollow tree. Even the room's three windows were made to look like natural holes in the tree's trunk. Looking around in amazement, Martina concluded that Dr. Renfrew was either obsessed with the fantasies of J.R.R. Tolkien or she had designed her office while tripping on LSD.

Although the two upholstered reclining chairs looked somewhat out of place inside of a tree, once Martina nestled into one of them she understood why they were there. After only a few minutes of reclining in the soft comfort of the chair, the illusion of being snug, safe, and protected inside the trunk of a mighty tree became real, and Martina felt as though she could stay there forever. She had even forgotten about why she was there in the first place, nor could she remember the last time she felt so relaxed. Suddenly, Martina became aware of the soft sounds of birds chirping and light rain falling outside the tree. A pleasant aroma, like spring flowers, filled the air. Dr. Renfrew, Martina noticed, was reclining in the other chair, looking as though she was about to fall asleep. Martina wondered if this was the extent of what people did in these sessions: simply relaxed and listened to the sounds of nature. But she was not left to wonder about it for long.

The first few sessions were spent talking about safe topics, such as clothes, hairstyles, school, movies, and the like. Just basically getting to

25

know each other. When Dr. Renfrew attempted to broach the subject of Martina's pregnancy, Martina clammed up. But Dr. Renfrew was an expert at gaining her patients' trust and breaking down barriers. Even though Dr. Renfrew had been thoroughly briefed by Shotgun Mitchell concerning all aspects of Martina's case, she had also taken the time to read all of the pertinent information in the voluminous court file. She wanted Martina to open up and talk about the death of her mother, the actual extent of her father's abuse, the shooting, the expected baby, everything. She could see the girl was holding it all inside and slowly suffocating herself.

Martina proved to be a hard nut to crack. It wasn't until five sessions into her counseling that Dr. Renfrew was able to get Martina talking about her plans for a career after the baby was born, that subject naturally gave way to more personal discussion.

"What about your baby's father?" Dr. Renfrew asked. "Wouldn't he like to participate in raising the child?"

In a clipped, almost emotionless voice, Martina responded, "He's dead. Martino...my father...shot him." That was when Martina finally broke down and cried—a long, soul wrenching cry. It was a major breakthrough for both the counselor and the patient, because Martina had kept those tears stuffed inside for such a long, long time.

Dr. Renfrew emitted a barely audible sigh of relief. As far as she knew, this was the first time Martina had opened up in front of anyone. She did not speak until after all of Martina's tears had dried up. Now that Martina had finally introduced the subject of her father, Dr. Renfrew intended to pursue it.

Then, deliberately staring up at the ceiling, she calmly asked, "Why do you suppose your father shot your husband, Rod?"

"Because he did not want me to be with Rod or have his baby," Martina answered.

Still staring upward, Dr. Renfrew nodded pensively. Then she said, "Did your father love you in a way that was more than just fatherly?"

"No— Not really."

Dr. Renfrew could feel that Martina seemed to be getting ready to say something else, so she remained quiet and closed her eyes.

"I think Martino was confused about things. I— I think I confused him."

When Martina didn't further explain herself immediately, Dr. Renfrew probed with a questioning "Oh?" She heard Martina draw in a deep, ragged breath.

"When Jacqui...my mother...died, Martino was very sad. I think he was really depressed. My parents were different from most parents, but they were a lot alike in their thinking...so Martino was really broken up over her death. One night...I heard him crying in his room and I felt so bad for him. I wanted to do something to make him feel better. So...I...uh...I found a nightgown that had been Jacqui's...it was Martino's favorite because it matched the green color of her eyes. I put on the gown and went to his room and...I got into bed with him. I put my arms around him...to...to comfort him. I think he thought I was Jacqui, because he called me by her name. When he began kissing me and touching me I did not stop him...I just wanted him to stop crying. I really didn't mean for it to happen...."

Her words abruptly stopped and she sounded as though she was going to cry again.

The psychologist and her patient sat quiet, each into their thoughts, for the next several minutes. Dr. Renfrew noted how the girl called her parents by their first names, instead of "Mom" or "Dad," as most children do. She wondered if the Fiasconis' were that new breed of parents who raised their child as an equal member of the family, as opposed to the usual parent-child structure. Dr. Renfrew had previously dealt with a few young patients who were the confused spawn of such progressive thinking.

When Dr. Renfrew finally broke the silence she did it with the softest, gentlest voice possible. "Do you think it was possible for your father not to know the difference between you and your mother?"

Martina jumped to Martino's defense. "I think he was in so much grief that he was confused. Jacqui and I were about the same size and we looked a lot alike."

It was not uncommon for abused children to defend their abuser, and Dr. Renfrew had experienced that phenomenon in her counseling many, many times before. It was a form of Stockholm syndrome – a condition experienced by some children, who, after having been abused for an extended period of time, begin to identify with and even feel sympathetic toward their abuser. No doubt Martina was assuming all of the guilt as well.

"Is that why you refused to tell the police about it? Because you felt responsible?"

"Yes. I confused him." Her mumbled words and lowered head conveyed the shame she felt.

"Did it only happen that one time?" asked the Doctor.

"No. There were other times."

"Do you think your father was confused those other times, too?"

"I don't know. I think he just wanted Jacqui back and I was the closest thing to her."

Dr. Renfrew was surprised by the intelligence of Martina's observation. "Did either you or your father attempt to stop it?"

"Yes. I did. About six months after we…afterward. That's when I met Rod and we started seeing each other…having regular dates…I told Martino that it wasn't right for us to be having…uh…to be so close. At first, he got upset but then he agreed that we needed to stop. That was just before he shot Rod and was arrested …and I came here to San Francisco. I don't think Martino really wanted to let go."

Now it was time to ask Martina the big question, and Dr. Renfrew needed to carefully couch it. "Martina…I need to ask you an important question. If you feel uncomfortable with answering it, then just tell me that you don't want to answer it. Okay?"

Martina nodded her head slowly, a wary expression coming across her face.

"How do you know your father is not the father of your baby?"

The tense expression on Martina's face visibly dissipated.

"That's an easy one, Dr. Renfrew," she said, almost smiling.

"How so?" Asked Dr. Renfrew, surprised by Martina's light-hearted, school-girlish response to such a serious subject.

The girl was so mature in many other ways it was easy to forget she was, after all, only a teenager.

"Because Martino had a vasectomy after I was born. He and Jacqui didn't want any more kids."

Now it was Dr. Renfrew's turn to relax. She had been really concerned about the medical and social ramifications of Martina having a child who was the offspring of an incestuous relationship. The Doctor masked her sigh of relief with a throat-clearing sound.

"But even if—" Martina cut off her words abruptly, not sure she wanted anyone to know the details of what happened between her and the man who was supposed to be her father.

Chloe Renfrew looked over at the girl, hoping she would finish the sentence. The Psychologist could easily read the changing expressions on Martina's face and knew the girl was struggling with her thoughts. Renfrew thought it best to remain quiet and let Martina process whatever it was that appeared to be troubling her. The strategy paid off when Martina suddenly blurted, "Even if he wasn't…uh…able …there was no chance of me getting pregnant because we didn't ever have real sex."

Dr. Renfrew stifled the impulse to spring forward in her chair. She was flummoxed by Martina's bombshell revelation. If they did not have "real" sex, then what variation of sexual contact did they engage in? Despite her peaked impulses, she maintained a calm, even tone when she said, "I'm not sure I understand what you mean by that."

Unfortunately, Dr. Renfrew would not get the clarification she hoped for during that particular session, because Martina flatly announced, "I don't feel comfortable with talking about what happened…with Martino."

The truth of the matter was that Martina's unwillingness to discuss "what happened with Martino" stemmed from her own confusion and self-loathing as the result of what did, or did not, happen with Martino. She wished she could blot it all from her mind, but the confusion and blame she felt was as strong as ever. Not even the passing of time diminished the intensity of guilt she felt from being the one who had initiated the affair with Martino, as well as the one who was responsible for Rod getting shot. Every night, she fell asleep under the weight of the guilt and when she awoke in the morning she still felt pressed down by it. All that kept her going was the baby that was growing inside of her. Rod's baby. A tiny glimmer of hope that grew bigger every day.

Dr. Renfrew understood that Martina was grappling with a two-headed tiger, but did not want to risk compromising the trust and confidence she had painstakingly built up with her patient by pushing too fast and too hard. In its own time, the Doctor hoped, the subject of her patient's relationship with her father would seamlessly open up for discussion.

Switching to what she knew was a safer topic with Martina, that being anything to do with her coming baby, she asked, "Did Rod McDonough know you were pregnant with his child?"

"No," Martina said, looking pathetically downcast. "I was going to tell him that same day…the day he was shot. We were supposed to get together in the afternoon. Rod was going to come over to my father's house and we were going to go riding on his motorcycle. But that morning I made the big mistake of telling Martino I was pregnant. I thought if he knew about the baby it would help him to put our…everything…in the past. I thought he would be okay with it because we had talked about…things, and Martino had even started dating a woman he'd met at school. Another professor. So I felt okay about telling him." She paused and emitted a deep sigh, then continued. "But instead of being happy about it, Martino went berserk and said I would have to get an abortion. He called some doctor he knew who had a clinic where they did abortions and made the arrangements for me to go in that same afternoon." She paused to get her emotions in check. She had not told anyone, other than Julie, who was her only close friend in Millborough, about Martino taking her to the abortion clinic. Not even her Aunt. And talking about it now brought back all of the raw feelings of the fear and anger she had felt that day.

Picking up the thread of her story, she went on. "I told him that he could not force me to have an abortion because Rod and I were married and it was Rod's baby, too. That only made Martino even madder since he had filed a Complaint with the court against Rod because I was a minor...Martino said my marriage to Rod wasn't legal. At that time, everything happening in my life was a big mess, Dr. Renfrew. And Martino...he didn't care about anything except getting me to the clinic that afternoon. There was no sense trying to argue with him because I could see that he was acting crazy. So, I went along with him as a way of getting out of the house and going someplace where I hoped I could get away from him. He drove me to the clinic and made sure I was signed in and then he left, saying he would pick me up when it was over."

It seemed that Martina had put herself into a terrible funk with the telling of her story, so Dr. Renfrew felt it would be a good time to end the session. But before doing so, she said, "I think you are a very brave and strong young woman, Martina. I don't believe I have ever before met anyone in my years of practice who has been through what you have encountered in your young life and managed to keep themselves so together."

Through her tears, Martina beamed at the Hobbit woman.

"Thank you, Dr. Renfrew, but I don't know how together I am."

"Do me a favor, kiddo. Drop the "Doctor Renfrew moniker and call me 'Chloe.' And trust me when I tell you that you are one together young lady."

Martina blushed, speechless. It just figured that Shotgun Mitchell would know someone like Chloe Renfrew, she thought. It was then Martina decided that she truly liked Chloe Renfrew and wanted to live up to Chloe's opinion of her: that of being a strong and together young lady. For the sake of her baby she would have to be.

3.

Over the past two and a half years a strong friendship had grown between Martina and Chloe Renfrew. Chloe tried to help Martina work through the "dating block," as Chloe called it, and offered to introduce Martina to a young man she knew who was the vice president of a bank, whom she touted as "hot and handsome," but Martina begged off. She just wasn't ready to date and didn't know when she would be. Right now, she was only interested in raising her son and pursuing her modeling career, which was really starting to take off, thanks to her Aunt Catherine.

Running her hand over the soft curls on Roddy's head, she said, "Let's go get lunch my little man." Roddy was now pulling at the front of her blouse with his pudgy little fingers, trying to get at the lunch that he knew awaited him under the layers of cloth that covered his mother's breasts. Martina knew what was on the boy's mind and she tried to distract him with his favorite stuffed toy. He wanted no part of the toy and continued with his quest to open the blouse. She removed his hand and stood up. "C'mon, Roddy-boy," she cajoled, "let's go get some lunch." She held a hand out to him but he slapped it away.

"No!" He cried, about to pitch a fit.

"Mama's got your favorite soup in the kitchen. Let's go get some soup and crackers."

Martina started to walk off toward the kitchen, hoping Roddy would follow along without a fuss, as he had done a few times in the past when she used the distraction tactic. Such would not be the case today. The little boy began to wail as though his heart was breaking. Roddy was almost eighteen months old and he still insisted on nursing. Martina was beginning to wonder if she would ever get him off her breast and onto a sippy cup. Her Aunt Catherine and Dr. Chloe were on her case about it all the time. "What are you going to do," Chloe chided her just the other day, "go off to kindergarten with him, so you'll be handy?"

And it was embarrassing when he went after her in public and then made a scene whenever she told him "no." She worried that there was something wrong with him, but both her Aunt and Chloe had assured her there was nothing wrong with Roddy; it was his mother who had the problem. And Martina knew they were right. She was indeed the problem. She couldn't stand to tell him "no" or to see him cry. After all, the poor little boy had no father and she felt obligated to make up for that deficit. It was her own feelings of guilt that misguided her judgment.

Once, about a month ago, when she and Roddy were having Sunday dinner at her Aunt's and Uncle's house, Roddy had thrown a tantrum at the table when she thwarted his attempts to nurse. Her Aunt Catherine was in the process of rendering her opinion that a child of Roddy's age should have long since been weaned from his mother's breast, when Shotgun Mitchell, who was sitting directly across the table from Martina, presented his own *ore tenis* motion in the defense of the irate boy, "It seems to me," Shotgun pontificated with his trademark authoritative, nasal tone, while he sucked the last shreds of meat from a rib bone, "the boy should be applauded for knowing where to go to get the best meal in town." Quickly adding, "And I mean no offense to your marvelous cooking, my dear Catherine."

Aunt Catherine gasped with dismay and Martina turned crimson with embarrassment.

As she now watched her son thrashing about on the sofa and turning a deep reddish-purple with anger, Martina suddenly thought of Shotgun's commentary about "the best meal in town" and burst out laughing. The sound of her laughter surprised the little boy and he ceased crying to look up at his mother in wonder. Scrambling down off the sofa, Roddy toddled over to where Martina was standing and threw his chubby little arms around her legs. "Mama! Mama!" he wailed.

Martina bent down and scooped him up, covering his inflamed wet cheeks with kisses.

"C'mon, baby," she crooned, pressing her cheek lovingly against his, "let's go lie down on Mommy's bed and take a nap. Roddy released a deep, shuddering sigh and rested his head against his mother's shoulder. He knew just from the comforting tone of her voice that he would soon get what he wanted.

The unopened envelope again came to mind as soon as Martina woke up from her nap. When it was hand-delivered that morning she feared reading the contents. No good news had ever come her way from the likes of Martino's attorney, Vittorio Travante. But now, inexplicably, her curiosity had taken hold and the strong urge to open the envelope made her want to get off the bed and go get it. Carefully, she inched away from her sleeping son and slowly swung her legs over the edge of the bed. As she walked past the dressing table mirror she caught a glimpse of her disheveled image and decided she needed a quick makeover before she did anything else. It would have been wonderful to take a long soak in a hot bubble bath right now, but with Roddy due to wake up at any moment a bath was out of the question. She'd have to settle for a cat bath with a soapy facecloth.

And as she predicted, by the time she had washed up, put on some fresh clothes, re-applied her makeup, and brushed her hair, Roddy was awake and rearing to go. She'd have to chase him down to change his diaper and get him washed up. Travante's envelope would have to wait for the moment.

Resorting to the electronic babysitter, Martina turned on the television. She often used the Sesame Street kid's show to entertain Roddy so she could get chores done around the house. After placing the boy in his highchair and giving him some banana slices and a sippy cup of apple juice, the one liquid he would take from a cup, Martina went to retrieve the envelope from Travante.

It was really very silly of her to be so affected, and Martina freely admitted that to herself, but she was just too paralyzed with fear to open the envelope. A dozen frightening thoughts crossed her mind about why her father's attorney would take the trouble to hand deliver an envelope to her, all the way from Millborough. Now that she was over eighteen, and no longer a minor under the law, Martina supposed that the protective order that had been put in place by the court some three years earlier no longer applied, and Travante was coming after her again for some legal purpose involving her father's case. Travante, she had heard, was handling the appeal of her father's conviction.

The sight of the envelope provoked a flood of old emotions that came upon her rapidly, swirling around and around inside, threatening to carry her off in their fearful current. First her throat, then her chest and her lungs felt constricted, like someone had her in a stranglehold and was squeezing the breath out of her. She began to hyperventilate.

Then a little voice on the other side of the room called out to her, "Mama." That one word was all Martina needed to hear over the pounding in her ears, and almost immediately a more dominant instinct took control and supplanted whatever demon it was that taunted her. Tossing the envelope aside on the sofa, she rose to go tend to her son.

Hoisting Roddy out of the high chair and onto her hip, Martina saw that he was wearing more of the banana and apple juice than what he probably ingested. Just the sight of his round angelic face, even if it was plastered with mashed banana, made her heart quicken with happiness. "I think my little boy needs a bath," she told him playfully, as she carried him into the kitchen. Sitting him on the counter next to the large porcelain sink she turned on the water to fill up the sink. The kitchen was filled with the mid-afternoon sunshine, which warmed the room, so she often took advantage of this natural solar warmth to give him a bath. The little boy recognized what was coming as he watched his mother go through the routine of pouring in the bubble bath mix and making sure the water was just the right temperature. He began waving his arms and wiggling his body with excitement.

"Bat! Bat! Bat!" He chanted and rocked back and forth with anticipation of playing in the water.

"Okay! Banana Boy! Hold still, so I can get you undressed," Martina said, laughing at his excitement and trying to avoid contact between her clean sweater and Roddy's banana caked face and hands. Suddenly, tears of joy pooled in her eyes.

How blessed she was to be given this beautiful, perfect, healthy little boy. Miraculously, in all of the madness that had surrounded her during the last months she lived in Millborough, this precious little child was taking form inside of her body, and she could no longer imagine her life without him. Her thoughts compelled her to spontaneously hug him with a maternal reverence that almost made her heart ache. How she wished that Rod was alive to be a father to their son.

Roddy, however, was not going to allow his mother to be sentimental when just a few inches away there was a sink full of bubbly water and a bunch of plastic toys floating around in it. "Bat!" He exclaimed, pointing with his little banana-caked index finger at the bubbles.

"Yes, Roddy," Martina assured the little boy, laughing at his excited jabber, "you're going to get a bath." After removing the last of his clothing and a soggy diaper, she helped him step down from the counter and into the deep sink. The little boy squealed with delight to finally be splashing in the water with his toys. She was amazed that this delightful little cherub, pudgy and rosy cheeked, was hers to love and cherish.

When she touched his pale, mottled skin the stark contrast of her own South Seas complexion was startling, and his fine curly hair, which transformed into tight ringlets when it became damp, was such a dark brown it almost appeared black. Studying Roddy's profile, Martina could see nothing of herself in his features. Through and through, the boy was a veritable miniature of Rod, and she just knew that when he grew into a young man he would look exactly the way she remembered his handsome father had looked the last time she saw him.

Martina watched, fascinated, while Roddy played in the water. Every so often she would attempt to scrub the smeared banana off of his face with a washcloth, but he protested the interference with his play. Eventually, she was able to get him banana free. The one thing he did not object to was her massaging his back with the soapy washcloth. Like father, like son Martina thought, remembering how Rod, too, loved her to rub his back when they bathed together after a long afternoon of lovemaking at his house. Her bittersweet memories of Rod segued into thoughts of the unopened envelope from Attorney Travante.

There was only one thing to do, she finally decided, she would call her Aunt and Uncle. She'd get Uncle Jack to read the letter and give her whatever advice he thought appropriate. And if he couldn't help her there was always Shotgun to turn to.

4.

When Jack and Catherine Denault arrived at Martina's apartment, in response to her call for help, they were loaded down with shopping bags full of new clothes and toys for Roddy and a few bags of groceries. They never came empty handed. Martina had just finished giving Roddy dinner and was getting him ready for bed. Once Roddy spied the bag of toys his grandparents had brought, any hopes of getting him to bed on schedule were dashed. And the boy was excited to see his "Ampa" and "Amma." Of course, Jack and Catherine were head over heels with their grandparenthood, and thought that Roddy was the most adorable, intelligent, lovable, talented, bright, and perfect child that ever walked the face of the earth, bar none.

Martina was amazed how her Uncle and Aunt were reduced to Silly Putty in the hands of her toddler son. She would have never believed her Uncle Jack was capable of crawling around on the floor in his custom-tailored trousers, and whole heartedly playing with Roddy. And her Aunt Catherine was not much better. Although her Aunt would actually sit on the floor with Roddy from time to time, she preferred to take him up on a chair with her and read the old Fairy Tales and Aesop's Fables to him. It was unbelievable how kid oriented they had become, and Martina was so happy that they were there for Roddy, to provide him with a sense of family, however small it was.

Of course, there was also "Aunt" Chloe and "Uncle" Shotgun to extend the family ties. All that was missing were a couple of playmates Roddy's age, but Martina was hoping to eventually meet mothers of other small children when she and Roddy were out walking in the neighborhood. But Pacific Heights was not exactly the place where most mothers walked around with their kids. In that upscale venue of expensive homes, staffed with butlers, maids and gardeners, she'd be more likely to run into children's nannies, who as a rule, were not very friendly toward strangers

After the frenzy over the new toys had settled, although Martina did not know who was really more excited, Uncle Jack or Roddy, she brought up the subject of the hand delivered letter. "I don't know what's wrong with me, Uncle Jack," Martina explained, "but I just cannot seem to bring myself to open the letter. I think I'm just scared of what's inside."

"I'll take a look at it for you," said Uncle Jack, who was now sitting in a chair and back to his usual dignified self.

Aunt Catherine had offered to get Roddy bedded down for the night and had enticed him to his bedroom with his new stuffed panda. Martina could hear Roddy's giggles coming from his bedroom down the hall as she walked over to her desk to retrieve the manila envelope.

"You say it was hand delivered to you here this morning?" Her uncle asked, somewhat surprised, as he took attorney Travante's envelope from Martina's hand. "I wonder how they were able to locate your latest residence?" Jokingly, he added, "Your Aunt and I can barely keep up with your frequent address changes ourselves."

"Oh! Please! Uncle Jack!" Martina kidded in response. "I've only moved five or six times since leaving your house last year." Actually, she had only moved three times and, obviously, her efforts to remain a jump or two ahead of Travante and the rest of the snarling pack were pointless.

Her Uncle Jack didn't even crack a smile at her joke. Unperturbed, he said, "Well— it still amazes me they were able to track you down. They must have hired the reincarnation of Sherlock Holmes to do so."

Even while Jack applauded Martina's desire to be independent and stand on her own two feet, he did not understand why she could not live under his roof and be independent at the same time. If she had been involved in a relationship he could certainly understand Martina would have a need for privacy. But that was not the case. The truth was he missed the nearness of them. Especially, Jack missed seeing the wonder on Roddy's face when the boy discovered some new facet of his environment, which seemed to occur on a daily basis. Witnessing Roddy's excitement over the simple occurrences adults take for granted, such as a bird flying overhead or an ant crawling on a leaf, seemed to refresh Jack's perspective. Recently, Jack had heard some of their friends talking about special seminars they attended, paying hundreds of dollars to learn how to awaken their inner child. He supposed that was what spending time with Roddy did for him – awakened his inner child, and all for the price of admission to the San Francisco Zoo. Jack was just happy that Martina had moved only several blocks away, rather than out of state.

Perhaps as a form of harmless retaliation for her teasing him, Jack made a drawn out production of first getting comfortable in his chair and then slowly opening the envelope before extracting what appeared to be only a letter. From the corner of his eye he noticed Martina was perched expectantly on the edge of the sofa. Once again, he shifted his position in the chair and then thrust his arms outward a couple of times

37

as if the sleeves of his shirt were constricting the movement of his arms. Finally, her Uncle asked, "Shall I read the letter aloud to you, or would you prefer I read it first to myself and then provide you with a summary of the salient points?" His expression entirely too serious for the occasion.

Martina knew her Uncle Jack had a very dry sense of humor and liked to taunt her for sheer sport. He was deliberately trying to exasperate her by taking his time and going through all of those unnecessary contortions in the chair. She sighed and rolled her eyes to let him know that he had succeeded.

"Please! Just read it to yourself and then give me a summary of what it says."

Jack perused the letter for barely a few seconds, when he suddenly exclaimed, "Oh! Dear God in heaven!" Martina could see her uncle looked genuinely stunned and knew he was no longer kidding her.

"What! What's wrong?" Alarmed, Martina sprung from her chair.

Jack placed the letter face down on his lap and looked up at Martina with a somber expression. "I'm so sorry, Martina. Your father has died."

The letter fell from his lap when Jack suddenly jumped out of his chair and rushed across the room to catch Martina before she collapsed to the floor in a dead faint. Jack had just placed Martina on the sofa when Catherine rushed into the room. She had overheard the commotion and came running. Seeing Jack slapping Martina's cheeks, she panicked.

"What happened, Jack?" Catherine cried out with alarm, as she ran over to the sofa and knelt down beside Martina.

"Keep an eye on her," Jack blurted, as he bolted to the kitchen for some cold water and a cloth to make a compress.

"Honestly, Jack!" Catherine scolded him when he returned to the room, carrying a pan of ice water and a washcloth. "Whatever did you say to the poor dear to make her faint?"

"I had to inform her that Martino died," Jack said with a matter of fact tone as he got right to the business of dabbing Martina's face with the cold washcloth.

Catherine gasped, stunned. "Martino is dead?" Her question was merely a rhetorical measure of her disbelief.

"That's what Travante's letter said. I didn't have the opportunity to read all of it," Jack confirmed, continuing to move the cool cloth around Martina's face. "A pity we don't have smelling salts," Jack added, with his usual aplomb. "Salts would bring her right out of it."

Catherine took hold of her niece's hand and began to vigorously slap her palm.

Jack gave her a questioning look. "What in God's name are you doing?"

"I'm trying to help revive her," Catherine answered.

"Good grief, Catherine! That only works in Victorian plays." Jack's tone conveyed his astonishment with Catherine's innocence. However, just as Jack made that comment Martina emitted a soft moan and seemed to be awakening from her faint. "Humph!" He huffed, defending his position. "Just a lucky happenstance."

Catherine merely looked up at him and smiled demurely.

As Martina regained consciousness, her body felt leaden and she could hardly lift her head. Then came flooding back the memory of her Uncle's last words before she had passed out, and suddenly she was sobbing. Jack and Catherine tried to comfort her, but they could offer no consolation for the confusing mix of emotions that took possession of her. They could not know that Martina was overcome with guilt.

Even though she and Dr. Chloe had devoted numerous counseling sessions to exploring and working through Martina's feelings of guilt concerning her role in the relationship she had with her father, hearing of his death instantaneously reopened the barely healed wounds. Her Aunt Catherine made a mental note to call Chloe Renfrew as soon as possible and advise her of what had happened, and ask Chloe to call and check on Martina later.

When Martina was finally able to speak, she asked her Aunt, "Is Roddy okay?"

Aunt Catherine nodded and patted the top of Martina's hand. "He's sound asleep, dear. Not to worry." Catherine was grateful she had taken the child out of the room prior to his mother fainting or, she was sure, he would have been traumatized by the incident.

Then, turning to her Uncle Jack, Martina's voice sounded weak when she asked, "Will you please read me all of Mr. Travante's letter?"

"Perhaps it would be best if you waited a few days," her Uncle advised, concerned for her emotional state.

Her Aunt Catherine nodded in agreement.

"No!" the young woman found the strength to assert. "I must know what it says or I won't be able to sleep tonight."

Her Aunt opened her mouth to say something, but her Uncle held up his hand to stop her. "If that is what you want," Jack said, wanting to respect Martina's decision. "I'm sure the worst of it is already known."

Martina nodded affirmatively. "Yes. That is what I want."

So, her Uncle retrieved Attorney Travante's letter from the floor and read it aloud:

"My Dear Ms. Fiasconi,

It is with great regret that I must advise you of your father's passing. It is my understanding that Doctor Fiasconi suffered a massive heart attack in his prison cell and died before he could be transported to the local hospital. Given the circumstances of your estranged relationship with your father, and at his prior written instructions, I have fulfilled his wishes and arranged for his immediate burial, as he specifically stated that he did not want you to be burdened in such an event.

However, there are various matters involving the disposal of your father's estate, including, but not limited to, the real property located in Millborough, which will require your decisions and disposition. As you are aware, the residence on the property has been vacant for some time and will require some renovation, regardless of what you want to do with it.

While I do hope it will not be an inconvenience to you, I would prefer that you be present in my office for the reading of your father's Last Will and Testament.

Although I am your father's attorney I can assure you that I am quite sensitive to your situation and I will certainly not require you to participate in any discussion that will cause you discomfort, nor will you be expected to enter onto the premises of the estate if you do not wish to. I have taken photographs of the various antiques and other personal property, as well as the anticipated repairs, so you will need only to advise me what you wish me to do in each instance. I would imagine that you may wish to list the house for sale and I will be more than happy to assist in that regard.

Please contact me at your earliest convenience to schedule our meeting. If you do not want to return for this purpose I will fully understand your reticence to do so. However, if that should be the case with you, I must advise you to immediately retain legal counsel here so that we can amicably resolve the outstanding matters and properly close your father's estate.

Thank you for your attention to this request.
Very truly yours,
Vittorio T."

5.

Martina wondered who could be ringing her door bell so early in the morning. It seemed as though she had only just fallen asleep after spending a restless night of tossing and turning, with her mind replaying the words of Vittorio Travante's letter over and over. Cocking a bleary eye at the bedside alarm clock, she saw that it was barely eight o'clock. Slowly getting up, she attempted to pull on her bathrobe and discovered it was upside down. Martina would whole heartedly agree that she was not the brightest bulb in the chandelier before ten o'clock in the morning, but she could tell that her bulb of a brain was particularly dim this morning.

Adjusting the thick terry robe, which she acquired complements of a Hilton Hotel photo shoot in Hawaii, she made her way down the hall toward the front door. Looking through the peep hole in the door she immediately recognized the wild crimson hair that could only belong to the top of Chloe Renfrew's head.

"Top O'the Morning," Chloe chirped brightly when Martina opened the door. She was holding a large brown bag with both hands. "Brought us some breakfast," she announced, and marched straight through the living room and into the kitchen, where she set the bag down on the table. Martina followed along behind like a zombie.

"Is Roddy still asleep?" Chloe asked, surprised.

Martina sleepily nodded a response.

"So…your Aunt Catherine called me last night," Chloe said, hoping that brief statement would suffice to explain why she was there so early.

Martina nodded dumbly and plopped into one of the kitchen chairs. Chloe removed her coat and draped it over the back of a chair, and then proceeded to remove fried egg and ham bagels from the bag, followed by containers of steaming coffee. The aromas seemed to stimulate Martina's awareness.

"Bless them," Martina said with a wide yawn, referring to her Aunt and Uncle. "I wish they wouldn't worry so much about me."

"They wouldn't if they didn't love you so darn much," Chloe said, in between sips of coffee. "They told me about your father dying." Her expression and tone turned sympathetic and she added, "I'm sorry, Martina. I know this has to be difficult for you."

Martina placed her hands around the hot container of coffee, absorbing the warmth through her palms, and simply nodded a response.

Chloe wouldn't let the subject die of neglect. "Any thoughts you'd like to share? Is there anything I can do?" Although, from Martina's red-rimmed, bloodshot eyes Chloe could pretty much surmise the young woman's thoughts. No doubt Martina was going through some changes.

Shrugging, Martina pulled her fingers through her long, tangled hair. "I feel a bit sad. We were a happy family when Jacqui was alive. It's hard to believe that they are both gone now."

Chloe nodded sympathetically. "It's good that you have chosen to remember those happier days, when you were a family."

"Except that those happy memories end up being a comparison to the bad things that happened later. It's like the bad cancels out the good." Martina paused and sipped her coffee. Then she said, "I can think of all of the wonderful moments…the times we went skiing in Austria and when we hiked the Grand Canyon. Things like that. But then my thoughts automatically turn to the last days I was with my father…when he was so crazy with jealousy that he—" Martina was cut off by a familiar morning time summons.

"Mama! Mama!" Roddy called to her from his bedroom down the hall. Martina immediately rose from her chair and jokingly said, "The king of the manor has arisen. Would you care to join me in his throne room while I change his royal diaper?"

"All hail to the little king," said Chloe in the manner of a royal court crier, but she was really anxious to see her precious godchild.

The two women headed down the hall. They found Roddy jumping in his crib, utilizing the mattress as a trampoline.

"Look whose here to see you, Roddy," Martina announced, with all of the excitement she was capable of mustering at eight-fifteen in the morning. "It's your Auntie Chloe."

The little boy squealed with excitement, and pointing toward Chloe he jabbered, "Ancho! Ancho!"

"He's trying to say 'Aunt Chloe,'" said Martina, laughing at the little boy's attempts to talk.

"Hey, angel face!" Chloe called out, as she ran to the crib and snatched up the excited child. She had been calling him "angel face" since the day he was born, mainly because that was how he looked to her. And, now, with a head full of curly hair he looked even more

43

angelic. "Wow! Look at you, little buddy. You're sure getting heavy for ole Aunt Chloe."

"Ancho!" The little boy cried out once more and then pressed his face against Chloe's cheek.

That was the be-all and end-all moment for the typically no-nonsense Doctor Renfrew, she fairly melted under the boy's touch. "Was that a kiss? Did he just give me a kiss?" Chloe asked Martina, unable to contain her own childlike excitement.

Martina smiled with pride. "He sure did. That was a Roddy kiss."

Chloe sat the little boy down on his changing table and embraced him lovingly. "Ah, my little man. You've stolen my heart, you have," she proclaimed. Her Irish brogue seemed more pronounced than usual. Turning to Martina, she said, "The boy is already quite the little charmer, isn't he? What on earth will he be up to when he's a young lad?"

"I shudder to think of it," answered Martina, laughing.

Later, as Martina helped Roddy eat his breakfast of oatmeal mixed with cinnamon apples, Chloe asked her, "Your uncle mentioned that Mr. Travante has asked you in his letter to return to Millborough to deal with your father's estate. Will you be going?"

Martina studied Chloe's face for a moment. "Is that something you want to know for yourself, or are you asking for the benefit of my Aunt and Uncle?"

"I'm sure all three of us would like to know, Martina. As your friend, I'm interested, certainly. But as your erstwhile counselor I am concerned about your well-being. Do you feel you are ready to go back to Millborough?"

Martina seemed to be looking inward and seriously mulling over Chloe's question. Finally, she said, "I guess I won't know unless I do go back, will I?"

"Indeed, that is true. But what if you go back and you have problems dealing with it?"

Martina shrugged. "Then I suppose I'll just have to call you."

Chloe laughed and slapped the table with both hands. "And I'll be there for you." Then Chloe's face became serious and she looked at Martina with a curious expression. She asked, "Would you like me to go with you? It would be strictly as a friend, though, and I wouldn't put on my doctor's hat unless you really needed me for counseling."

"That's so nice of you, Chloe. Really. But the thing is that a psychologist I know named Doctor Chloe Renfrew once told me that I cannot live my life in a glass bubble. And I can't. I'll never be a whole person if I don't go back and face up to things. Right?"

Chloe affected a mock grimace. "Well, that Doctor Renfrew is right...in theory. But you know," she joked, "those blowhard shrinks don't know what their talking about half the time."

Martina laughed at Chloe's self-deprecating humor.

Handing Roddy his little spoon, so he could scrape the little bit of cereal left in his bowl and learn to feed himself without decorating the kitchen with oatmeal, Martina got up from her chair and went to the stove to make a pot of coffee.

Chloe observed Martina as she went about the process of filling the coffeemaker with grounds and then water. When did the young girl become a woman? She asked herself. It pleased Chloe immeasurably to see how Martina had grown into mature young woman and a wonderful, responsible parent. But she had always known Martina would be that kind of quality person.

Then, getting back the reason for her visit, she asked Martina, "Would you mind if I had a look at the attorney's letter?"

"Not at all, Chloe. I'll go get it."

6.

Jack and Catherine held the hope that the death of their brother-in-law would miraculously, and finally, free Martina from her constant need to move to new locations. In their minds, they attributed Martina's frequent moves to a neurotic fear she had that her father would somehow get out of jail and try to reclaim her. They worried that the climate of fear and constant moving would negatively affect little Roddy. The Denaults unloaded their own fears on Chloe Renfrew, in her capacity as Martina's one-time counselor, and hoped Chloe could give them instant relief from their worries.

Chloe tried to be reassuring to the Denaults, but she knew that Martino Fiasconi's death would not provide an instant panacea for Martina, or them. Without revealing any of the confidential conversations she had had with Martina during their recent early morning visit, Chloe informed the Denaults, as nicely as she could, that the fear Martina held for her father was burrowed deep into the young woman's bones and would not be dispelled simply by a letter advising he had been found dead in his jail cell.

Furthermore, Chloe could not tell the Denaults that the onus for Martina's neurotic behavior was not all riding on the life or death of their brother-in-law. For, mainly, Martina blamed herself for being the instigator of all of the ugliness that precipitated. That, in a good measure, Martina was moving around frequently because she was attempting to outrun herself.

And, now, added to the Denaults' frustrations and concerns, was the letter received from Attorney Travante, suggesting Martina return to Millborough. They were beside themselves with worry that she might actually go, taking Roddy with her, and who knew how she would handle being back in the epicenter of the horrific events that drove her to them for help, and how, at her young age, was she competent to make important decisions in legal matters involving her father's estate.

The Denaults appealed to Chloe to use her influence with Martina to suggest that they accompany her, should she decide to return to Millborough. The anxieties of the Denaults over Martina's possible return to Millborough, coupled with her own, placed Chloe Renfrew in a very tenuous situation. As a friend to both the Denaults and Martina, she wanted to be loyal to all parties. Chloe knew she was walking on a tightrope, trying to pull off a very delicate balancing act.

After Chloe had left that morning, Martina tried to interest Roddy in going for a walk. The boy had been shadowing her around the kitchen as she cleared the dishes from her impromptu breakfast with Chloe, and now clung to her bathrobe as she stood at the sink rinsing and stacking the dishes for washing later. "Let's get dressed and go out for a walk, Roddy," she coaxed, trying to pump up her words with excitement.

Roddy's response was a simple, but emphatic, "No!" Raising his arms upward to her, he whined, "Up! Up! Mamma. Up!"

As soon as Martina lifted him into her arms he went right to the business of pulling the front of her robe open and fumbling with the bodice of her nightgown. Martina sighed with resignation and smiled at him knowingly. Hugging him tightly against her, she walked into the living room where she could be more comfortable on the sofa while she attended to her maternal duties. She knew Roddy would soon enough outgrow his desire for her breast. So why, she reasoned, try to force him to stop? He only pitched a fit if she denied him access, and what was the advantage of that? She had tried using the repertoire of distraction tactics that Chloe had suggested and none of them worked on the tenacious little boy. At least when he was nursing, they were spending quiet time together and bonding. And she had always loved the feeling of the closeness between them that those moments created. How could that possibly be detrimental? So, there she sat on the sofa, with her son blissfully curled up against the warmth of her body, as she softly stroked his curly head, a living tableau of the Madonna and her child.

In the quiet of the moment, Roddy drifted off into a peaceful sleep, his perfect little bow-shaped lips now slightly parted and resting against caramel colored skin her breast. Rather than disturb him by attempting a move to his crib, she eased into a more comfortable, reclining position. It was unusual for Roddy to be napping so early in the day. She looked over at the clock on the mantel above the small brick fireplace and saw that it was just a few minutes shy of eleven. No doubt he was zonked from being up so late the night before, when her Aunt and Uncle came over with the large bag of toys.

Thinking about last night naturally brought Martina's thoughts straight to the letter from Vittorio Travante. It was still hard for her to get her mind around the fact that Martino was now dead. As in permanently gone from the world. And, yes, she did feel a deep sadness. While she would never admit it to anyone, even to Chloe, there was a part of her that still deeply loved the man. Maybe it was the part that was imprinted during the happy years of her childhood, when no child could have had two more loving and supportive parents. Or maybe it was the part that came much later, after Jacqui died, when she and Martino became closer than they should have. There was a time, and it lasted many months, when she truly, deeply loved him as just a man and not as her father. Now, of course, she knew that such feelings were forbidden in the eyes of society and the law, but the moral standards imposed by a society could not erase from Martina's memory those feelings. It was the outrage of society over the relationship that made her feel guilt and shame, and even tried to intimidate her into hating Martino.

But she did not hate him for the closeness they once shared. How could she hate him for something she alone had initiated? Something that, at the time, felt to her like an act of unselfish love and kindness. She saw Martino suffering and simply reacted. She had no idea, at her young age, of the long term consequences for both herself and Martino. Society called it "sexual abuse," but she knew there was nothing abusive, or even lustful, about what went on between her and Martino in the early months of their closeness. The hate and the abuse would come much later.

During Martina's counseling sessions, Chloe helped her to see that even though her motivation to help Martino over the loss of his mate was a pure act of kindness, that he, as the adult and the parent, knew it was crossing the line and he should not have allowed it to happen. There was no condemnation or disgust in Chloe's voice. Chloe's attitude, Martina saw, was just the opposite. "What is, just is," Chloe once told her after a very emotional session, when Martina finally bared to the Doctor the terrible guilt she felt about what she had done. "Life sometimes gets complicated. We are not here to point fingers and wallow in guilt. We are here to fix and heal." Those comforting words did more to set Martina on the path of resolving her conflicted feelings than almost anything else that transpired between Chloe and Martina as the months and sessions went on. Without that context, nothing else they would later discuss would have made any sense to Martina. And it was Chloe who pointed out to her that the very unusual, partnership type of relationship that both of her parents fostered with her, where they had always encouraged her to address them by their first names and participate as an equal in all family decisions, may have been the underlying reason she felt such a strong need to "help your father overcome his grief."

48

The ultimate break-through occurred for Martina when Chloe pointed out to her, "In the egalitarian atmosphere in which you were raised, you would have naturally concluded that it was your place, if not your duty, to step up and take your mother's place. So, I ask then, why do you feel guilt?"

Chloe's question had given Martina a lot to think about between sessions, and eventually she was able to work through her feelings of guilt and come to a point where, although she could not forgive herself entirely, she at least had a greater understanding of why she responded to her father's grief as she had. Chloe once told her, "You are a natural born nurturer, Martina. You must be careful to whom you give your nurturing energy. For, with it, you give away a huge piece of your heart and soul." Indeed, how true that statement was.

Now, reclining on the sofa and protectively holding Roddy snug against her body, Martina smiled down at the sleeping child, remembering Chloe's words. Unless Rod McDonough miraculously came back into her life there would be no other man for her to nurture. And Rod was dead, or so she thought.

There was only one person she was interested in nurturing these days and that was Roddy. There were already three large pieces of her heart and soul missing—pieces representing Jacqui, Martino, and Rod—she could not afford to lose any more pieces.

7.

Normally, Martina cherished the quiet time she spent with her son, but today her mind was running at top speed. While Roddy was sleeping peacefully in her arms, she was thinking about all the things she should be doing at that moment. But, lately, she had gotten into the bad habit of negotiating with her "To-Do" list, to see what things could be put off for another day. The consequence of her procrastination was an oppressive accrual of errands and other matters now needing her immediate attention.

One such task obviously needing her immediate attention was her apartment. As she glanced around the room she saw how her good intentions to be neater and more organized had fallen by the wayside. Then it caught her eye—the manila envelope containing Attorney Travante's letter. It was lying on the seat of the armchair directly across the room from where she was sitting, where Chloe had left it that morning. Definitely, she would have to contact the attorney with her decision within the next couple of days. The matters involving her father's estate could not be put off for weeks, like the dry cleaning.

Despite her psychological breakthroughs under the guidance of Chloe Renfrew, somehow it didn't seem fair to Martina that her father should escape his full punishment by dying. Her father, after whom she was named and the one person she should have been able to trust completely, had forever altered her life by killing the man she loved, and depriving her son of his father. And she had no doubt that if Martino had gotten his way, he would also have seen to it that her precious child was aborted. It was for those reasons alone that Martina had turned her back on her father, and they were reasons enough given the heinous nature of his acts and intentions. There were other cruelties that occurred during those last months, when it seemed to her that Martino had completely lost his mind, but those acts paled in comparison to taking Rod's life and wanting to kill his child.

It crossed her mind that Martino was just diabolical enough to find some way to appear as though he was dead, and once his body was transported outside of the prison, he would revive himself, and then possibly come looking for her. He knew she had fled to San Francisco, and the thought of his being on the loose caused a cold shiver to ripple through her body. She looked down at her son as he peacefully slept and gathered him closer. The child felt her sudden movement and stirred. Martina hoped he would awaken, as he had napped for over an hour and her arms were getting stiff from holding him for so long. When his thick dark eyelashes fluttered open she was relieved, but she continued to hold him for a few more moments to allow him to fully wake up. Suddenly, he reached up and gently touched her cheek. "Mama," he said, with his sweet, angelic baby voice. It was worth being held captive on the sofa for over an hour, with her arms aching, just to experience that moment. She squeezed him tight against her and smothered his face with kisses, her heart bursting with love for him.

Roddy may have finally awakened, but getting him washed up and dressed to go out was like grappling with a wisp of smoke. It took another hour for Martina to get themselves both presentable for a public outing, then she hauled Roddy, his stroller, and the bundles of laundry and dry cleaning out to her Saab coupe, which was parked at the curb in front of her apartment, and off they went to deal with a few of the critical items on Martina's "To-Do" list.

It was nearing five o'clock when Martina returned home, hauling Roddy, several bags of groceries, and a plastic garment bag of dry cleaned clothing into the apartment. She had hoped she would get home early enough to call Vittorio Travante, but since Millborough was three hours ahead of San Francisco time her call would have to wait for tomorrow.

That night, after putting Roddy to bed, Martina set about tidying and re-organizing her apartment. Coming across Vittorio's letter on the chair, she picked it up and was about to take it to her desk, when it occurred to her to read it for herself. She wasn't prepared for the sadness that overcame her and the tears that followed when she read the brief account of Martino's death, but she had been putting off those emotions, too, as though they were simply another item on her list of "To-Dos," and now they had reached critical mass. There was no bargaining with sorrow. Despite the bitter ending of their father-daughter relationship there were still many years of history between them, and most of that consisted of happy, loving memories. It was for those good memories she mourned, but her tears were also for what could have been.

After reading and rereading Vittorio's letter, Martina had pretty much decided that she would handle her father's estate matters by telephone, or find an attorney in Millborough to deal with it for her. She could just imagine the wave of gossip her appearance in Millborough would create, not to mention the stares when she walked down the street with Roddy. It was unthinkable to put her child or herself through that. Although, she thought about how nice it would be to see her old best friend Julie. They had met in junior high and were fast friends up until the day Martina left Millborough. Where Martina had light brown hair and caramel-colored skin, Julie was blonde and fair complexioned. They were both about the same height and both had Barbie doll figures. Martina wondered if Julie still looked like a Barbie doll and what she was doing with her life these days? Was she still married to Freebird? Sadly, she hadn't been in touch with Julie since the night she fled Millborough, even though they had pledged to keep in touch. It was Julie who came to her rescue after she had slipped away from the abortion clinic. With only a learner's permit to her credit, Julie raced across town, using Freebird's car without his permission, to pick up Martina and drive her to the airport. If it were not for Julie's daredevil driving Martina didn't know how else she would have made her flight to San Francisco, as she did not even have enough money for bus fare at the time.

8.

"What a day!" Martina commented aloud to herself, thinking about Chloe's early morning wake up visit and all of the errands she managed to get accomplished that afternoon. Placing Vittorio Travante's letter on the mahogany writing table that served as her desk, she vowed to call the attorney first thing in the morning and switched off the faux Tiffany desk lamp.

It was only 9:15 but she felt like it should be midnight. Earlier in the day, Martina had promised herself a hot bubble bath as her last official act of the day and now it was time to make good on that promise. As her tired, achy body parts seemed to dissolve in the hot, sudsy water, Martina's thoughts ricocheted like a pinball until they settled on Julie. How wonderful it would be to see her friend again. But they had missed so much of each other's lives. Would they be able to pick up the thread of their friendship? Of course they would, she scolded herself. What a stupid thought. How could she and Julie not go on being friends; there was too much history between them that time could not erase.

It would be impossible to write off all of the silly, if not just plain crazy, stunts she and Julie used to dream up and pull off. It was on one of their double-dare adventures that Martina first met Rod McDonough. They were supposed to have been at the library that afternoon, studying for a history test, but Julie had heard about a bunch of guys who had a motorcycle club over in North Hampton, a kind of other-side-of-the-tracks town that was way down on its luck. When Julie got excited about something she had a way of making her eyes grow wide and light up like there was a tiny bulb implanted in each orb that emitted a bright ray. It was in just that kind of excited, bright-eyed way that Julie related to Martina what she had heard about the "motorcycle guys" over in North Hampton, who hung out in an old converted storefront clubhouse. According to Julie's older brother, Donny, the clubhouse was painted all black and red inside and decorated with "bad-ass black light posters, and the biker dudes hung around there smoking pot all day and night and the cops were afraid to even go near the place."

Julie's blue eyes fairly glowed as she excitedly double-dared Martina to go with her to "check out the clubhouse and the biker dudes." Not even considering for a fleeting moment the danger they might be putting themselves into, the two giddy young girls, all scrubbed and color-coordinated, with their perfect little Barbie doll figures, hopped on the gleaming cross-town bus that would take them to the Millborough township line of demarcation with North Hampton.

It was not a case of upper crust Millborough running smack into lower crust North Hampton. Heaven forbid. When the City Commissioners of Millborough saw how the misfortunes of time were wreaking havoc on the neighboring town of North Hampton, they created a buffer zone to protect the aesthetic sensibilities of good citizens of Millborough from even the slightest view of the bleak, used-to-be mill town of abandoned shoe factories. If it were legally possible, the Millborough Commissioners would have erected a giant wall around their town to prevent any form of encroachment by the unwashed masses who populated North Hampton, not that there really was much of a population left after all of the factories moved south and then, eventually, to China.

The last stop for the gleaming bus was on the Millborough side of the buffer zone, where it pulled up in front of a long line of multiple rows of tall Poplar trees. Martina and Julie exited the bus and walked across the buffer to a beat up, graffiti covered bus that would take them to their destination in North Hampton.

The further the rattletrap bus took them into North Hampton the more abandoned and squalid the buildings on either side of the litter-filled streets became. Martina looked out the cracked window at the passing scenery with some alarm, but Julie chatted on excitedly about their escapade, seemingly unaffected by the dilapidated, burned-out ghetto they were traveling further into. When Julie nudged her arm and declared, "The next stop is ours," Martina nodded dumbly. She had never before been to such a creepy place and wondered how Julie could be so blasé about it. And how did Julie know which stop to get off at, anyway?

The bus driver, a peculiar-looking fellow with a droopy expression, eyed them suspiciously when they walked up to the front of the bus to stand next to the door, in anticipation of getting off. With their neatly pressed jeans and shoes that perfectly matched the color of their Orlon sweaters and leather purses, they were obviously not from North Hampton. Martina surreptitiously eyed the bus driver with equal suspicion and figured he was hired for that job because he fit in so perfectly with the general look and feel of the place—weird and spooky.

When the bus lurched to a stop in front of mostly boarded up stores and other run-down shops, Julie jumped out and bounded onto the littered sidewalk. Martina hesitated in the doorway like a frightened paratrooper, her heart pumping in her chest. Behind her, the gruff voice of the bus driver snarled, "Let's go, girlie!" So she jumped from the bus. What else could she do?

Looking up and down the street, Martina noticed there were few people actually walking on the grimy sidewalk. All pedestrian commerce seemed to be occurring in the doorways of the abandoned buildings, where groups of rough-looking, jittery men huddled, smoking cigarettes, talking in low conspiratorial tones, and casting furtive glances over their shoulders. Martina had the distinct impression that these men were up to no good but she wasn't sure what sort of illegal enterprises they were plotting. Noticeably, there no women out and about, which seemed somewhat strange. Of course, with just about all of the storefronts and other buildings deserted or boarded up, with the exception of a narrow gage liquor store with a roll-down metal door that would completely barricade the place when it was closed, there was no practical reason for any woman to be on that street as far as Martina could see. And she knew that she and Julie stuck out like the two uptown girls that they were.

So as not to encourage any unwanted advances, Julie didn't waste any time standing around. She grabbed Martina's arm and, speaking out of the side of her mouth in a hushed tone, said, "C'mon, let's keep moving." Leading Martina up the street, in the same direction the bus had disappeared, Julie pointed to an old, weather beaten sign, with now unreadable lettering, that extended over the sidewalk. "The clubhouse is down the side street that's just beyond that sign."

Martina wondered how Julie knew exactly where to find the clubhouse and how her friend got to be so street smart all of a sudden? It was a side of Julie that Martina did not know existed until now. "Have you been here before?" She asked Julie.

"No. Of course not. This is not the kind of place I would just come to as a normal thing. Donny told me how to get here."

"Donny gives really good directions," Martina commented, wondering why Donny would be hanging around in such a place himself. "How did Donny find out about the clubhouse?"

"Donny has a motorcycle. An old Indian Chief he bought from some weird little guy named DeLuca. DeLuca was the one who told him about the clubhouse and even brought him here once to…you know…introduce him to the guys. Donny said they were all 'righteous brothers.' Whatever that means. But it sounds okay to me."

When they got to the corner of the street they were to turn into, Julie pulled her into the unoccupied doorway of the long-gone store. The once gold lettering on the grimy plate glass windows had been sloppily scraped off and what remained of the gold was discolored. "Let's fix our lipstick and hair before we go scoopin'," said Julie. The word "scoopin'", as used by Julie, was synonymous with the phrase "picking up guys."

Julie was brushing Martina's hair to perfection when they heard the unmistakable chug-a-chug-a-chug of a Harley Davidson somewhere in the vicinity. They looked at each other with wicked, Cheshire grins, and their respective levels of excitement amped up a notch or three.

The two girls giggled conspiratorially as they primped for their walk down the street where the clubhouse was situated, with all of its reputed blacklit, pot smoky, testosteronic mystique. According to their pre-formulated plan, they were to "perambulate" down the sidewalk on the opposite side of the street from the clubhouse, look straight ahead as if they were on their way to someplace important, and pretend to not even notice the clubhouse, with its habitual cluster of motorcycles and gaggle of bikers out front. When they arrived at the other end of the street, if any of the "motorcycle guys" (Julie's designation for the club members) came after them, there were only two possible courses of action: if the guys were cute, then they would flirt with them for a while and maybe even give them their telephone numbers for future dates; if the guys were "onky" (translation: ugly), then they would just be friendly, tell the guys they had to go somewhere to meet someone and they were late, then immediately split the scene, giving no phone numbers.

The girls usually planned their forays of this nature to the utmost degree, and they had developed over the course of their long friendship an abbreviated vocabulary to characterize certain aspects of their escapades. Of course, some of their friends at school thought they were talking gibberish just to keep everyone else in the dark about what they were saying, but that was not the case. Martina and Julie just had a thing for making up words. When they went walking around town, all decked out in their fancy outfits, trying to meet new guys, they were out "scoopin'." They didn't just walk, they "perambulated." When they let some lucky guys pick them up, they were then "scooped." If they thought a guy was ugly, he was termed "onky." If they went out on a date with a guy and he was too touchy-feely, they would say he "mauldigated" them. And for someone they really didn't like they reserved the nomenclature of "low class clientele." They had concocted numerous other derivations of words that made no sense to the uninitiated, but the cryptography came natural to the two fast friends.

So, after passing each other's critical inspections in the grimy, littered doorway, the two friends excitedly stepped out onto the sidewalk and scampered around the corner. Crossing the street to the opposite sidewalk they began their perambulation down the narrow street, which was hardly more than an alleyway, but made a bit more attractive than most by fresh coats of paint on the facades of a few buildings.

Julie pointed to the bent over street sign and started giggling uncontrollably. Between Julie's snickering, she managed to say, "I wonder if that's why the motorcycle guys chose this street for their clubhouse?"

Martina looked up at the faded street sign to see what had struck Julie so funny. Reading the street name, she, too, cracked up. "Alcock Way," Julie repeated. "And from the way it's leaning over toward the clubhouse it looks like it's pointing us in the right direction." The two conspirators dallied under the sign for a few moments while they laughed hysterically.

Further down the alley, several bikers were gathered at the curb in front of their clubhouse, admiring a club member's new Harley, when peels of girlish laughter drifted their way. Ever alert, as young men on the prowl are likely to be, their respective male antennae rotated in near synchronized motion toward the direction of the laughter. Two fresh-faced girls, one wearing a bright pink jersey and the other a turquoise sweater, both wearing tight jeans, were headed in their direction.

Wondering what two tender young chicks like that were doing in a neighborhood like theirs, the bikers gave each other silent, questioning glances, while their collective pheromones kicked into high gear.

"Holy Christmas!" One of the bikers, who was known to the club as "Dirty Dan," exclaimed in disbelief. "Santa Claus has come to town."

"Fucking jail bait!" Said another, whom they called "Preacher," because he was always throwing a damp blanket on anything that looked like fun, but might lead to trouble with the law.

"Who's checkin' IDs," someone in the pack rebutted.

"Fuckin' A!" Came another response to the comment about the IDs.

Only one of the bikers refrained from indulging in commentary. It was the club member who had just arrived to show off his new Harley, and he was still sitting on it. From the moment Rod McDonough set his

57

eyes on the exotic beauty of the girl with the long honey brown hair, who seemed to glide down the sidewalk with such an easy elegance and graceful sensuality, he knew he wanted her. His eyes zeroed in on Martina, taking a mental snapshot of her almond-shaped eyes, the profile of her aristocratic nose, the fullness of her ruby colored lips, and he felt a deep stirring in his soul. As his eyes continued their downward scan, Rod McDonough noted how her turquoise sweater clung to her young girl's body, and the way her tight jeans accented her marvelously rounded rear end and long, slender legs, all of which stirred his more carnal nature. "Hot damn!" he whispered under his breath.

Clearly distracted by the swaying hips and sexy visage of the two lovelies, the bikers quietly ogled as the girls walked on by. It was obvious from their polished, jewel-like appearances they did not live in that neighborhood. Most likely, they did not even live in North Hampton. And even though the chicks appeared to be on an important mission, their eyes seemingly riveted on some important destination at the other end of Alcock Way, and acting as though they did not notice the leather clad gaggle of bikers standing just several feet away in the narrow alley, the horny bikers knew exactly why those two girls just happened to be sashaying down that particular alley. Such perambulations of provocatively dressed young women were getting to be quite the phenomenon on Alcock Way, ever since The Vikings Motorcycle Club had established their clubhouse in the middle of the block.

After Martina and Julie strutted past the clubhouse and the young bikers had ample opportunity to examine the girls from all angles, there was a collective low rumbling of exhalations. Then, Rod McDonough, one of the founding members of the Vikings, immediately grabbed the handlebars of his new bike and knocked out the kick start pedal with the toe of his glossy engineer boot. "See you hosers later," he quietly announced, "I'm going after that sweetie in the turquoise sweater."

McDonough, who was clean cut and well built, was accustomed to the ladies pursuing him. But he knew that if he did not stake his claim to that beauty with the long, honey hair and fine rear-end one of his brother Vikings would. So he immediately declared his intentions and prepared to take off after her.

"Hold up, Rod!" called his sidekick, Freebird, a sinewy, dark-skinned Viking clubber with long, straight black hair that proclaimed his Native American heritage. Quickly staking his own claim, Freebird added, "I'll take that cute little blond."

Ever since meeting Rod about a year ago, Freebird stuck pretty much by his side. Rod didn't mind the attachment; he liked Freebird's amiable company and considered him a younger brother from a different mother. They were definitely brothers of the saddle and frequently spent long hours riding together out into the country, amongst the outlying dairy farms and horse pastures. Both men preferred being surrounded by nature and regularly sought it out. But right now, they had their sights set on those two extremely curvaceous young ladies and were anxious to explore their hills and valleys.

When Martina and Julie heard the motorcycles kick over behind them they were sure they had provoked the interest they had hoped for, but they continued to play it cool and kept on walking. Although, they had to resist the acute temptation to turn around to see what their pursuers looked like. When the two bikers roared past them, as though taking a cue from the girls' own playbook and pretending the girls did not exist either, Martina and Julie looked at each other, crestfallen.

Julie squeezed Martina's arm, and said, "Did you see that one with the long black hair? He looked really hot." Martina merely nodded, thinking the bikers were leaving.

The bikers appeared to be making a right turn at the end of the alley when, suddenly, they whipped their machines around in tight U-turns and came roaring back up the alley toward them. The fierce rumbling of their engines reverberated off of the brick and mortar structures lining either side of the alley, and it was a wonder the antiquated buildings didn't come tumbling down like the walls of Jericho. Suddenly, one of the bikers was up on the sidewalk and aiming straight at Martina and Julie. His buddy was clipping down the street, next to the curb, giving the girls no where to run without getting mowed down by one or the other fast approaching motorcycles.

Screaming, the girls grabbed hold of each other and flattened their backs against the brick facade of a grim looking building, their hearts pumping double-time and their chests heaving with fearful gasps. Amazingly, each biker came to a lurching halt, just inches away from the terrified girls, and revved their engines for good measure.

Martina was sure that she and Julie had finally succeeded in putting themselves in the ultimate of dangerous situations. They were in a strange town, miles from the safety of their homes, and surrounded by a gang of merciless barbarians. Running through Martina's mind were horrific visions of her and Julie being dragged into a biker clubhouse full of dirty mattresses, where they would be mauled and savaged by the entire gang of hairy, leather-clad Vikings. And there was no point of screaming for help. Julie's brother had said that not even the cops would dare to venture into the alley of The Vikings, so Martina knew that she and Julie were strictly on their own.

Apparently, Julie's thoughts were running pretty much along the same lines; just at that moment she clutched her friend's arm so tightly that her fingernails dug painfully into Martina's skin.

The two young men continued to sit on their bikes and brazenly stare at the girls, whose pretty young faces were locked in mutual expressions of stark fear. Rod McDonough switched off his engine and Freebird followed suit. But that did not end the cacophony. The girls could now hear the raucous laughter and vulgar comments being shouted by the gaggle of bikers who were standing behind them, back at the clubhouse, and their escalating rowdiness was even more frightening. It was evident to Rod that the girls were scared shitless; the blonde one now looked like she was about ready to cry, but the other one stood firm and her expression had become defiant.

Rod noticed that she had the most incredible green eyes; the color reminded him of the ocean off the coast of Oahu, where he surfed as a young teenager. As he studied the beauty of her face and her flawless caramel complexion, his gaze gravitated back to her amazing sea-green eyes, which now leveled their defiant glare directly at him. Rod caught his breath. God, how she turned him on. Not wanting to piss her off and ruin the chances of coaxing her onto the back of his bike, Rod decided to let a little bit of his cultured self show through his biker image.

"So...," he intro'd, "what are two visions of loveliness...such as yourselves...doing in a rank and rodent infested place like this." He punctuated his statement by gesturing with open arms, encompassing the entire alley. His attempt at eloquence seemed to work. The girls relaxed just a fraction but remained guarded.

Of course, Martina and Julie, who had previously scripted their possible responses to any query about what they were doing in that particular neighborhood, had not anticipated such a well-articulated sentence. And certainly not one that referred to them as "visions of loveliness." They had only planned their responses to accommodate mere grunts and monosyllables.

Taken aback by this well-spoken, Galahadian approach they could only look at each other, surprised and tongue tied. After a few seconds,

Julie managed a feeble, "We were trying to find a cousin's house and got lost."

Rod looked at Freebird and the two bikers started laughing heartily. It was the lamest of all of the excuses they had heard from the various girls that were as of late venturing into their alley.

Freebird turned to Julie with a sly smile, and said, "Where does your cousin live? Maybe we can help you find the house?"

For once, Julie was caught short of a quick response. But Martina jumped to the fore with a ready answer, "She lives on Upton Road. We thought it was down this way."

Rod gave Martina an indulgent smile and folded his arms across his chest. He pretended to wrack his brain for a recollection of any Upton Road in his travels around North Hampton, although he was almost positive there was no such street. Carrying the charade a bit further, he looked over at Freebird and asked him if he'd ever heard of a street named "Upton." But Freebird had already made eye contact with the little blond honey, and she with him, and the two were in the process of conversing with body language. Distractedly, Freebird merely answered with a laconic "no."

Martina could sense the interest of the biker with the dark curly hair from the way he seemed to drink her in with the intensity of his brown eyes. It wasn't that his gaze made her feel threatened in any way. On the contrary, she could feel her body uncoiling and her adrenalin receding to a near normal level. There was something about his stare that, instead, made her feel admired and appreciated, like he was looking at a fine piece of art. At least, that was the feeling he was conveying to her at the moment with his soft, almost caressing, eyes, as they scanned and gently touched on every feature of her face and then her body.

Martina was aware that her exotic appearance, passed down by her South Seas island grandmother, was the constant source of curious stares. As it was with her mother, people were naturally intrigued by the unusual combination of her sea-green eyes radiating from deeply tanned skin. She had learned from her mother not to be taken in by this endless attention. Some of the stares she received in public were so frank and invasive they made her feel uncomfortable. But not the stare of the young man on the motorcycle. She could only describe the feeling he aroused in her as *thrilling*.

Exactly why this young biker, whom she knew nothing about, was so easily stirring up the nerve endings of her body with only his gaze, she wondered. Perhaps it was because she, too, was attracted by his handsome features. There was a raw sexiness about him, yet his face still retained a hint of the little boy he had grown from. Maybe it was his smooth, pale skin that made him look youthful, but she knew he had to be much older than he looked because he had the well-developed body of a man. Probably, she speculated, he was in his early twenties, because there was a quiet maturity about him. He seemed to have long since shed the ungainly frame of the unsure teenager and settled into his man's lean, muscular body, quite comfortable with himself. And rather than being put off because he was older, Martina was fully intrigued and attracted by his sexy manliness.

In a less obvious manner, Martina had conducted her own inventory of the curly-headed biker and took notice of all his finer attributes, such as the way his muscular arms stretched the sleeves of his black T-shirt, and the well-developed chest that ballooned his black leather vest. Even his jeans, which she noted looked freshly laundered and pressed, were stretched tight around his solidly muscled thighs and legs. And as he sat astride his motorcycle, Martina absorbed and assimilated in her seventeen-year-old mind all of the visual details about him that she could see and imagined a few that were not quite so visible. Not even the sexual innuendo of the metal and chrome jutting out from between his muscled thighs was lost on her, even though she might not be able to put those feelings into precise words.

When Rod had eyed his fill of the young girl's exotica, he reached over and gave Freebird a nudge that seemed to bring the smitten Indian to his senses. "I think these ladies are lost," Rod told his friend.

"Wh— What?" Freebird asked, suddenly snapping to attention.

"I said...I think these ladies are lost," Rod repeated, and then added, "and the proper thing for gentlemen to do would be to take them where they want to go."

Knowing Rod McDonough as well as he did, Freebird estimated that it was about time for Rod to zero in on the two girls for the big score. Having been in similar situations with Rod many times before, Freebird knew what a smooth operator he was with the ladies and almost always made the score with them. While Freebird was not a fancy talker like Rod, he knew the chicks found him attractive, and he preferred to use his tongue to impress the women in other ways. So, Freebird just smiled at the little blonde and nodded enthusiastically. And she smiled back at him, with equal enthusiasm. Amazingly, the two had not exchanged one word, yet a connection of some sort had formed between them.

Beaming his most winning and humblest smile at the green-eyed beauty standing before him, Rod qualified, "That is...if these two dazzling ladies will consent to hopping on our scooters and letting us take them wherever they want to go."

Martina and Julie stared at each other, dumbstruck. They were completely bowled over by the flowery way the curly haired biker was talking, but that was Rod's general intention. Of course, the girls were young and easily impressed.

Then Martina thought to say, "But we don't even know who you are...so I don't think it would be a good idea for us to go anywhere with you guys." Just then, she felt Julie poke her disapprovingly in the back.

"That can be easily corrected," Rod assured. Pointing to Freebird, he said, "This fine fellow is my long-time good buddy Freebird. His real name is Clayton T. Terry the Third, and my name is Rod McDonough. So...now you know who we are, but we don't know who you ladies are."

Not wanting to waste anymore valuable time, Julie extended her hand to Rod, "I'm Julie Owens." After quickly shaking Rod's hand, Julie turned her full attention to Freebird. When she put her hand out toward him, Freebird latched on to it and pulled her to his side, looking at her like he had just won the First Prize in a lottery.

It was now Martina's turn to introduce herself and Rod was eagerly awaiting the touch of her hand and knowing her name. She saw his eagerness and devised a ruse to keep him waiting. In the same manner that Rod had a flare for flowery speech to impress the ladies, Martina had an equal flare for the dramatic pause, and in this case she used it to draw out the anticipation of the moment: As Martina pretended to step forward to introduce herself, she faked a stumble, and cried out in pain. "There must be something in my shoe...." Using the handlebar of Rod's bike for support, she bent down and removed her turquoise patent leather slipper and shook it out. While Rod was otherwise distracted by the drawn out routine, he failed to notice that there was absolutely nothing in Martina's shoe. Julie had to bite her tongue to keep from laughing; she had seen Martina's improvisational acts numerous times before and knew she was just being coy.

Finally, after reinstalling the shoe on her foot and wiping the imaginary dust off of her hands, the verbal part of her drama ensued,

"Sorry…it felt like a piece of glass but it was only a little pebble," Martina explained, addressing no one in particular.

Unwittingly, Rod called her bluff. "Would you like me to look at your foot?" He asked, concerned.

"Oh— It's okay now. Just a pebble," she said, begging off.

Rod felt himself growing impatient. Usually, by now, he had already talked the chick onto his bike and was half way to where he wanted to take her. This one, though, she was different. She was young, probably no more than sixteen or seventeen, and much too young for him to be fooling around with. But her eyes told him a totally different story: that of maturity and intelligence beyond her years. "So, are you going to tell me your name or talk about pebbles?" He asked, trying to get back on track.

Extending her hand graciously, she finally said, "I'm Martina Fiasconi."

Rod took hold of her hand and clutched it as though he were afraid it might flutter away. He liked the soft, smooth feel of her skin and the caramel color of it. "Martina…" Rod repeated aloud, just to hear the sound of her name and test its resonance on his tongue. He smiled at her and his expression was rather like she had given him the key to her front door instead of just her name. When Martina tried to withdraw her hand, he clutched it tighter. "Not so fast!" Rod exclaimed, "You made me wait about five minutes before I could shake your hand. Now, let me hold it for five more."

Martina laughed and politely removed her hand from Rod's, so that she could acknowledge Freebird. Freebird merely nodded and smiled when she shook his hand. She noticed that Julie had already ensconced herself on the buddy seat of Freebird's motorcycle and Martina wondered how that had happened so fast when she had not heard any conversation between them, other than telling each other their names.

"I think we'd better head home," Martina reminded Julie

"Mar…tina!" Rod called to her. He seemed to be playing with the sound of her name and trying it out in different verbal formats. "Or shall I call you Marty or Tina.

She turned to look at him and saw that he was only teasing her to get her attention. "No. Please. I'm definitely not a Marty? Or a Tina? No way. Just call me Martina."

"Okay, Mar…tina, where's home?" Rod asked, reaching down and pulling out the bike's kick pedal.

"Millborough," she answered, wondering if they would want to take her and Julie that far out of their way.

"Millborough!" Rod exclaimed, surprised at the distance they had traveled just to walk down a funky alley and not look at what they really wanted to see. Looking over at Freebird, he said, "I told you these two little chickadees didn't come from this side of the tracks."

His friend nodded, and said, "Yep. Definitely not from this side of the tracks."

"You don't have to take us all the way back to Millborough," Julie bargained, "How about just as far as the transfer station?"

Frightened that his cute little passenger would slip away and he'd never be able to find her again, Freebird patted Julie's knee reassuringly and said, "It's no hassle. We'll take you to Millborough."

Surprised by the soft, mellow tone of Freebird's voice, Martina reappraised the young man. She could see why Julie was instantly attracted to Clayton T. Terry the Third. He was handsome. Half of his long, shiny black Indian hair, which hung down past his shoulder blades, was pulled away from his face and fastened high on the back of his head by a length of leather thong decorated with red, yellow, green, and black crow beads on each end. With his high cheek bones, keen dark eyes, broad rounded nose, and the determined set of his mouth and jaw, Freebird looked every bit the intrepid warrior, albeit wearing a Harley T-shirt, a pair of faded jeans, and riding on an Iron Horse. He was just the sort of swarthy, wiry guy that Martina had always seen Julie eyeballing whenever they were out and about and scoopin'. The only thing that concerned Martina about the two of them hitting it off was that Freebird seemed very quiet and unassuming, while Julie could be somewhat on the rowdy side when she decided to cut loose, which was often enough. Martina didn't think Freebird would go for Julie's wild antics but, then, he might be just the one to calm her down. After all, if opposites do attract each other there must be a good reason.

Martina looked at Rod to see if he was in agreement with Freebird about taking them all the way to Millborough but, just then, someone back at the clubhouse yelled in their direction,

"You're losin' your charm, McDonough. It's been over five minutes and you still haven't got the broad on your scooter."

Martina nervously looked over her shoulder, wondering what the shouter meant by that remark. Was this biker, whose motorcycle she was about to climb on, some kind of a record-breaking ladies' man?

65

Rod McDonough ignored the shouted comment, and flashed a boyish grin at Martina. "Millborough sounds like a fine ride to me. That's why we live to ride and ride to live."

Rod stood astride his bike and smoothly kicked it over. "The bus for Millborough is leaving," he shouted to Martina over the roar of the motor. "You getting on?"

9.

Never having been on a motorcycle before, Martina wasn't quite sure of how to mount it gracefully. Luckily, she was tall and agile enough to balance herself on one leg while she launched her other leg over the seat. Holding on to Rod's shoulder for good measure, she then slid easily into the space between his body and a chrome back rest. It was a snug fit and she searched about for handles under the seat or something else to hold onto while they were moving. Rod solved her dilemma by reaching back, taking both of her hands in his, and pulling her arms around his body. She was struck by the strangeness of her arms being suddenly wrapped around the midsection of a man she hadn't known for even an hour, but then she realized that her inner thighs were also more or less wrapped around this man's body, and that in itself was an extremely intimate posture. But such was the nature of riding on a motorcycle with another person, whether or not you knew each other very well.

To add to the bizarre turn of the afternoon, the other members of the Vikings, who had been steadily milling about the alley and exhibiting their basest Neanderthal behavior in an all-out attempt to scare off the girls, had amassed in the middle of the narrow street to block Rod's and Freebird's passage. Of course, it was all in good brotherly fun but Martina and Julie did not know that was how biker brothers horsed around with each other. The girls hung on, equally terrified, as Rod and Freebird ran the feral gauntlet of fisted salutes, raised third fingers, hoots, howls, and a fair measure of crude suggestions that, thankfully, the girls could not hear over the roar of two motorcycle engines reverberating in a narrow alley. Once breaking free of the melee, Rod and Freebird accelerated to the end of the alley, and then stopped abruptly. Laughing wildly, the two bikers looked at each other and signaled their next move with only a nod of agreement. Quickly executing a U-turn, they then positioned themselves for another run at the jeering mob of Vikings.

Martina gave Julie a quizzical look; the girls had no inkling of what was to happen next since the biker lifestyle was an entirely new experience for them. Suddenly, Rod yelled, "Hang on tight, ladies!" Instantly, the bikes lurched forward and accelerated down the alley, with each of the girls pressed flat against the backs of their respective drivers. This time, the element of high speed was in their favor and the awaiting gauntlet of tattooed and leather-clad bodies was forced to scatter in all directions when it became apparent that Rod and Freebird had no intention of slowing down. Martina and Julie were quick to realize that they had just participated in some sort of biker sporting event, but at that moment they were too petrified to be amused.

Once out on the highway, however, Martina quickly forgot about the frightening chicken race in the alley and the strangeness of clinging to a stranger, as they became one with the motorcycle and leaned into the dips and turns. Almost immediately, she fell in love with the feel of roaring through the streets, with nothing between her and the currents of wind created by their own motion. She had never known such exhilaration, so it was easy to forget about the present complications of her life and how they might affect her future.

Cruising into the Millborough city limits, Martina directed Rod to the public library on the assumption Rod did not know his way around the town. Freebird, who had donned a pair of aviator's goggles for the ride, followed close behind, with Julie clinging to his back and smiling dreamily. When they came to a stop, Martina felt a weird sadness that the ride had ended, although her whole body was still vibrating. Martina and Julie were then instructed by their respective chauffeurs to hop off, while the guys switched off their motors and maneuvered their bikes backward and carefully positioned their back tires against the curb in front of the library.

When Rod dismounted from the bike, Martina saw that he was about six feet tall and very well proportioned, with a sturdy build. She wondered what it would feel like to be embraced by his strong, muscular arms. As though Martina's thoughts had sent out a vibration into the surrounding ozone, Rod looked straight into her eyes and gave her a smile she was never to forget. It was almost as though he had heard her thoughts and was inviting her to sample the wonderfulness of his embrace. But, then, Rod needed no vibes or prodding to tune into this exotic beauty with the dazzling green eyes. Somewhere, back on the highway into Millborough, Rod had already made up his mind that he wanted to be with this woman for a lot longer than just one of his usual encounters. And, yes, she was indeed a woman, despite her obvious youth. It was not just her body language that conveyed to him that she was no flighty schoolgirl. There was some age on her soul, and he could see it deep in those penetrating green eyes of hers. How or what, he could not fathom. But he could tell from the way she talked and handled herself that she was not a street type, or what the guys at the clubhouse called a "knock-around broad." Rod could sense a classiness and maturity about her that he found lacking in the other young women he was used to dating. If he had any idea of how she had acquired the "age" he saw accumulated in the depths of her eyes, even he might have been shocked.

At that moment, however, as they stood on the street in front of the Millborough Library, Rod was looking for a way to stay in Martina's company a while longer. He wasn't ready to let loose of her and hoped to detain her until she felt comfortable enough to give him her telephone number. Just across the street the opportunity presented itself. Pointing to a quaint coffee shop, with a *faux* cottage facade, he polled: "Hey! Anyone up for coffee or something to eat?" Smiling down at Martina, he took one of her hands in his, and coaxed, "I'd really like it if we could get to know each other a little better."

Martina couldn't help being taken in by the intensity of his dark eyes and the sexy, crooked grin, but her instincts detected a certain well-polished charm and sensuality about him that triggered alarm bells in her head. She knew how the pick-up game was played. Sure, he was standing there smiling his sexy smile and acting all polite, but in his head he was calculating how long it would take him to get her into bed. Martina did not intend to be anyone's frivolity. And bikers did, after all, have a certain reputation for sexual conquest. She had no doubt Rod McDonough was all about conquest. His muscular body was in itself a statement about his sexuality, and in spite of her convictions about bikers and the warning bells, Martina had a difficult time keeping her eyes from wanting to absorb every inch of his physicality. So when Rod suggested they all go for a cup of coffee she didn't need a whole lot of coaxing. But she wasn't going to give Rod the benefit of an easy "yes."

Rendering her most enigmatic, Cheshire smile, Martina made a big production of consulting her watch to determine if she could possibly spare him any more of her valuable time. The truth of it was that both girls had parents who were mostly out of the house all day and sometimes until the late evening, and they were pretty much free to keep the same hours. Martina noted that it was only five-thirty and she had hours to spare, since her father was teaching a class that evening and wouldn't be home until after nine o'clock. But wanting to play it coy, she said to Julie, "I can probably hang out for a half hour, what about you?"

"Okay with me," answered Julie, who was half way sitting on the saddle of Freebird's bike, her claim already staked. Then looking at Freebird, she added in a flirty voice, "Who wouldn't want to."

Towering over her, Freebird smiled down at Julie and pressed his brown lips to her white forehead. Her arms automatically circled around his waist and her hands found their way into the back pockets of his jeans, where they squeezed his butt. The two seemed struck on each other already, and signals passed back and forth between them by way of facial expressions. Martina envied Julie's ability to simply take things at face value, whereas she always had to examine motives and meanings and nuances.

"Well...let's not waste anymore time," said Rod, seizing the moment. Gently squeezing Martina's hand a few times, he led her across the street. As they approached the front door of the coffee shop, he remarked, "I've always liked the look of Millborough, but the people who live here need a major attitude adjustment."

Martina laughed at his observation. "You are so right-on about that," she averred, having already seen a few people giving them strange looks. Bikers and guys with long hair, like Freebird, were not often seen on the streets of Millborough. It wasn't that the police or anyone else overtly discouraged them from living or visiting there. It was just the kind of a town that bikers, hippies, and people with limited means intuitively avoided. It was the negative attitudinal pall hanging over the place that put them off, like Rod had said.

"Have you spent much time in Millborough to know that much about it?" Martina asked Rod.

He laughed at her remark. "I'd say so," he responded, his expression turning into a wry smirk, "I grew up here."

Martina stopped in mid-stride and looked up at him with surprise. "You did?"

Rod pulled open the front door of the restaurant and stood back, to allow Martina, Freebird, and Julie to enter ahead of him, he said, "Sure did. I even went to Millborough Prep." Martina gave him a wide-eyed look of disbelief.

There were only a handful of people in the coffee shop, but they all looked up and gawked when the two young girls entered with their older biker escorts. If it were not for the fact that Maybelle Oaks, the proprietress of the "Millborough Chat and Chew," had known Martina and Julie for several years, she probably would have tossed them all out. As it was, she gave the girls one of her sternest of looks and

70

Martina could almost hear her preaching one of her pet phrases, "If you lie down with the dogs, you're sure to get up with their fleas."

Martina pursed her lips to keep from laughing at Maybelle's expression. If only Maybelle knew what was going on in the Fiasconi house late at night she'd be happy to see Martina in the company of Rod McDonough, even if he was one of those dreaded bikers.

Taking a booth in the back corner, where they could talk in private, Martina and Rod took one of the bench seats and Julie and Freebird molded together on the other. Freebird had his arm around Julie's shoulder and kissed her on the cheek frequently. The two became rapidly lost in each other's mooning gazes.

Martina commented to Rod, "You went to Millborough Prep?"

"For four of the toughest years of my life," he answered. "My father threatened to send me to a military academy if I got tossed out of prep school. So, I hung with it and actually managed to get all As and Bs."

"Really?" Martina asked, not sure if she should believe him. Because Rod was so much older, she would not have any knowledge of the raucous acts he and his young friends committed around town when he was in his early teens.

"Really!" He answered. "I graduated in the top ten of my class. Of course, in those days the school was filled with all of Millborough's juvenile delinquents and quite a few from around the country. It was like a high-priced boarding school for kids who probably should have been in a juvenile detention center, but their parents had the money to send them to a prep school instead."

Martina laughed at his depiction of the revered Millborough Prep. "How old were you then?" she probed.

"About your age," he responded.

"Seventeen?" She said, realizing he had cleverly set her up to find out her age and now she could not say she was older.

"Actually, I was about fifteen," he said.

The waitress came to take their order, so Martina held her next question until the waitress left.

"So," Martina asked, as soon as the waitress was out of earshot, "how old are you now?"

"Whoa! You get right to the point, don't you?" Rod said, laughing at her boldness. He stared at her for a few seconds, wondering whether she would be put off by their age difference. May as well tell her the truth, he thought, she's the type who would dig around until she found out anyway. Besides, he did not want to lie to her. It would be best if she accepted him regardless of his age. He did not consciously go out looking to pick up a seventeen-year-old girl. He didn't have to, because there were plenty young girls who showed up at the clubhouse, and after a few minutes they didn't hold his interest. But this girl-woman was different. She definitely held his interest, and more so than a lot of the women his own age that he had dated. Finally, he answered, "I'm twenty-two."

"That's not so bad," she said.

Rod took her response to mean that she felt the difference between their ages was not that big of a deal to her. He had the feeling she had already considered the matter and put it to rest in her mind. He smiled down at her, automatically taking her hand in his. What he really wanted to do was take her in his arms and kiss those full, red lips, explore the inside of her mouth with his tongue, and maybe pull off that clingy turquoise sweater and kiss her spectacular breasts. But all of that would have to wait for another day. He sure as hell could not do that here in the coffee shop. But he knew it would have to be one day soon, because he didn't think he could stand to just simply look at her much longer.

Like a jungle cat circling its prey, he sprung. "Would you like to go riding with me tomorrow afternoon?" He noticed that, at first, she looked excited about his offer, but then the brightness of her eyes seemed to cloud up with cumulous panic. He wondered what that was about. Probably her parents, he thought.

"Uh...I'd love to go riding with you again...but I just don't know about tomorrow." Without thinking, she blurted, "Martino gets home early tomorrow afternoon and he likes me to come home right after school when he's there."

"Who's 'Martino?'" Rod asked.

"Oh— My father."

Rod made the connection between the names: Martina and Martino. "You call you father by his first name?"

She nodded, not really wanting to go any further with that subject, which was fine with Rod. His only interest was in finding out from her when he could see her again.

"Then when can I see you again?" He pressed her, but so gently it was almost like he whined the question.

Surprisingly, she upstaged him by asking for his telephone number. "That way," she reasoned, "I can call you and let you know."

Rod was almost shocked to hear himself say, "But how do I know you'll call me?" Even Freebird turned to look over at Rod when he heard him ask the question; he had never known Rod to be insecure with any woman before. Martina gave Rod a questioning look, like she couldn't believe he would be concerned with such a thing. Squeezing his hand, she said, "Why would I not want to call you? I think you're a pretty cool guy."

Rod caught hold of his emotions and got them back under wraps. He now had no choice but to acquiesce and give her his phone number.

10.

For two days Rod McDonough stayed close to his telephone waiting for Martina's call. At the end of the second day he was ready to concede that she wasn't going to call him. Then, at eight o'clock that night, his phone rang. Picking it up, he heard her say, "Hi, Rod. It's Martina." So relieved to hear her voice he dropped into a chair like a sack of wet cement. He hadn't realized how wired he had become over the last two days while waiting and wondering if she would call him.

"Martina! How are you?" He faked nonchalance.

"Fine," she said. But she was not at all fine. She was nervous and upset. Last night she had brought up the subject of dating to her father and his response scared her. He threw the book he was reading across the room, knocking over a framed photograph of her mother, and breaking the glass. Slamming his fist down on his desk, he said, "Don't be ridiculous! I didn't raise you to date."

She was shocked by the violence of his actions and the tone of contemptuous anger in his voice. It was completely out of character for Martino to get angry. And what did he mean when he said she was not raised to date? His statement did not make any sense to Martina. Although he later made a big show of apologizing to her, his words did not sound sincere, and she was left even more unsettled by the incident. Now, she had two men to assuage. "I wanted to call you last night but Martino and I had a…a disagreement, and I couldn't use the phone."

"He's not violent or anything, is he?" Rod asked, concerned about her safety.

Martina laughed. "Martino? Violent? No. He'd never lay a hand on me." She thought about the book he had thrown last night and how it barely cleared her head before crashing into the photograph of her mother. Just to be certain Rod didn't get any wrong ideas, she added, "He's just being a typical protective father."

"I can understand that," Rod said, wondering how many young guys her father probably had to run off in the course of a week due to Martina's beautiful face and hot little body. He immediately recognized the odd feeling that had just kicked him in the gut. It was jealousy, and he hadn't felt that emotion in years. A minute ago he was ready to kick Martino's ass if he was being mean to Martina; now, he was grateful to Martino for keeping the guys away from her. Curious about her home life, he probed, "What was the fight about…if you don't mind me asking?"

Martina was forthcoming in her answer. "Dating you… basically."

"You told him about me?" He hoped she had not told her father about him, or the man would lock her up in a cage for sure.

"No. Not exactly about you. I just told him I wanted to date."

"And he didn't like the idea, no doubt."

"Let's just say he was less than thrilled." She emitted a deep sigh.

"Where is he now?" Rod asked, fearing she might get in trouble for talking to him.

"He had to go back to school," she said.

"Your father goes to school?"

Laughing at his question, she clarified, "No. He doesn't go to school as in being a student. He's a professor at Wingate U. He lectures on philosophy mostly."

"Ah!" Rod exclaimed. "No wonder you are so smart."

Martina laughed at his remark, but said nothing further on the subject.

So far, Rod had not heard her mention anything about her mother, so he came back at her with a question designed to probe that aspect of her life. "And how does your mother feel about you wanting to date?" He heard her take a deep breath and then release it.

"My mother passed away…several months ago."

Hearing the sadness in her voice, Rod was immediately sorry he had asked the question, especially over the phone.

"Oh— Geez," He said, exhaling the words. "I'm sorry to hear that, Martina…." Unsure of what else to say about it, his words faltered. Thinking it best to steer away from such an awkward subject, Rod commented, "I guess that explains why your father is so protective of you."

She, too, thought it best to move away from the subject of her personal life, so instead of responding to Rod's last comment about her father, she seamlessly redirected the conversation by asking him, "So…have you been out scaring any more girls lately?" She tried to make it sound like she was just kidding, but she wasn't. Over the last two days she had given considerable time to thoughts about what Rod might be doing and wondering if he was going out with other women.

Rod, of course, understood the real intent of her question. Women used that backdoor approach all the time to find out if a guy's been out screwing around. He took heart from it, although. She wouldn't have asked if she didn't care. He was really tempted to tell her that he had been sitting around the house for two days, holding onto his dick and waiting for her to call, but he instinctively knew he couldn't talk to her like that. Nor did he want her to know that she had him all hung up.

Instead, he calmly said, "What would be the point of that...now that I know you?"

The directness of his answer caught her off guard and left her flustered. And while her tongue was temporarily immobilized, Rod decided it was time to cut to the chase and pin her down. The last forty-eight hours had brought an interesting turn of events for the usually self-assured Rod McDonough, who sometimes had two or three women clinging to his muscular arms at one time, and all of them vying for his attention. It wasn't Rod who made an issue of his sex appeal, it was the women he came into contact with. It seemed that no matter what juke joint he and his fellow pack of Vikings invaded, an often treacherous competition brewed among the ladies on the premises to see who was going to hang out with him for the night. If he selected anyone for a one-night saddle ornament, he usually sought out the one chick that didn't make a fuss, because she didn't think she had a snowball's chance in hell of getting his interest. Most times he preferred to ride alone, as it seemed less of a hassle. His buddies always teased him about his taste for the "Lee sisters—Ug-Lee and Unsight-Lee." But his biker brothers certainly liked having him in their company because he was a chick magnet, and they were always assured of profiting nicely from the fallout. Rod was beginning to tire of the repetition that hanging out with The Vikings had become, and he wondered where these same old scenes of flesh pillage, replayed in bar after bar they rode up on, were going. It was all so predictable and meaningless to him anymore.

Then, two days ago, a softly sauntering breath of fresh air wandered down a North Hampton alley in the lithe, shapely form of Martina Fiasconi, an incredible collage of caramel skin sculpted over a fine-boned face, bejeweled with ruby lips that made his mouth water, and glowing green eyes that pierced his soul. The second he saw her it was as though he had been sucker punched in the gut with a velvet fist, and his gut had been sending shock waves throughout his body ever since. His brain was seemingly locked on the vision of her walking past the clubhouse, his stomach too knotted for food, and his dick was in total rebellion. In the hours since reluctantly leaving Martina in front of the Millborough Library, after detaining her in the coffee shop for over an hour, he ranged through his house like a nomad high on speed: not wanting to be anywhere in particular, but just needing to keep moving.

And it was worse at night, when his rebellious organ really acted up and his eyelids refused to stay closed. All he could think of was the feel of her warm body leaning against his back when had she sat behind him on his motorcycle the day they met. Then his active mind would conjure images of a more sexual nature akin to the close proximity of her body and he would find himself standing in the shower in the middle of the night, washing away the effects of such thoughts. He couldn't even remember acting so pathetic when he was a sexually awakening teenager.

And, now, here he was finally connected by telephone with the source of his past hours of dysfunction, wanting to charm and impress in his usual manner, but the smooth talking, macho persona he had honed to perfection in the bars with his fellow Vikings no longer seemed an appropriate companion for this delicate, exotic flower of beauty. So, on the spot, he had no alternative but to resort to being himself and hope she would like him in his as-is condition.

"Martina?" he asked, sounding tentative, unsure.. "When can I see you again?" He thought the inaugural outing of the real Rod McDonough was as shaky as a newborn colt.

"How about tomorrow afternoon, after I get out of school?" she said.

Rod jumped up from his chair and began pacing back and forth, as far as the length of the phone cord would allow. "Great! Great!" He said, trying to control his excitement. "Do you want me to pick you up at school?"

"No!" She said emphatically, a hint of panic in her voice. Rod thought her tone suggested there would be dire consequences if he showed his face around the high school.

And she was probably right about that. An older guy on a motorcycle picking up a seventeen-year-old girl was sure to be noticed, and word might get back to her father about it. Then her father would see to it that she was strictly supervised for the next five years to prevent any further contact with him, or maybe even take more stringent measures and ship her off to The House of Good Shepherd, that cloistered convent on the outskirts of Millborough, which was surrounded by an impenetrable concrete wall and governed by wizened-faced nuns, who looked meaner than junkyard dogs and capable of performing ritual castrations.

With the convent scenario now graphically etched in his brain, he quickly backtracked, "You're right. That would not be a good idea.

We're going to have to find our own private little meeting place. But where?" He paused to think of a likely spot, but the circuits in his brain were jammed. "Maybe you can think of someplace?" he asked.

"How about the transfer station?" She suggested., thinking it would be between her school and North Hampton, where she thought he lived.

"Wouldn't that be too far away? We'd end up spending the whole afternoon getting to the place where we're going to meet," he said.

"I suppose," she said, confused. Maybe he didn't live in North Hampton after all, she thought. "Well...then...if I knew where you were coming from, then maybe we could meet somewhere in the middle," she said.

"I'd be coming from Scenic Drive," said Rod, still trying to think of a convenient meeting place in between his house and her school.

"Scenic Drive?" Now, Martina was really confused. Scenic Drive was located on the west side of Millborough and, as far as she knew, was a very exclusive enclave of million dollar mansions. And the most exclusive of those were the large estates nestled in the trees along Scenic Drive, which were at the very top of Mulberry Hill, and overlooking the entire town of Millborough. As the street name implied, the view from Scenic Drive was spectacularly scenic.

But Martina was sure he must be pulling her leg. "You live on Scenic Drive?" She asked him again, clearly incredulous.

Laughing at her tone of disbelief, he affirmed, "Yes, Martina. I live on Scenic Drive. But you're the first person who has ever made me feel ashamed of it."

"Well...I didn't mean it that way, Rod. I just didn't think it would be the kind of place where you would want to live."

"Why not? Is there something going on up here that will affect the property values?" Rod tried to pull off a serious tone of voice, but he was too amused by her reaction.

Martina knew he was making fun of her, so she decided to go along with the joke. "Yes. Actually, there is something going on up there that will absolutely destroy the value of the properties."

"Oh, really? What's that?" He asked, playing along.

"Bikers are moving in," she said. "Haven't you heard?"

Rod laughed heartily at her silliness. Continuing to play along with her, he said, "Good heavens! I'd better warn the neighbors to lock up their daughters."

Then she switched the subject to a more personal level. "Do you live with anyone?" It had suddenly occurred to her that he might be married, with children of his own.

"No. I live alone for the present."

"For the present?" She asked. "What does that mean?"

"What it means is that I live in my parents' house and take care of it when they're away. They stay in the Bahamas most of the year. My dad is sort of retired, but not completely."

"Oh."

"What are you getting at, Martina? Do you think I'm married or something?"

"Don't you think I should know about it, if you are?"

"Hmmm. Would it make a difference?" He asked, curious to hear her response.

"Yes," was all she would say, leaving Rod to guess that she would probably not want to get involved with him if he was married.

"It doesn't matter anyway. I'm not married and never have been," he said, ready to end the parrying and get back to deciding on a place to meet tomorrow afternoon. "Where should we meet tomorrow? If it will make it easier, I'll pick you up in my car?"

"Okay. In that case, how about the parking lot of Mulberry Mall? I can be there at three o'clock. I'll be sitting on a bench by the fountain near the main entrance, wearing a red scarf and dark sunglasses," she said, dramatically affecting a strange accent.

"I doubt that a red scarf and sunglasses would be any kind of disguise," he laughed at the image it conjured in his head.

"You'd stick out like a sore thumb."

"That's the idea, Rod. Then you won't have any trouble finding me."

"Like I couldn't pick you out of a line up of a dozen women wearing red scarves and sunglasses. I'd have to be blind."

"What does that mean," she fished.

"I'll tell you when I see you tomorrow."

11.

Ending his conversation with Martina, when Rod set down the phone he found himself too restless and wired to hang around the house. He went out to the big garage, where his Harley was parked, cranked on the music, and began to polish the chrome with a fury. Freebird, who now lived in Rod's old apartment above the garage, usually came down to hang with him and also tinker with his bike, or read old issues of *Penthouse* and *Easyriders* that were lying around. But ever since he met up with that little blonde, Julie, he was missing in action. Rod chuckled to himself as he thought of Freebird and his new fox. He loved Freebird like a brother and was happy that he found himself a nice chick. Except, Julie was not even old enough to have a driver's license and Rod hoped Freebird would play it cool. He cautioned his saddle brother, "Keep it in your pants, Bro, 'cause they don't let you take your scooter to the joint, and you'll be in there for a long fuckin' time if you get caught screwin' a minor."

Of course, Rod realized that he was stuck in the same pickle jar with Freebird. Martina might be old enough to have a license, but she was sure as hell still jail bait. Rod knew that prison time would extinguish his soul, if not his life. With all the legal and free stuff running the streets, he wondered why the hell he was getting himself involved with a seventeen-year old minor. He had no answer for it, other than she was the most beautiful woman he'd ever seen and he wanted her. What was really weird to him was that he knew his desire for Martina was not all about her looks and body; there was something about her manner and personality that he also found attractive. Rod would admit his first attraction was to her looks. She was like a work of art—a DaVinci painting or a Michelangelo sculpture. He could close his eyes and see every feature of her face, especially her piercing green eyes, like the color of phosphorous glowing under the ocean waters. But the more he talked with her, the more he saw her as a person, and he easily became interested in her thoughts, feelings, opinions, and ideas.

Like a man possessed, Rod briskly polished the chrome of his exhaust pipes and thought about the long telephone conversation he just had with Martina. It was probably the longest conversation he ever had with any woman, with the exception of his mother. Not only was the girl intelligent, she had a way of making him laugh. He felt he could be himself with her. Recalling her sultry voice, Rod wished she were there with him now. If he knew where the hell she lived he'd go see her; she had said her father was not at home. How was it, he suddenly realized, that he did not know Martina's address? The address was always the second thing he asked for whenever he met a good looking chick. The telephone number was the first, and he didn't have her number, either. This Martina seemed to have him all turned around and upside down. How did he let that happen, Rod wondered? Did she have some bewitching powers or was he losing his edge?

* * * * *

After her long conversation with Rod, Martina stretched out on her bed, staring up at the ceiling and recalling the sound of his voice. She tried to remember everything he had said, and marveled at the fact he lived up on Scenic Drive, which was quite a far cry from the scruffy alley in North Hampton, where she met him. She wondered why a good looking guy of twenty-two would be interested in her. There was a big gap between them in more than just age, like, for instance, experience, education, music, and lots of other things.

She considered that he might be just interested in having sex with a young girl. A lot of older men, she was aware, were attracted to young girls for that reason alone. Isn't that what all guys want from women, anyway? But, in her heart, or wherever it was inside of her that instinct lived, she didn't feel that Rod's interest in her was mainly for sex. After all, she was a minor. A guy like Rod wouldn't risk going to jail just to have sex with her. She was sure that Rod could probably just snap his fingers and half a dozen women would come running from six directions. So, what exactly it was that he saw in her, she didn't know. But she sure wanted to find out. And one thing Martina knew for certain was that Rod McDonough was the sexiest guy she had ever set eyes on.

Having pondered every aspect of her conversation with Rod to the point of exhaustion, Martina went down the hall to the spare bedroom her mother once used as both a dressing room and "get away" space. All of her mother's clothing and other possessions were still in the room, just the way she had left them before her death. Martino refused to remove anything from the room, as though Jacqui might walk through the front door at any minute and resume wearing her old clothes. Even if by some miracle Jacqui did come back from the dead, Martina was certain her mother would insist upon an entirely new

81

wardrobe, since all of her clothes were now out of fashion. Jacqui never wore anything that was past season.

Martina went to her mother's bureau and riffled through the drawers. Somewhere, she knew, in one of those drawers there was a red silk scarf. And sitting right on top of the dusty bureau were her mother's Dior sunglasses. Jacqui loved those sunglasses because the lenses were so big they practically covered her whole face and, that way, people did not stare at her.

Martina took the scarf and sunglasses to her room and stuffed them into her book bag, to take with her to school the following day.

12.

"Get married!" Martina exclaimed, shocked by Julie's latest revelation. "But you've only just met Freebird...don't you think you should give yourselves some time to get to know each other before you even think of getting married?"

The two girls were at school, in between their first and second period classes, and it was the first time they had seen each other that day, so there was much news and gossip to catch up on. Sitting together on a bench at the end of a quiet corridor, where their privacy was assured, Julie had just finished telling Martina the story of her first real date with Freebird, which had occurred the night before. Since Julie's mother was divorced and spent a lot of time running around in search of her next husband, Julie had an inordinate amount of unsupervised time. And even though Julie did not get home until close to two o'clock that morning, she had still beaten her mother home by at least a full hour.

Since there was only a ten minute break between classes, Julie had to give Martina an abbreviated version of how she met Freebird outside of the library about seven o'clock last night, went riding on his motorcycle, stopping at Raccoon Lake to talk and make out. She described to Martina how passionate Freebird had become while they were French-kissing.

"Poor Freebird." Julie sighed with earnest pity. "He was so hot and horny that we had to get back on the bike and go riding just to keep from doing it right there and then." Martina shook her head, dismayed by the graphic details of her friend's fast-moving love life. Julie sped on with her narrative.

"Then he took me to see where he lived and it was this really cute little house...like a gardener's cottage or something...on someone's big fancy estate up on Scenic Drive."

Martina's antennae cocked right up as soon as Julie uttered the words "Scenic Drive," and immediately made the connection. "Ohmygod, Julie! Rod lives up on Scenic Drive too. Freebird must live up there with Rod."

Julie looked at Martina with a puzzled expression. "How did you find out where Rod lives? I thought you had decided not to call him because he's too old?"

"I changed my mind. I didn't see the harm in just talking with him on the phone. And twenty-two is not really too old. Besides, you know I can't stand guys our age…they're so immature."

"That's for sure. After being with Freebird I will never be able to date any of these nerds around here," Julie declared with an expression of distaste and gestured toward the school hallway, where three of the so-called nerds were horsing around about twenty-feet from where the girls were sitting.

Martina gave her friend a sudden look of alarm. "What do you mean 'after being with Freebird?' How 'with' him were you?"

Julie rolled her eyes and emitted an impatient sigh. "Martina! I promised you I wouldn't do it with him. We just laid on his bed with our clothes on and dry-fucked."

"Julie!" Martina exclaimed, shocked by her friend's vulgar language and the matter of fact way she used it. "Where did you pick up that expression…or should I even ask?"

"It's just an expression, Martina. But that's how Freebird described what we were doing. But he said he didn't know how long we could continue doing it that way because it was against the laws of nature and we could go blind or insane."

"Oh— Please, Julie! Get a grip! No one goes blind or insane from that sort of thing."

"I was just kidding about that part," Julie laughed, her blue eyes sparkling.

"Get serious, Julie. You're playing with fire. And what's worse…you could end up getting pregnant?" Martina's voice conveyed a tone of great dread.

"But Freebird loves kids," Julie said, affecting a dreamy expression, and deliberately trying to exasperate her too-serious friend.

"Not funny, Julie. You'd ruin your life."

Julie scrunched her face, looking truly perplexed.

"Well…what are we going to do, Martina? Freebird says Rod gave him the same lecture about not having sex with me because he'd go to jail. It really put the fear in him. Freebird says that the only way to get around it is to go over the state line and get married by a justice of the peace. They can't send him to jail for having sex with me if we're married."

Martina looked at Julie like she had three heads. "Girl! I think you and Freebird have already gone blind and insane over this whole thing. That's the nuttiest thing I've ever heard you come up with."

Just then, the warning bell sounded for the second period class. Martina jumped up and grabbed her book bag off the floor. Julie wished she could go someplace and take a nap.

"So...," Julie said. "When are you and Rod going to get together and do some dry-fucking yourselves?"

"Julie!" Martina gave Julie a look of mock disgust.

"See!" Julie chided. "You know you will do the same thing as us, the first chance you get."

Martina laughed at Julie's comment. Her friend might possibly be right. "I'll let you know later, because I have a date with him today, after school."

"Oh! Really! Well thanks for telling me sooner."

"You didn't give me much of a chance, what with all your talk about getting married and dry you know what-ing," answered Martina, pretending to be exasperated.

Julie cracked up laughing at Martina's prudish inability to say the "F" word. "See you at lunch," Julie said, still laughing, and took off running down the hall toward her classroom, which was way over on the other side of the building.

13.

After eating lunch with Julie later that afternoon, the last one-and-a-half hours of the school day seemed to drag on interminably for Martina. Perhaps the fact that she had been checking her wristwatch every few minutes had something to do with it, but her eagerness to hop the bus to the Mulberry Mall was all-consuming. She had even checked three or four times to make certain the red scarf and sunglasses were in her book bag and, of course, they were snug in their place each time.

Finally, the last bell of the day rang at two-thirty and she shot out of the class room, merely flashing a quick goodbye to Julie, as she ran past her in the hallway. As she neared the end of the bus ride to the Mall, she put on the red scarf and the sun glasses, so that when she exited the bus she would already be in disguise.

Martina surreptitiously glanced around as she walked from the bus stop toward the fountain, which was about 50-feet from the entrance to the rambling one-story mall. She quickly scanned the area but did not see Rod anywhere in sight. She pretended to be doing something with her book bag in order to steal a glance at her watch. It was precisely two fifty-five. If he was watching her from some vantage point she certainly did not want him to think she was anxious. But she was anxious. What if something happened and he could not come? What if he changed his mind? A half a dozen "what ifs" nipped at her heels as she walked toward the circle of benches spaced around the fountain. Choosing the bench that would allow her the best view of the parking lot, she sat down to wait for Rod. Since she had forgotten to ask him last night what kind of car he would be driving, she had no idea what to watch for, other than for him physically. To calm her nerves, she took one of the books out of her bag and opened it to a random page, and actually tried to read. Suddenly, a muscular arm reached over her shoulder and placed a single, long-stemmed red rose across the pages of the book, and a familiar voice recited, "*Gather ye rosebuds while ye may....*"

Smiling, she slowly picked up the rose and finished the poem's verse, "*Old time is still a-flying....*"

"Aaah! So you know your Robert Herrick?" said Rod, slipping onto the bench beside her, impressed that she knew the old poem.

"Aaah!" She mimicked. "So you're a biker and a poet."

Although, she thought it curious that he chose that particular verse to recite, since it was supposed to be an ode to virgins to make the most of their youth to find someone to marry before they got too old to attract a husband. As he sat down beside her she noted how neat and sexy he looked in a black polo shirt and black jeans that accentuated his muscular build. The sensual manliness of his body, so close to hers, suddenly frightened her.

"I'm much more than just a biker or a poet, my lady in the sunglasses and red scarf." His voice was soft and mellow, as his eyes bored into the lenses of her sunglasses. Martina found the intensity of his stare unnerving, and suddenly regretted she had agreed to meet him like this, by herself. His muscular physique, which she found so attractive the day they met now seemed threatening to her. With such strong arms he could easily overpower her. Her mind raced on with thoughts of him taking her to a remote location where no one would hear her screams for help. She thought herself stupid and silly for even considering an involvement with such an older guy. Yet, she found him so magnetic. It was the very danger about him that she found exciting. With her mind so occupied she didn't realize that her body had become rigid and tense.

"I sense that you're uptight about something," Rod gently probed, his tone was serious and concerned. He wondered what he had said or done that was a turn-off. Then, drawing on his wry sense of humor, he added, "Is it the choice of poem...or me?"

The accuracy of his question in both categories, along with the ultra-seriousness of his expression completely dissipated Martina's *noire* mood and she burst into laughter. It was the convulsive kind of laughter that came from down deep inside, where it had been stored for a long time, just waiting for something or someone special to set it free. Rod took her laughter as a good sign that the tension he sensed had been broken. It took several minutes for Martina to get herself under control, as every time she looked at Rod's amused face she was seized with another spasm of hysterics. In the end, she wondered how she could have ever thought he was dangerous.

"Do you feel better now?" Rod asked when she had finally calmed down.

"Uh-huh!" She nodded and smiled reassuringly.

"What a relief!" He sighed. "For a minute I was worried you were going to jump up and run away."

"For a minute...I was thinking about it," admitted Martina.

"Why?" He asked, barely concealing his bruised ego. After their phone conversation last night Rod was sure he had scored some high points with her. "I hope you don't think I'd take advantage of you or do anything to hurt you…if that's what you're worried about."

Martina studied his expression and knew he was telling her the stone truth. "I know that…now."

She thought he was reaching over to remove the sunglasses.

Instead, he placed his index finger on the bridge of her nose and began gently tracing its profile, his eyes intently following along the sensual trail, moving down onto the fullness of her lips, where he briefly paused to feel their satin softness, and continuing over the roundness of her chin. Lifting her face upward toward his, he then slid off the sunglasses, so he could see those striking green eyes that had haunted his days and nights since meeting her. He slipped the sunglasses into the front pocket of his polo shirt. Without the dark lenses to hide behind, she self-consciously lowered her head to avoid the intensity of his gaze. Again, he lifted her face upward and began untying the loose knot of the scarf under her chin, letting the silky cloth slide down her hair onto her shoulders, and eventually onto his lap. He saw that she was still clutching the rose he had given her.

He was captivated by the sensual fullness of her lips and felt a strong desire to kiss her. At such an early stage of their relationship he didn't think it would be a good idea to act on his impulses, so he asked, "I'd really like to kiss those delicious looking lips of yours, Martina."

When Rod didn't move in on her right away, she realized that he was waiting for her approval. Shyly, she made a quick nod and that was good enough for Rod. Although he had been visualizing this moment for days he did an admirable job of checking the full force of the passion he had stirred up inside of himself. Martina, however, was totally unprepared for the intensity of the emotions that surged in her body when Rod encircled her with his strong, protective arms and his lips came so softly down upon hers. Surprisingly, she felt herself responding to his touch and the movement of his lips, giving herself over to the sweet sensations of his kiss, the feel of his body touching hers, and the manly scent of his skin. All of these sensations were new to her and she marveled in them.

And, yet, it was just a sweet, first time kiss, exchanged on a bench at a Mall. There was not contained in it the raging lust of two impassioned lovers, but Martina glimpsed the possibilities and, now, the genie had been let out of the bottle.

It was Rod who reluctantly ended the kiss. He, too, glimpsed numerous possibilities, but he didn't want to explore them on a bench in the middle of a public thoroughfare. Needing a few moments to cool off, he looked down at the book on her lap and asked, "What were you reading when I sneaked up on you?"

"Greek mythology," she answered, understanding his need for diversion. She almost felt sorry for him.

"Those Greeks. They had quite the culture. Aristotle. Socrates. All those philosophers in one place around the same period of time. There must have been something in the water in Athens back then." He paused, looking around for a moment at the people who were walking by, then continued. "I suppose your father lectures on the Greek philosophers in his classes at Wingate?"

Martina, who was folding the red scarf to put back into her book bag, almost visibly recoiled to hear Rod mention her father. Turning to look at him, she said, "I don't want to talk about my father." Her tone wasn't harsh, but certainly did convey her seriousness.

Rod studied her face for a second and nodded. "Are you still mad at him about the fight...that you told me about on the phone?"

"No. I just don't want to talk about him when I'm with you," she said. Her tone was flat and suggested no further discussion on the matter was welcome.

"Fine with me," he said, wondering what all that was about.

"Would you like to go get something to eat?"

"Maybe just a cold drink," she answered, now wedging the book in her bag.

"Well...let's hit it, Little Mama. I know a place where we can go to...out on the way to Summerville." He stood up and offered her his hand, which she readily took hold of, and pulled herself up. He had noticed earlier she was wearing a black and white flowered skirt with a matching black short-sleeved jersey, but it wasn't until she stood up that he saw how short the skirt was. The flared style of the skirt showed off her narrow hips and slender, shapely legs to perfection. "I guess we won't be going bike riding today," Rod commented.

Martina gave him a puzzled look.

"You're wearing a skirt," he reminded her.

"Oh— I'm sorry. I didn't even think of it," she apologized, flustered.

Looking her up and down with obvious admiration, Rod said, "I guess I can't have it both ways."

Martina gave Rod a quick, considered look. "Humph!" she remarked, as she took the lead. "Nor will you."

Rod stopped in his tracks, smiling with appreciation as her skirt swished from side to side with the sway of her hips. "I guess not," he said with a grin, more to himself than to her.

When they approached the end of the sidewalk, Martina stopped and pointed in the general direction of the Mall parking lot. "Which way do we go?" she asked.

Rod took hold of her arm and escorted her toward a white Corvette convertible, which was parked near the end of the first row of cars. Opening the passenger door for her, he gestured to the low-slung seat with an exaggerated flourish of his hand. "Your chariot awaits!"

Martina looked down at the custom rolled red leather upholstery and all of the accessories and ornaments that were, no doubt, added to the car's interior once it left the dealer, such as the grotesque little skull fitted to the top of the gear shift lever and the furry red dice with black dots that hung from the rear view mirror, and shook her head in disbelief. Turning to look up at Rod, she kidded, "This is supposed to be less conspicuous than your motorcycle?"

"Actually," he said with a sheepish grin, "I've been looking for just one more…very hard to find accessory…to give it a real look of class."

Looking around at the general flashiness of the blazing red interior, Martina remarked, "I can't imagine what that could be?"

Pointing to the sun visor in front of her, he said, "Pull down that visor and you'll see a picture of what I'm looking for."

Unaware of what he was up to, she pulled down the visor and was surprised to see her own image staring back at her from a mirror that was embedded in the plush leather. Either it was the reflection of the surrounding red upholstery or her face had turned beat red from blushing. Then she wondered if he was just poking fun at her, but when he climbed into the driver's seat beside her, she saw that his expression was quite serious.

The road to Summerville had probably once been a cow path, but was now a picturesque, tree-covered two lane black top that wound its way through pastures of grazing horses and staring, masticating cows. Martina had never been out that way before and was taken by the clusters of colorful wild flowers along the sides of the road and old barns with sleepy expressions, rendered by the symmetrical placement of eye-like windows and gaping mouth-like doors. Riding in the Corvette with the top down reminded her of the many times she rode in her mother's Jaguar convertible, but her mother would never trifle with a scenic ride into the country unless there was a shopping mall with exclusive stores to be found there.

When they came to the little town of Summerville, which seemed to consist only of an antiquated gas station, a storefront post office, and a combination hardware and feed store, Rod down-shifted to a slow roll and nosed the road-hugging, "pregnant roller skate" (Martina's description) into the side yard of what appeared to be a quaint, two story clapboard house. On closer inspection, Martina saw the downstairs of the house had been converted into a restaurant and the gold lettering on the picture window of what used to be a living room indicated it was now "Katie's Korner."

Switching off the engine, Rod turned to Martina and said, "This is a great little restaurant. I think you'll like it."

"How did you ever find this place...way out here in the middle of nowhere?" Martina asked, scanning the front of the house-restaurant and wondering how many girlfriends he had brought here to eat.

Rod heard the real question behind her question and decided a silly response was what she needed. Affecting a highly effeminate voice and limp-wristed posture, he lisped, "Actually, Freebird and I found it when we were out on one of our long rides together. We come out here a lot. Just the two of us. It's our special place."

The image of Rod and Freebird sitting up against each other in a booth at Katie's restaurant immediately conjured in her mind and she started laughing so hard she could not stop. When she tried to stop, Rod would swish his wrist at her or make a silly face and she would be overcome with another spasm of laughter. Rod enjoyed seeing her laugh; he had a feeling that she did not do much of it, because she was so adept at seriousness. Finally, when her sides began to ache and her face started to hurt, she drew herself to a stop. He saw that tears had streamed from the corners of her eyes and he brushed them away with his fingertips.

"Don't ever do that to me again," she giggled, still trying to keep from laughing.

"Do what?" He asked, putting on his most innocent, boyish expression. He would have loved to continue teasing her but his stomach was now growling, and he was eager to put away one of Katie's hot roast beef sandwiches on crispy French bread, smothered with gravy. Extricating himself from the low-profile roadster, Rod went around to the passenger side and opened the door for Martina. Once he had occasion to take hold of her hand, to help her out of the car, he was not about to let it go. When she stood up next to him, he gently pulled her close and asked, "How about another one of those kisses?"

This time, when their lips came together, so did the length of their bodies. This time he could fully embrace her, but the bounds of public decency restricted him from kissing her the way he really wanted. Backing off before his reaction to her nearness became embarrassingly obvious, Rod gave Martina a look that told her he'd be back for more later, and then he led her into Katie's.

14.

"Where are we going, now?" Martina asked Rod, as he smoothly navigated the Corvette through the streets of Millborough. They were now in a section of the town that was unfamiliar to her, having taken a network of back roads on the drive homeward after leaving Katie's Korner in Summerville.

"I thought maybe you'd like to see where I live...since you didn't believe a biker could possibly live up on Scenic Drive."

Martina tried to conceal the panic she felt about going with him to his house, where the two of them might be alone. From the way he kissed her in the parking lot at the restaurant a couple of hours ago, compared to the innocent kiss he had given her at the mall, she knew that his urges were getting stronger and bolder. And she was certainly feeling her own excitement rising by degrees, especially whenever he gave her that look of boyish innocence. Sometimes, if she caught it just right, there would be an expression in his eyes that made her want to just cover him with her body and protect him from the world. Martina was not able to understand what it was she saw in his eyes at those moments, or even give it a name. It seemed a look of multiple needs, like he was hurting inside and not able to find whatever it was he needed to relieve the pain. Maybe that was why he had a fancy new motorcycle and a Corvette, and no telling what other diversions he accumulated at his house in his search for relief. Or, maybe, what Martina really saw were her own needs reflecting back at her in his dark brown eyes.

Martina was certain of one thing: there was a fiery chemistry between her and Rod. There was only one possible outcome if she allowed him to kiss her again and again, especially if they were alone together at his house. But a relationship with Rod was not the cause of her panic. It was the complications that were sure to follow should Rod, or anyone else for that matter, find out about her secret life. And, right now, she was already dealing with enough complication. Just last week, Julie commented: "Martino is awfully possessive of you these days." The fact that Julie, whose mind was almost always locked on some "sexy hunk" or the latest outfit she has to have, even noticed Martino's changed behavior meant that others who knew him even better were also sure to notice. And these were the thoughts that bounced around Martina's troubled mind, as Rod wound around this corner and that, to finally make the ascent up Scenic Drive just as the sun was dipping toward the horizon.

Close to the top of the hill he turned into a blacktop driveway that was flanked at the entrance by fieldstone pillars, adorned with large bronze coach lights. Rod maneuvered the Corvette along the narrow, curvy blacktop with a precision and timing that suggested he could probably negotiate it while blindfolded. The rambling, two story house with its fieldstone carapace suddenly loomed through the leafy filter of ancient oak and pine trees that seemed to encircle the home like verdant, impervious guards. Looking upward at the imposing structure, Martina noticed a sizeable balcony, enclosed with a black wrought iron railing. The balcony sat on top of the roof of what appeared to be a semi-circular solarium that jutted out toward the driveway. The French doors leading from an upstairs room, probably a bedroom, out onto the balcony were wide open. Martina remembered Rod saying he lived alone in the house, but now she wondered if there was someone else in the house after all. She couldn't imagine that Rod would go out for the day and leave doors wide open.

Rod accelerated between two of the giant oaks and headed for a stone-encrusted three car garage, which appeared to have an apartment or studio above it, which stood at the end of the long driveway. Lurching to a stop in front of one of the garage doors, Rod pulled himself out of the car and walked around to the passenger side to open the door for Martina, who was staring around in disbelief. It was hard for her to imagine that the young man she had met in a scruffy alley in North Hampton actually lived in such a grand and beautiful house. She also liked the inviting look of the back lawn, which had groupings of Adirondack chairs and recliners placed at strategic locations. The lush, bucolic setting belied the closeness of neighbors and the burgeoning town of Millborough, which clamored at the base of the hill.

"Well? What d'ya think?" Rod kidded. "Doesn't this place make a great biker pad?"

Martina laughed and nodded, going along with his joke. "Yeh! It'll do. No telling how many bodies are buried in the backyard."

Rod took Martina by the arm and led her to a huge back porch that had the look of an open air pub, complete with a built-in bar and a dart board. Rod opened the back door and stepped aside to allow her to enter the house first. Martina hesitated. He noted the expression of worry on her face.

"What's wrong?" Rod asked, concerned.

Martina shrugged. "I don't know...maybe I shouldn't go in."

"Why not?" He asked. The tone of his voice was soft and serious when he added, "Are you afraid to be alone with me?"

She looked up at him, surprised he guessed her thoughts. But before she could respond to his questions, he placed his hands on both of her shoulders and, staring deep into her worried green eyes, he assured, "Don't you know by now that I would never do anything that would make you feel scared to be with me? I'm sure not going to force myself on you. If you don't want to be with me, then we can end it all...right here and now."

They stood staring into each other's eyes for a moment. Martina searched for the slightest flinch of insincerity in Rod's expression, but his gaze remained rock steady. And at that moment, whether Martina realized the full extent of it or not, she sealed her commitment to Rod when she plainly told him, "I'm not afraid of you." Rod couldn't help but smile when he saw the tiniest flash of defiance in her phosphorescent, sea green eyes, and he was reminded of that day he met her in the alley, when she had given him a much stronger look of defiance. He almost groaned aloud from the mere pleasure of now simply having her in his house and watching her skirt sway in time with her hips, as she walked ahead of him into the kitchen.

Rod took two sodas out of the refrigerator and handed one to Martina, who was clearly absorbed with examining every detail of the kitchen's architecture and design. The room was generous in its size and its appointments. The interior wall of the kitchen, which divided the room from the rest of the house, was long and constructed entirely of the same stone that was used to construct the outside shell of the house. Here and there the stone wall seemed ablaze with glinting copper accents, such as a highly polished range hood, which descended from the ceiling, and other unique, shiny bric-a-brac. To the left of where Martina stood, just inside the back door, was a dining area containing a large, heavy-looking round table and several equally solid chairs, positioned in front of a picture window overlooking the idyllic backyard.

Martina was particularly taken with a wide, arched stone hearth built into the opposite end of the long stone wall. The cave like opening made the wall appear as though it was in a perpetual, semi-circular yawn. From copper hooks somehow affixed to the stone wall next to the hearth, hung a huge copper ladle and a matching spoon, as if to be at the ready when the family prepared its cauldrons of wild game soups or venison stew. There was a huge stone-based island built in the center of the kitchen floor and one side of it was used as a snack bar, with six wooden stools lined up alongside of it. The top of the island was fitted with a thick solid piece of butcher block that bore the scars of much use. Just past the hearth, was an arched doorway leading to a formal dining room of grandiose proportions, and at the far end of the kitchen was another arched doorway that led to an enormous living room and study.

"This is a fabulous kitchen," she said, as her eyes scanned the dark wood cabinetry and high-end appliances. She was even more impressed when Rod told her that he helped his father build it.

It took over an hour for Rod to tour Martina around the enormous house, mainly because he had a funny story or two to go with every room. Later, when they were kicked back on the living room sofa, she realized that she had not seen the room with the French doors that opened onto the upstairs balcony. She was driven to ask, "Which room is the one that opens on to that cool balcony upstairs? You didn't show me that room."

Rod gave her a look of surprise. He didn't think she would notice the omission of viewing his room when there were so many others to look at. "Oh— That's my room. I didn't take you in there because I didn't want you to get the wrong idea."

"Wrong idea?" She said, looking puzzled. "About what?"

"About what?" He countered. "About why I was taking you in there...especially after you were afraid to come inside the house at all."

"But I...I want to see your room," she coaxed. She had read somewhere that a person's bedroom can tell you a lot about their personality.

Rod immediately stood up and extended his hand, "Well, then...let me take you back upstairs to see it."

Opening the door to the bedroom, Rod stepped aside while Martina slowly entered. He remained standing in the doorway while she gawked in disbelief at the canopy bed, with its matching lacey white bedspread and canopy. She gave Rod a sly look and shook her head, not sure of what to think about Rod's personality.

"What can I say? This was my parents' bedroom and I just left it as is for when...or if...they ever return. Though they seem to like their boat life in the Caribbean much better."

Martina started to laugh. "I would have never thought you'd be sleeping in such a frilly room." She walked over to the bed to touch the lacey spread and then looked up at the lacey web stretched over the wooden canopy frame. "It's very beautiful," she commented, admiring the patterns in the lace.

"My father was a little bent about it too, but he put up with it because it was easier to give in than go against my mother once she had her mind made up about what she wanted to do. And I'm not about to bring down the wrath of my mother, either, by changing it."

"You're still afraid of your mother?" she asked through her increasing laughter.

"You don't know my mother," Rod qualified, as he watched her admiring the design in the lace.

Suddenly, before Rod even knew what had come over him, he was pulling her into his arms and trying to kiss her sensual lips. Alarmed by his sudden movement, Martina tried to get away but he had her secured in his powerful arms and she could not move. Holding her tight against his body, he calmed her with his soft, pleading words. "I just want to hold you and kiss you…don't be afraid." He felt her body relax, so he continued to hold her and gently stroke as much of her body as he felt he could appropriately touch. Then, unexpectedly, he felt her hand responding in kind. He hoped that meant he had finally gained her trust.

After many moments of gentle touching, where each became familiar with the feel of the other's skin: the shape of an ear; the hardness of a muscled arm; and the curve of a hip or thigh, there came the sweetness of their tender kisses. When Rod felt his passion escalating to a level where puckish thoughts of removing Martina's clothing began interfering with his attempts to keep his contact light he reluctantly pulled his lips away from hers. Martina was almost disappointed that he was able to exercise such great restraint, but she understood the need to do so. He continued to hold her close and she felt his chest expand with a deep breath and then deflate with a heavy sigh. Martina looked up into his eyes and gave him a questioning look. She wondered if he was sorry about getting involved with someone who was too young to have sex with him. Was he now thinking about the older women he could be with at this moment, who could do anything he wanted them to? A sudden mix of odd emotions left Martina feeling useless and threatened by the numerous available women she was sure he could have on a whim.

Martina heard herself ask him, "Are you wishing you were with someone else right now?"

Surprised by her question, Rod loosened his embrace and looked down at her. His tone was quite serious when he answered her with a simple, "No." Then he asked, "Do you think that all I am interested in is having sex with you?"

She looked up at him and shrugged her shoulders. "I'm sure it has crossed your mind, Rod."

Rod, who was trying to be serious, had to laugh at her comment. "Oh, yah! I won't deny that thoughts of making it with you have crossed my mind a time or two…and I'm probably holding on right now by just a thread…but I'm not going to risk what I hope will in its own time be something real by being a jerk now." Pulling her close against his chest again, he said, "I don't know how I'm going to do it…but I want to do this thing right with you."

The complete sincerity in Rod's voice brought tears to Martina's eyes. She tried to blink them away but they spilled out and rolled down her tanned cheeks and she was embarrassed by them. Rod did not see her tears but he sensed from her movements that she was crying. He held her close, saying nothing, until the early evening shadows began to darken the room and he knew it was time to take her home.

15.

Professor Martino Fiasconi was waiting somewhat impatiently in his study, eyeing the hands of the clock on his desk, when he heard the front door of the house open and close.

He heard Martina's footsteps tapping across the hardwood floor of the foyer and then become muffled by the hall rug. When she appeared in the doorway of the study, Martino gave her a curious, if not sullen, stare.

"Where have you been until this hour?" He asked, trying unsuccessfully not to sound annoyed.

"I'm sorry. I had dinner at the Mall with Julie," she lied, "and I guess we lost track of time." Martina walked over to him and automatically kissed his cheek. She noticed the soft puffiness of his face and the fine lines at the corners of his eyes. He seemed to look suddenly older to her. She felt guilty for lying to him about where she had been and her throat began to constrict.

"You look flushed," Martino commented. Then, in an attempt to be poetic, he added, "Like a maiden in love."

"Really?" She said, cool and detached. Changing the subject, she asked, "How was your day?"

He, too, changed the subject. "Shall I draw your bath?"

"Okay," she said, trying to sound enthusiastic, and even mustering a convincing smile. Although, she wasn't feeling very happy about the prospect of a bath. The familiar line about drawing a bath was Martino's way of signaling he wanted her attention tonight. But, really, she just wanted to go to her room and be left alone to relive her day with Rod, and then write it all down in her journal. If she was lucky, Martino would fall asleep early, leaving her to enjoy her thoughts of Rod until she, too, fell asleep.

Lately, all Martino wanted to do was watch her take a bubble bath and maybe, if he was in a good mood, massage her back with a loofah sponge. After the bath routine, he would pick out one of her mother's nightgowns for her to wear. Then he might want her to simply lie next to him until he fell asleep. Other times he would want more physical attention. But Martina was tired of playing the body-double of her mother. She had not intended for Martino to become so dependent upon her for diversion and pleasure. By now, she thought Martino would have found another female interest. Certainly, there were many unattached women at the college he could have connected with. But a young woman of Martina's age and limited experience could not know of the innate laziness of some people, when their immediate needs are being met, leaving them no desire to seek alternative pleasures on their own.

Martino stood, extending his hand to Martina, "Come then...," he said, now warmed by her presence. "Let's go upstairs." She took his hand and followed him, resigned. It was at that moment Martina knew she would soon have to have a serious talk with Martino and let him know she was ready to move on. Especially now that she had met Rod.

16.

Looking at the calendar one day, Martina could hardly believe that three months had slipped by since her first date with Rod. And nearly every day of those three months had proven to be a fine balancing act for her. Keeping Martino pacified, while at the same time trying to develop a relationship with Rod, took up a lot of her creative energies. Even though she was managing to keep up with her dual roles, there were changes taking place at the deepest level of her awareness that would eventually upset the fine balance she had so painstakingly arrived at. Quite simply, she was falling deeply in love with Rod McDonough and wanted only to be with him.

She knew she could not carry on with her pretense much longer. Each time Rod got excited and pulled away from her, whether out of respect for her young age or the law, Martina felt ashamed and hypocritical. She wondered how he was going to react when he found out she was not quite a virgin.

To his credit, Rod was extremely patient with the constraints on Martina's time. After all, he reasoned, she was only seventeen and still in high school. He understood that she could not spend as much time with him as he would like her to.

And it was probably just as well their time together was limited; it was difficult enough to keep his promise not to force himself on her. If they were together more often it would really be an impossible situation for him. But she would be graduating in several months and then, if all went according to his hoped for plan, he would ask her to marry him. He just hoped he could hang on that long without bursting a blood vessel.

Martino, on the other hand, was not at all understanding of the young woman's need to socialize. Martino resented all of the time she spent away from him to be with "her friends" and freely voiced his resentment to Martina. At first, she felt sorry for him and responded with special pampering, such as cooking his favorite meals and buying him little presents. But her efforts only caused him to be more complaining about her future absences. Finally, one day Martina cracked. She simply could not take the dual roles any longer. Waiting until after dinner, Martina summoned the nerve to have a talk with Martino. She had no idea how he would react but at this point she did not care. Her feelings for Rod had been steadily growing and she knew it was time to cut Martino loose. So, as she cleaned up the kitchen,

Martina mentally practiced her speech. Then, afterward, she went to the study, where she knew he was preparing for the next day's classes.

Martino looked up and smiled at Martina when she sat in the chair opposite his desk. He initially thought she had come into the study to keep him company while he worked, but then he saw the troubled expression on her face. "Is there something wrong?" he asked, getting right to the point.

"Actually— Yes. There is. I think it's time for me to start dating," she blurted, feeling her face growing hot. "And I think it's time you started dating, too."

Martino sighed with exasperation. He studied her for a moment, trying to get a grasp on what was really going on with her. "I see," he said, continuing to stare at her as though he could see into her mind and divine what she was thinking. Then he asked, "Are you tired of our closeness?"

Martina did not flinch under his stare nor did she mince her words when she answered, "Our closeness…as you call it…is not the right thing for us to do. When Jacqui died I wanted to help you get over losing her and…I think you have. But I cannot be her substitute anymore." Martina lowered her head as tears came into her intense green eyes. "I just can't anymore."

The stately professor of philosophy looked as though he had just come loose from his moorings, lost and adrift, momentarily. He immediately realized he did not have many, if any, options under the circumstances. It was not as though he could have her declared a disobedient juvenile for refusing to sleep with her own father. Leaning back in his chair and steepling his hands under his chin, he looked almost as though he was in complete agreement with Martina. But then he lurched forward and pounded his fist on the top of his desk. "No!" He shouted, angrily. "No! You cannot date. It's out of the question."

Martina stood up and gave him a fierce, defiant look, which seemed to fuel her tone when she said, "I will date and you cannot stop me. The truth is that I've already met someone I care about very much and I plan on seeing him every chance I get."

Martino was stung by her admission of having already met someone she cared about but he was not shocked. He had for a while suspected, from all of her late night's at the mall, she was seeing someone other than Julie. If it is a young man from her school, Martino felt certain she would soon tire of whoever it was, especially since she was used to the company of an older, more sophisticated, man. In a split second, he decided he'd best tread lightly with her. He was sure she would come around in due time, and it would be to his advantage to back off and let her current interest run its course. But before Martino could make a conciliatory gesture, she had run upstairs and locked herself in her bedroom. He thought it best to leave her alone for now.

17.

"When am I going to meet your father?" Rod asked Martina one night, after a session of particularly heavy petting in his Corvette. They had been to dinner and a movie and were now parked at an overlook at the top of Scenic Drive. "We've been dating for three months, Martina...don't you think it's time I met him?"

At this point in their relationship, Rod's desire for Martina was growing stronger and he was miserable from his unprecedented sexual frustration. He didn't know what good meeting her father would do in that respect but he felt that it was just time he met the man. It had crossed Rod's mind more than a few times how odd it was that Martina had not once invited him to her house during the past several months they had been dating. Was she afraid to introduce him to her father because he was so much older than her? Or maybe, Rod fretted, he was just a passing infatuation and, in that case, meeting her father would not be necessary, since she wasn't planning on a long-term relationship with him anyway. Nagging doubts about his role in Martina's life preyed on his insecurities and somehow Rod came to link the validation of her commitment to him with the meeting of her father, as though one was incumbent upon the other.

Martina instinctively knew that introducing Rod to Martino at this time would be a disaster. Ever since the night she told Martino she was dating he seemed depressed and insecure about it. Even though Martino had approached her the day after their confrontation over her dating and apologized for his "childish behavior", she knew he was still steaming inside. If she chanced bringing Rod to her house to meet Martino just now, there would definitely be an explosion of some sort. Martino was sure to notice that Rod was no weak-kneed teenager.

And, now, Rod was making demands of his own upon her. Martina tried to think of something neutral to say in order to put Rod off without arousing his suspicions.

"C'mon, Martina, when am I going to meet that daddy of yours?" Rod pressed her, while they kissed and stroked each other.

"It's not a good time right now," she told him.

"Why not?" He was now nibbling her ear.

"Because he has still not gotten over my mother's death," she answered, thinking that would be a satisfactory explanation.

Rod stopped in mid-nibble. "It's been long enough now for him to get a grip on it. You've had to pick up the pieces of your life and go on."

"It's different for him, Rod. He's lost the love of his life," she said, convincingly.

Rod pulled her close against him. "I guess I can understand that," he said, and rested his cheek on the top of her head, thinking how empty his life would be if he lost her.

"Just let me decide when the time is right, Okay?" she asked, with a soft, throaty voice. Rod could hardly say "no."

"Okay. You get to call the shots on this one because you know your father better than I do. But as soon as you think the time is right I want to meet him," he conceded, somewhat disappointed.

"What's the big deal?" Martina asked, laughing at Rod's sulky tone.

Rod tilted her head upward, so he could look her straight in her moonlit eyes, and answered, "Because I want to ask him for his permission to marry you before you turn eighteen."

"Rod!" gasped Martina. "Are you serious?"

"Serious as a heart attack," he affirmed.

"Martino would never go for that," she said, her mind whirling at the idea of being married to Rod.

"Why not? I'd take good care of you."

"Because he wants me to go to college," she said, sounding a bit sulky herself.

"You can be married to me and still go to college. I'll even carry your books to class for you." As he spoke, Rod opened his door and climbed out of the car.

"Where're you going?" she called after him, but he did not answer.

The next thing Martina knew, the passenger door was yanked open and Rod knelt down on the ground beside her. Taking her hands in his, he said, "I love you, Martina. I know you're young and need to do your thing…and I'm willing to wait as long as I know you want me to." Under the brightness of the moon, Rod intently searched her face for a sign of encouragement. This was the first time he told Martina he loved her and now, as he knelt in front of her, he felt exposed and vulnerable. He saw the glistening tears well up in her eyes and then run down her face; he held his breath while he waited for her to respond.

When she heard him say he loved her, Martina's heart seemed to explode in her chest, leaving her momentarily tongue-tied. Pulling her hands free from his grasp, she threw her arms around his neck and began sobbing on his shoulder.

All of her emotions – her anxieties about Martino, her worries and fears about Rod finding out about her secret life, and her own desires and frustrations – seemed to tear loose in that instant and flood out of her. Overcome with an intense mixture of happiness, sadness, relief, and apprehension she could no longer control, she could only cry until the welter of these feelings was exhausted.

Rod soon sensed that there was something more going on with Martina other than a reaction to his words of love and marriage. He could almost feel the mixture of pain her sobbing conveyed. He held her as tight as he could without choking off her breath and comforted her. When he felt her wracking sobs subside, he whispered in a gentle voice, "It's going to be okay, Baby. Talk to me, Martina. I need to know what's happening."

And Rod really did need to know what it was that made her cry so hard. He wanted her to share something of herself with him.

"Please...Martina," he practically begged her, "Please tell me what's making you hurt so much."

Hearing his words, Martina caught her breath. Keeping her face buried in the embrace of his warm and comfortable body, she said, "How do you know its hurt?"

"I can feel it, Babe," Rod answered. "I'm holding you in my arms and I'm kind of tuned in."

Martina reached up and placed her palm on his face and softly, gently caressed him. "I guess I am just being silly."

The rocky ground was digging painfully into Rod's knees. "C'mon," he said, standing up. "Let's go sit on that bench over there." He pointed to one of the benches placed in front of the low wall surrounding the lookout's parking area, and then helped her out of the Corvette. When she stood up beside him he put his arms around her and gently cradled her. She threaded her arms under his and around his waist.

"Rod...I love you so much—" She was barely able to finish her own declaration of love before breaking into another round of sobs.

Rocking her gently in his arms, he again felt it coming up with her sobs, from someplace deep inside of her – the pain.

All he could do was to hold her and wait for her to stop crying. When her sobbing finally ended, he led her over to the bench, where they sat down. Rod held her close and wished she would tell him what was causing her such hurt. Perhaps it had something to do with her mother's death.

"Tell me what's wrong, Martina," he again asked her, keeping his voice soft and unassertive. He heard and felt her emit a deep, ragged sigh in response. He could tell she was on the verge of wanting to tell him something but, for some reason, could not. Just a moment ago, when she said she loved him, he had the feeling she was about to say something further but, instead, broke into tears. He had to know what was making her sad at a time like this. He had just expressed his love for her and she said she loved him, too. He had been looking forward to hearing those words from her. If anything, they should both be crying tears of joy.

"How can we hope to have a close and trusting relationship if you don't feel you can tell me what's going on with you? You are upset about something." Martina shook her head in denial. Rod tried begging her again. "Please, Martina. There's nothing you can tell me that will freak me out. Whatever it is, we'll work it out."

Tempting as Rod made it sound to her, Martina could not tell him the real cause of her sadness. It was far too complicated. What could she tell him: that she had seduced her own father and now he did not want to let her go? Would Rod still love her after hearing that? He would probably never want to see her again. Yet, what kind of a life together could she and Rod have if she started it off by lying to him. Just thinking about the possibility of losing him made her sick to her stomach. She could not lie to this loving, trusting man, who held her so protectively and had just opened his heart to her.

Perhaps she did not deserve his love but she was powerless to walk away from it, as she loved him with all of her heart. And his love, in return, made her feel whole and a part of something special. She hoped they would be able to work out what was troubling her, if she ever found the nerve to tell him. If not, she just didn't know what would become of her.

So, finally, it came to her to say, "Even though we've only been together for a few months I feel like I can trust you with my life, Rod. I'm so lucky to have met you." She looked up at him and tried to smile, more so to put him at ease. For her own part, inside her nerves were all twisted in knots. "You are right...I am upset about something but I need more time to work things out."

All of Rod's senses immediately went on high alert. "Is it another guy?" He asked, hoping for some bit of a clue to the cause of her upset.

"No. There's no other guy. Please…Rod…don't ask me a bunch of questions about it. Let's just enjoy the rest of the night."

"Baby, I really care about you…I just don't like seeing you cry that way," he said, pressing his lips against hers.

"Just keep holding and kissing me the way you do and I'll be fine," she whispered.

"You love me, Baby?" He asked, his breathing already affected by her touch.

"I do love you, Rod…more than anything." She could feel the heat of his body as he pressed his chest against her and the palms of his hands were hot on her back. Even his tongue, when it breached her lips and entered her mouth, was hot and frenzied. She, too, felt her own body warming as she grooved along with him and before she could even think to stop herself her hand automatically gravitated to the hardness of his body.

Surprised by her touch, Rod stopped his kissing and succumbed fully to the pleasurable sensations aroused by the gentle intimacy of her massage. He was almost to the point of no return when it struck him that a bench off the side of the road was hardly the practical venue for what was certain to follow if Martina continued with her massage. The image of his lacey canopy bed suddenly formed in his mind along with the wish that they could automatically transport themselves there without missing a stroke of her hand. With a long, low moan of resignation Rod smothered her hand with his and the pleasurable spell of the moment was extinguished, although it took several more moments before their heavy breathing and wildly beating hearts to return to normal.

"Why'd you stop me?" She was obviously disappointed that he had.

"You know what's going to happen if you touch me like that?"

"Yes," she said. Her tone conveyed that she had already thought the matter through and had made up her mind about it.

And she had. For too many nights Martina lie awake, aching to be cuddled against his strong body, protected in his arms while he made love to her. Even when she was supposed to be comforting Martino, she thought only of Rod. It seemed foolish for her and Rod to deny themselves the fulfillment of their sexual feelings, nor could she stand the falsity of the pretense any longer. She was no longer a virgin, neither physically or mentally, and she did not want to be treated like one.

"Martina— We can't. You're only seventeen. You know what the law will do to me for laying a hand on you?"

"But I'll be eighteen in a few months."

"Not good enough, Babe. The age of consent is eighteen...you know that."

"The law needs to be revised, Rod. I know what I want."

Pulling her up against him, his voice was raw with emotion when he asked, "What do you want, Martina?"

Without hesitation, she answered, "I want to be with you."

"Then there is only one thing for us to do." His expression suddenly grew even more serious than it had been. "Martina...will you marry me?"

"Oh— Rod...." It was all Martina could say, as his sudden proposal left her stunned.

"Is that a 'yes' or a 'no?'" He asked, laughing at the shocked expression on her face.

"Yes," she managed to say before she burst into tears again.

Rod cradled her against his chest. "I hope those are tears of joy," he said, half joking, wondering if her crying was a continuation of her earlier episodes.

"But Martino will never give his consent," she said, wiping her tears.

"We won't need his consent, Baby. There's a justice of peace over in Clanton County that will be happy to marry us without his consent," he assured her, rubbing her arm. "We'll drive over there tomorrow night if you're ready to do it that soon?"

"I'm ready," she affirmed, and placed her hand back on his groin.

"It's time for me to take you home," he reminded her, sighing, as he removed her hand before his eager body could react.

18.

After taking Martina home, Rod waited outside the iron gate to the Georgian fortress for her signal that all was okay.

When he saw her bedroom light flash on and off twice he reluctantly went back to his car. If only there was a tree or trellis near her bedroom window, he'd be up inside of her room in a flash. Only one more night, he told himself, and Martina would be his wife. Then he would not have to take her back to that mausoleum of a house anymore. He studied the high wall with its overgrown vines that surrounded the large white stucco house. Other than the dim light glowing through the window in Martina's bedroom the rest of the house was in darkness and looked bleak and depressing. Suddenly, he saw the curtain-muted outline of a person standing in Martina's bedroom window. Rod could deduce from the shape of the outline that it was not Martina. No doubt it was her father who was staring out the window. Rod started up the Corvette, revved the engine a few times, popped the clutch, and then burned a little rubber off his tires as he took off. He knew it was a completely juvenile thing for him to do, but he felt like doing it.

The lights were on in Freebird's apartment when Rod pulled into his garage stall, so he decided to go knock on the door. He felt the need to talk with his friend. Freebird may not have had a college education but he possessed a wealth of wisdom that could not be learned from books. And, too, Rod simply enjoyed his company.

It took Freebird almost a full minute to open the door and Rod could see that he had obviously interrupted something. Freebird had come to the door wearing only a pair of hastily pulled on jeans, which were not completely zipped up, and his usually braided hair hung loose and was uncharacteristically tangled.

"Hey, man!" Freebird exclaimed, happy to see his friend.

The two men greeted each other with the traditional biker brothers' embrace.

"Jesus, Bro! You smell like a French whore," Rod kidded, after catching a whiff of woman's perfume emanating from Freebird's body.

Freebird smiled sheepishly, as Julie walked out of the bedroom wearing one of Freebird's Black Harley T-shirts, which hung down to her knees.

"Shit! Man! I came at the wrong time. I'll catch you later," said Rod, starting to back out of the door.

110

"No! Come in! It's never the wrong time for my Brother to stop by," Freebird motioned Rod to come back inside.

"Hey, Rod," Julie called out. "How about a beer?"

"I don't want to interrupt a good time," Rod joked, but meant it.

"Huh!" Julie commented, wryly. "Forget that. All we can do is masturbate each other."

"Julie!" Freebird scolded. "Go get my Bro a beer...please!" Freebird gave Rod a helpless look. "What can I say? She's an outspoken little chick."

Rod laughed. "Leave her be. I like the way she handles herself...and you must like it too or she wouldn't be up here with you every night."

Clearing some cast off clothing from a chair, Freebird said, "Sit down, Bro. Where's Martina?"

"I just brought her home," Rod said disappointedly as he lowered himself into the black leather armchair. Julie handed him a cold beer. "Thanks, Julie."

Freebird lowered himself to the floor, and sat cross-legged, with his back resting against the bottom of the black leather sofa. Julie stretched out on the sofa behind him and began playing with his hair. From under the sofa, Freebird slid out an aluminum pie plate that contained a four-finger baggie of pot and a package of Zig-Zags and began rolling a joint. "What's up?" Freebird asked, sensing Rod was uptight about something.

"I don't know what's up, Bro. Tonight...Martina...she just broke down and cried like something is really upsetting her."

Never one to miss an opportunity to tease his friend, Freebird kidded, "She must have discovered what a little pecker you have and that's what upset her."

Rod ignored the teasing and went on. "I told her how much I love her and she just cried. Something's going on with her. I asked her what she was upset about and she says she can't talk about it right now. What the hell could it be? I asked her if there was another guy involved and she said there wasn't...."

Rod's voice trailed off, as he thought about Martina's words.

Suddenly, Julie piped up, "It's not another guy, Rod. It's more like another man."

Rod jumped forward in his chair. "What? She said there was no one else."

"I don't mean another lover," said Julie, now sitting up and looking very serious. "I mean her father. Martino is obsessed with her or something. Ever since her mother died he's been real weird…like he wants to keep her for himself."

"Tell me more about this Martino dude, Julie," Rod pressed, now looking concerned. The image of a man's form standing in Martina's bedroom window earlier that evening was still burning in his mind.

Julie fiddled with her fingernails for a moment, unsure of what to tell Rod. Martina was her best friend and she didn't want to say anything that would cause trouble for her friend or hurt her in any way.

"C'mon, Julie," Freebird urged. "You started it…now tell my Bro what you know."

"I really don't know all that much. I mean…I don't go over to Martina's house a lot anymore. But when Martina's mother was alive she used to take us riding in her car…she had this red Jaguar convertible—"

Rod jumped up and interrupted Julie. "Wait a minute! I remember seeing that red Jaguar. That was Martina's mother?

That woman who wore the big sunglasses. Jesus."

He lowered himself back into the chair, remembering the beautiful woman in the red convertible. It was about two years ago that he first saw her, when he pulled up next to her at a light. He was riding his old Harley back then. She had looked over at him and smiled. At the time, he was sure she was flirting with him. When the light changed, she sped off. He followed her for a few blocks and then lost her. Catching himself, Rod said, "I'm sorry, Julie. Go on."

"Anyway," Julie continued, "Martina's parents always treated her like she was the third partner in their marriage. She even called them by their first names, which always seemed weird to me, because no other kids I knew of ever did that. And her mother treated her like she was her best friend…like once when we were out with her mother and her mother was shopping for a dress for a fancy cocktail party at the college. Jacqui—that was her mother's name—kept asking Martina for advice about what kind of a dress she should get. I thought it was cool in a way…because that'd be the day when my mother would ask me for an opinion like that. But the thing is that they never really let Martina just be a kid…she was always treated like an adult." She paused for a moment, as if she was viewing something in her mind's eye. After a moment, Julie continued.

"And Martino! That dude is something else…always reciting poetry to Martina…sometimes even in foreign languages…and expecting her to know what the heck he was saying. I just felt kind of sorry for her. That's all."

Needing to hear more about this young woman he loved, but whom he really did not know, Rod probed further, "Did you ever see him…her father…touch Martina? You know…in a way he shouldn't?"

"Are you kidding, Rod. Jacqui and Martino—at least when Jacqui was alive—and Martina were always hugging and kissing each other. And there was this time when I was over there…it was before Jacqui got sick… when Jacqui said something about Martina's boobs…how they were going to be bigger than Jacqui's. Martino was standing there and he went over and lifted up the front of Martina's blouse…I guess he wanted to see for himself if they were bigger. Martina wasn't wearing a bra. I was so embarrassed. Then Martino had Jacqui stand next to Martina and lift up her shirt and— Oh God!" Julie's cheeks turned red with sudden embarrassment. "This is too much…he took one of Martina's boobs in one hand and one of Jacqui's in his other hand and sort of weighed them up, like you would melons at the supermarket. And then he like did this formal announcement that Martina's were bigger. He told Martina that he hoped they didn't get too much bigger because he thought big boobs on women were vulgar. That's the word he used…vulgar. I was shocked by the whole thing. I mean…I'd die if my father ever did that to me. I mean…parents shouldn't do things like that to their kids."

Rod sprung up from his chair, obviously outraged by Julie's boob measuring story. "Was Martina upset about her father doing that to her?"

Julie shook her head. "Not that I noticed. I was the only one who was embarrassed about it. They all acted like it was an everyday thing at their house. God only knows what else they compared between each other. I mean…I'm not saying anything bad about Martina. She's the nicest friend I've ever had. It's just that her parents were really different and Martina grew up in their world. She can't help the way she was raised. That's why I kindda stopped going over to her house like I used to. Especially after her mother died. That Martino gives me the creeps the way he looks you over and up and down."

"Jesus! I'm sorry I took her back there tonight," Rod said, running his hands through his hair, and looking anguished. "No telling what that sonofabitchin' Martino is doing to her right now. I saw him

113

standing in her bedroom window tonight after Martina went into the house. That miserable fuck!" Rod suddenly turned pale and exclaimed, "That's what she's upset about!"

Freebird noted the wild look in Rod's eyes and became worried. He'd seen that look once before, when he and Rod first became riding buddies. It was back when Rod was living with a chick named Penny, and they were renting a little house in Devonshire, an older subdivision on the east side of Millborough. Rod had brought Freebird to his house one day to work on their bikes. Apparently, Rod's girlfriend Penny wasn't expecting him to come home so early, and Rod caught her and some other dude naked in the pool. Rod didn't lay a hand on Penny; he just threw her out on the street the way he found her in the pool — naked. But the unfortunate dude he caught Penny with got a serious ass whipping and was hauled off in an ambulance. Realizing he was lucky to be left alive, the dude refused to press charges against Rod. Freebird knew what Rod was capable of doing to Martina's father and he sure didn't want to see his friend get into any trouble. A guy like Martina's father would surely press charges.

Raising his hand, Freebird cautioned, "Whoa! Don't get crazy, Bro, We don't know what he's doing. Sometimes the mind imagines more than what is real."

Rod turned back to Julie. "Has she told you anything about Martino? Like him touching her?"

Julie wasn't sure Martina would tell her about such a thing even if it were true. But she saw the wild-eyed look on Rod's face and didn't want to further inflame him by saying so. Instead, she told him, "That's what was really weird after Jacqui died. All that touchy feely stuff just stopped. I never saw Martino ever hug or kiss Martina again after that, but he was always watching her. Like he watched every move she made. And God forbid if he ever got home and she wasn't there waiting for him, with his cocktail in her hand and his fancy gourmet dinner cooking on the stove. She told me that he would get just about spastic if she wasn't home when he got there. He really changed a lot. Now he acts more like a jealous boyfriend...not that he ever acted like a real father to Martina."

Rod, who had been pacing around the room while Julie was talking, suddenly said, "That perverted son of a bitch!"

"Ohmygod— Rod! Please! Don't ever tell Martina I told you any of this. She'll really be mad at me for saying anything."

"Don't worry, Julie. I won't blow it," said Rod, now sounding preoccupied. Freebird, who had been quietly rolling joints, gave Julie some sort of signal with his eyes and she obediently left the room. Lighting one of the joints, Freebird passed it over to Rod, who had returned to his chair and seemed to be in a somber mood. The two men smoked quietly, each deep into their thoughts.

Finally, Freebird asked, "Shall we go get her out of there?"

"You're reading my mind," Rod said, and then added, "but what do we really know? The last thing we need is a kidnapping beef...especially involving a minor."

Freebird nodded. "Whatever you decide, Brother. I'm right there with you."

"Then how about riding over to Clanton County tomorrow night?"

"Clanton County?" Freebird asked, confused.

"Yeh. I asked Martina to marry me and we're supposed to drive over to Clanton tomorrow night and do it."

"Whoa, man. That's heavy. Are you shittin' me?"

Running his hands through his hair, Rod shook his head.

"No. It's real. I asked Martina to marry me, and I don't know diddly squat about her. Am I fucked up or what?"

Freebird looked at his friend and asked, "Do you like what you do know about her?"

"Hell— I love what I know of her," Rod affirmed.

"Then what more do you need to know?" Freebird said with finality.

19.

Life could have gone terribly wrong for Clayton Terry the III, who would become known as "Freebird". For one thing, he had been abandoned on the night he was born in June of 1954 and spent the first night of his existence in a water trough. Any number of horrendous things could befall a defenseless infant left outdoors and alone all night, even in the cradle-like confines of a trough. But luckily for Freebird the trough in which he was so unceremoniously deposited just so happened to be on the property of Hayward and Selma Terry on the Mashantucket Pequot Indian Reservation in Ledyard, Connecticut. When Selma Terry went outside one morning to put water in the trough, as was her daily ritual, she was surprised to find what she at first thought was a discarded old blanket. As she investigated further she saw the spiky black hair on the top of the infant's head. Selma Terry was a very pragmatic woman; she was at that time 38-years old and had not been blessed with any children of her own. So when she carefully peeled away the folds of the blanket and saw the scrawny Indian infant she knew her prayers had finally been answered.

Since the abandoned baby was obviously Indian, numerous inquiries were made by the Tribal Council to determine who the biological mother of the abandoned infant might be, all to no avail. No one on the reservation would admit to knowing any woman who recently gave birth. In the end, the Terrys legally adopted the baby and named him Clayton Terry the III, even though there never had been any Clayton Terry the I or the II. Hayward and Selma simply wanted to give the child an instant, seeming lineage since his actual ancestry was unknown.

And it was of no consequence to Hayward and Selma that they were not the actual progenitors of little Clayton, as far as they were concerned the child was even more special to them because of his mysterious appearance, and they could not have loved him more if he was their own flesh and blood. To the barren couple, little Clayton was nothing short of a miracle and in their loving care he flourished.

As it turned out, the Terrys were not just honest and hardworking good people, they were highly respected members of the Mashantucket Pequot nation. Hayward was descended from a long line of medicine men and carried in his head a vast knowledge of herbal medicine, verbally transmitted from one generation to another since the origin of the tribe. Hayward was able to identify hundreds of roots, barks, berries, plants, seeds and other botanicals of numerous varieties and knew the exact healing properties of each and every one. And now he had a son to whom he could pass down his knowledge. Selma, too, was a gifted healer and knew the ways of preserving and preparing the herbs. Their small parcel of property was given over to propagating herbs, and their house was a veritable apothecary, with shelves containing rows of glass jars for storing the precious leaves, roots, and barks they painstakingly gathered, and the various compounds they ground into powders in the ancient granite mortar and pestle that had been in Hayward's family for as long as anyone could remember.

And to their wonder and delight, the sweet-tempered, intelligent little boy, who came to them as a mysterious gift, showed great interest in the herbs and retained everything they told him from day-to-day about them. As Clayton grew older he acquired an encyclopedic knowledge of the botanicals, and while there were other young men and women on the reservation who were selected for Hayward's tutelage, Clayton had a supernatural acumen for herbal medicine. And there were other things the Terrys noticed about Clayton that were also supernatural; he was able to predict events before they occurred and he often had visions wherein he was "shown" the location of missing items or given the answer to a perplexing questions.

Once during a vision he was shown the face of a young woman and he knew immediately she was his blood mother, but he was "told" that their paths were meant to be separate. Clayton accepted the information he received through his visions as the truth and never tried to dispel or second guess it. He simply had a knowing the visions came from a pure source.

Over the years Clayton formulated his own spiritual beliefs. He eschewed the Christian principles that were absorbed by the Pequot people from the preaching of the mid-eighteenth century missionaries, who considered the Pequot ceremonies as heathen and devil inspired. He assiduously studied the history and culture of his people and became fluent in the Mohegan-Pequot dialect, taking to heart the words of Chief Big Eagle, who had said that it was the "sacred obligation" of the Indian people to keep their language alive. In order to learn the old ways it was essential that Clayton learn the old language.

It was while he was in high school that Clayton became interested in motorcycles; at the time he was merely looking for economical transportation. He bought a used Kawasaki for two hundred dollars and learned everything he needed to know about the mechanics of its engine. He was pretty contented with his Kawasaki until the day a hard core biker riding a chopped, chrome-bedazzled Harley Davidson passed him on the highway. From that moment on Clayton's mission was to own a Harley just like the one he saw. He worked longer hours after school and on weekends in the Reservation grocery store, and saved more. In the meantime, he picked up a copy of a Harley mechanic's manual and read it from cover to cover. By the time he had graduated from high school and was about to turn eighteen he had saved enough to buy the Harley of his dreams, a chopper with a custom paint job and lots of gleaming chrome.

The minute he sat in the saddle of his new Harley he became "Freebird", it was his new Indian name.

It wasn't easy for Freebird to tell his parents that he wanted to leave the Reservation and see something of the world beyond. At first, Hayward and Selma were beside themselves with worry that they would never see their son again, and what of his legacy as the tribe's medicine man? What of the dangers and temptations he would face in his travels? Freebird felt their sadness, even though Hayward and Selma tried to maintain buoyant attitudes, but the pull of the outside world was just too strong for him to ignore. Before strapping his bedroll onto his Harley, Freebird sat down with his parents and stated his case for leaving. He told them that visions he had seen compelled him to leave, that there were other things he needed to learn that were not available to him on the Reservation, and he assured them that he would come back to them when he had completed his journey. When Freebird saw that his parents were comforted by his assurances he left.

20.

On the day after Rod's marriage proposal to Martina, a Friday, Rod woke up in his lacey canopy bed, feeling edgy. After what Julie had related to him the night before he now had a clearer picture of why Martina was so upset when they were parked up at the lookout last night. Rod knew that whatever was upsetting her had everything to do with her father. Just thinking about the possible bum trips Martino Fiasconi might be laying on Martina angered him to the point of frustration. He jumped out of bed and stomped into the bathroom to relieve his aching bladder.

He thought about driving over to Martina's house that morning and having it out with her father. The only problem with that idea, he realized, was that Fiasconi was holding all of the trump cards. First and foremost, he is Martina's father and her legal guardian; she is a minor; Rod had no proof her father had done anything illegal; and if Rod went over there and Fiasconi called the cops, Rod knew he'd be the one to get hauled off the premises. And, most likely, he'd be taken to jail.

Then there would be no trip to the justice of the peace in Clanton County that night. And there was always the possibility that Martina might get mad at him if he caused her any trouble, in which case there would definitely be no trip to Clanton County tonight, or maybe ever. As much as Rod hated to admit it to himself, he was hogtied by circumstances over which he had no control. And the mere thought of that was enough to put him in a bad frame of mind.

Having to bow to the superior advantage of Martino Fiasconi was a bitter pill for Rod to swallow so early in the morning. But as the day wore on and there was no telephone call from Martina, as she had promised, he plagued himself with a host of paranoid worries. Did she change her mind about marrying him? Maybe she really didn't mean it in the first place. Perhaps her father locked her in the basement, so that she could not contact him. He shouldn't have peeled his tires in front of her house last night. No doubt her father is pissed off at him and will not allow Martina to see him anymore. After going through the anguish of concocting all of the various reasons why he would never see Martina again, he then went back over each one and attempted to debunk them all. Mostly, his thoughts kept curving back to last night, the feel of her hand and the sound of her voice when she said she wanted to be with him. Deep in his heart he knew she really meant it.

All day, he wandered blindly around the house, unable to eat, shower, or shave, and not daring to venture out of earshot of the telephone in case Martina called him. He was just about as miserable as any hogtied man in love could be. Not even Freebird was available to give him any of his pithy, if not cryptic, shamanic insights; he had gone to pick up Julie at school and then bring her over to her house to get a dress to wear when they all went over to Clanton later on that evening.

Lucky Freebird. With Julie's divorced mother constantly on the prowl for a new husband, Julie could spend all kinds of time with him. Sometimes she spent the entire weekend up in his apartment. Rod thought of how he had to be content with seeing Martina for only a few hours after school and maybe a Friday or Saturday night dinner and movie. And she always had to be home before midnight. He felt like he was in a relationship with Cinderella.

After stewing all morning over the incurable situation with Martina's father, and then worrying about why she had not called him after school, Rod felt wasted. Stretching out on the sofa in the family room, with his forearm slung across his eyes to block out the light, he was deep into bemoaning his star crossed love life when he heard the back door open and close. Thinking it was either Freebird or his older brother Travis, stopping by to visit and talk shop, he didn't bother to move.

"Rod?" Martina called out.

Rod jumped up off the sofa so fast he banged his knee on the corner of the coffee table. Uttering a few choice epithets, he ran limping toward the kitchen and found Martina standing by the door. She was wearing a low cut white tank top that showed off her slender, defined arms and caramel skin, a long red skirt, red satin slippers, and a red straw hat with a wide brim. Her dark hair hung loose down her back. The sight of her completely reversed his dark mood and kicked up his pulse.

"What happened? Why are you limping?" she asked, concerned, when she saw him hobbling toward her.

"It's nothing," he said, gesturing with his hand "What's really bothering me is why you didn't call me. I was kind of getting worried...." Taking her into his arms, he hugged her as though he hadn't seen her for months, and let loose with a deep sigh of relief. "Baby...I'm so happy to see you."

"Did you think I wouldn't come?" She asked, wondering why he would doubt her.

"I thought maybe your father would lock you in the basement after I brought you home so late last night and then burned rubber when I drove off."

Martina threw her head back and laughed. "Martino did ask me how old you were after he heard your tires squealing. He said I should not be wasting my time with such a sophomoric young man."

"Did he, now," said Rod, happy to see her laughing. Then it suddenly occurred to him to ask, "How did you get here? I was supposed to pick you up after school."

"I drove," she said, a note of pride in her voice.

"What? When did you get your license?" Rod said, surprised.

"About a week ago."

"Why didn't you tell me?" He was hurt that she hadn't.

"I wanted to surprise you," she said. "But Martino is going to kill me when he discovers my mother's car is gone and me with it."

Rod envisioned the red Jaguar parked in his driveway and shook his head in disbelief. "Why didn't you call me to come get you?"

"Because Martino is in one of his moods and said I should not go out tonight since I was out late last night. I just pretended to agree with him. When he left to go play racquetball I threw my suitcase in the Jag and took off while I could."

Rod laughed, imagining her stealthy escape from Martino's House of Detention. "You are something else, Baby. I'd better keep my eye on you."

"I'd never run away from you, Rod," she murmured, in a soft, sexy voice that zeroed right in on Rod's heart like a direct injection of high intensity voodoo love potion.

"And I'm going to make sure you'll never want to," he whispered, his voice already tremulous from the excitement of simply holding her in his arms. All of his previous misery and anguish were now completely forgotten. Kissing her forehead, the tip of her nose, and then locking onto her lips, he moaned with pleasure as she gently sucked his tongue into the sweetness of her mouth. For all of Rod's muscle and brawn, this slender, young, wisp of a woman was capable of controlling his mind and body with only the soft pliability of her tongue. He knew it, but willingly succumbed to the power she had over him.

Martina sensed the strong affect she had on Rod, but instead of being corrupted by it she felt the need to protect him from his own vulnerability. Rod was the perfect outlet for her nurturing disposition.

Being loved by Rod and feeling the depth of her own love for him was a completely new experience for Martina. She had only been out on a few "dates" since turning fourteen, when Jacqui and Martino allowed her to go school dances or sports events. None of the boys at school interested her in the least, and it wasn't until she met Rod that she understood why. She liked, and truly needed, the security of a self-assured man, someone with the experience of life. And she was too used to the companionship and conversation of adults to ever find contentment with gangly teenaged boys, whose interests seldom went beyond their clumsy groping.

It was the sound of Freebird's motorcycle coming up the driveway that distracted them from their moments of pleasure. Slowly and unwillingly, they disconnected their bodies and headed out the back door. Martina was surprised to see Julie hop off the back of Freebird's bike, and ran over to greet her friend.

"So— this is where you've been hiding out," Martina yelled to Julie, as she ran across the back lawn toward the driveway.

"Martina!" Julie called to her, excitedly, adjusting a plastic garment bag that was draped over her arm. Running toward each other, the two friends embraced. "Ohmygod, Martina! You and Rod are getting married tonight. I can't believe it's really happening. Freebird and I decided to make it a double wedding." When the two young women began shrieking with their mutual joy and practically jumping up and down in their excitement, Rod and Freebird shrugged at each other and headed for the manly sanctity of the garage.

Rod eyed the red Jaguar convertible parked in the driveway and thought about the last time he saw it, when Martina's gorgeous mother was sitting at the wheel. Thinking about the conversation they had had about it the night before, he commented, "A freakin' small world,"

Freebird looked at the Jag, admiring its sleek design, and commented, "Amen, Bro. But I wouldn't want to have to paint it."

"Paint what? The Jaguar?" Rod asked, confused.

"No. The world," Freebird said, with his usual dry wit.

Rod knuckled his friend on the arm. "Man! You've got a weird sense of humor."

Once they were secluded inside the garage, the two men dropped their cool facades and embraced just as excitedly as their girlfriends were doing, without the jumping up and down.

"Man!" exclaimed Freebird, "Julie and I decided that since we are going over to Clanton with you guys, we're going to get married, too.

We've been talking about it for a while, so now we're going to finally do it. Tonight's the night, Bro."

Hearing that, Rod slapped Freebird on the back affectionately. "I hope we're not blowing it…but I'm sure in love with Martina and miserable as hell when I'm not with her," Rod freely admitted. He walked over to an old, grease smeared refrigerator in the back corner of the garage and pulled out two beers, handing one of them to Freebird.

"Listen to them out there," Freebird commented. "They are so excited…we can't back out now even if we wanted to."

After taking a couple of swigs from his beer, Freebird's expression grew serious, and he added, "I had a vision last night and my Spirit Guide took me to a ledge on our sacred mountain at the reservation. Julie was there waiting for me and she was wearing the white doeskin wedding dress of my tribe. The vision confirms that she is the woman that the Creator made for me."

Rod knew that Freebird was heavy into his tribal beliefs and Native American spirituality, but he couldn't resist teasing him.

"Are you sure that your vision wasn't inspired by what you were smoking last night?"

Freebird smiled at Rod, and said, "It makes no difference how the vision is inspired. Fasting and prayer are best. But the herb is much quicker."

Rod, who was now leaning against his Harley, broke up laughing at his friend's rationalization. "Well, Bro," he said, holding his beer bottle aloft, "here's to visions and our last day as single men."

Tapping his beer bottle against Rod's, Freebird observed, "Yeh! And no more keeping company with freakin' Rosie Palm and her five sisters."

"What are you guys doing in here?" said a curious voice behind them. It was Julie, standing in the wide entrance to the garage. She seemed unwilling to enter. Martina walked up and stood next to her, her eyes ingesting the spectacle of the garage: a black leather sofa against the back wall, odds and ends of other cast off furniture, an old recliner parked next to a refrigerator. Her eyes came to rest on a large, boldly colored poster on the wall above the sofa—a large-breasted blonde wearing nothing but black leather chaps and standing astride a wildly painted custom chopped motorcycle. "Humph!" Martina snorted, casting a glance of mild disapproval in Rod's general direction.

Rod watched the girls' expressions and smiled indulgently, knowing they were unfamiliar with the biker lifestyle. He was not the least bit ashamed of his taste in pin-up girls.

The girls looked at each other quizzically, both still not daring to enter upon this seeming hallowed shrine of polished chrome machines that could roar to life with deafening thunder, although they could not articulate their reticence in such terms.

Wide-eyed, they looked around at the collection of unidentifiable bike parts and emergency inventory crammed on the metal shelving that took up most of a side wall and then up at the array of items suspended from the ceiling joists, such as a dented gas tank, a salvaged front fender, a pair of mangled handlebars, a helmet that had obviously skidded a long distance across pavement, and a six-foot tall cardboard skeleton, the kind people decorated their house with at Halloween, which swayed and pirouetted delicately in the breeze. There was even a bentwood coat tree in the corner, just inside the door, that was heaped with black leather and denim jackets and vests. After taking in all of the trappings of a biker garage, the two young women looked at each other, perplexed, as though they had ventured into a strange land and encountered two of its aborigines. And the two men looked at them as though it was the first time they had ever seen such two fine looking sweeties.

Instinctively, Martina and Julie refrained from entering the garage, preferring, for some subconscious reason, to simply hang back at the entrance and view it as though it was a diorama in a museum.

Martina gave Rod an indulgent smile and then said, "We need to get dressed for our big event."

"My house is your house, ladies," said Rod, making a sweeping gesture with his arm toward the house.

To Martina, he said, "I'll go get your suitcase out of your car."

Turning to Freebird, Rod affected a sepulchral tone and announced, "The hour of doom is upon us, my good Brother. Let us go to our slaughter like men of honor, with our heads held high." It seemed the perfect thing to say to dissipate the strangeness of the moment, and they all laughed as they walked from the garage together. Rod stopped at Martina's car to retrieve her suitcase. It seemed very light considering he did not expect her to return to her father's house to live after tonight.

Freebird went up to his apartment to shower and dress, while Rod followed the girls into the house and ushered them upstairs to the master bathroom, which was the largest of the four full bathrooms in the house. He placed Martina's suitcase on the bed and, after removing from his closet the dark blue pin-striped suit and light blue shirt he planned to wear for his wedding, he immediately left the room, allowing the girls their privacy to get ready. They were all to meet in the living room at six o'clock for some quick photos, and then start off for Clanton, in order to be there by seven o'clock. If Rod had managed to do a couple of things earlier that day while moping about, it was to order flowers and call ahead to the justice of the peace, a fellow named J. Winslow Torpy, and confirm his hours of operation. The JP's wife told him to be there anytime before nine o'clock in the evening, because Justice Torpy liked to retire promptly at nine-thirty every evening.

In and out of the shower in record time, Rod was dressed in his wedding attire and pacing excitedly around the living room by a quarter to five. Freebird soon joined him; he was wearing neatly pressed loden green khaki pants, a tribal shirt that was trimmed with red, green, yellow, and black ceremonial ribbons, and his shiny black hair hung loose. The two grooms acknowledged each other with a nod, but did not entrust their nervous tongues with speech. When they heard footsteps descending the steps, from upstairs, the two nervous men looked up expectantly.

Julie was the first to come into the living room. Freebird caught his breath when he saw her. She wore a light pink gown that looked like spun sugar: it had a fitted satin top that was held up with skinny rhinestone straps and its flouncy knee length skirt was wound with layer upon layer of frothy ruffles. Pink high heels adorned her tiny feet. With her blonde hair swept up into a pony tail that cascaded from the top of her head, her big blue eyes, and the pink gown, Rod thought she looked like an adorable Barbie doll that had somehow magically come to life. Freebird merely stood looking at her, misty eyed, and smiling appreciatively. He wanted to hug and kiss her, but her dress looked too delicate for him to even brush against.

"Where's my wife?" Rod asked, purposely sounding like a kid who didn't get his share of dessert.

Julie giggled. "Maybe you'd better go upstairs and talk to her. I think she's having a panic attack."

Rod flew out of the room and took the stairs two at a time. He found Martina standing stalk still, holding on to one of the posts at the foot of his bed for support. He could hardly believe his eyes when he saw how beautiful she looked. She had on a pale blue silk jacquard

125

Oriental dress, the same color as his shirt. The dress was sleeveless, with a Mandarin collar, and its elegant fabric sheathed her slender body all the way to her ankles. Thigh high slits on either side of its skirt offered tantalizing glimpses of her tanned, shapely legs. The dress was trimmed with dark blue braided cord and frogs, the same color as his suit. Her long hair had been woven into an intricate bun on the top of her head and fastened with combs hand-carved from Abalone that had once been her mother's. Behind her left ear she had pinned a spray of tiny blue silk flowers and baby's breath, and wore dangling earrings that looked like blue sapphires.

Releasing the deep breath that had stuck in his throat at the sight of her in that incredible blue dress, he said, "You look amazing...like a beautiful Oriental princess." She flashed him a wan smile and he could see she had a death grip on the bedpost. "Are you okay, Baby?"

Nodding her head slightly, her voice was barely audible when she answered him. "I'm scared, Rod."

Determined not to let her go off the deep end like she did last night, he took hold of her free hand and comforted her. "All brides are nervous and scared on their wedding day. Come on, Baby, let's go get our pictures taken."

Reluctantly, she released her grip on the bedpost. "How do you know so much about nervous brides?" she asked, giving him a curious stare.

"It's a known fact," he told her, caressing her bare arm and studying the fullness of her ruby glossed lips. To further assuage her jitters, he added, "Brides have been known to do some pretty weird things just before their weddings." He started leading her slowly out of the room as he talked.

"Like what?" She asked, moving along with him toward the door.

"Oh— Terrible, unspeakable things...like blowing up their wedding cakes and setting fire to the would-be groom's tuxedo.

Once, I even heard of a bride who called in a bomb threat at the church just minutes before her wedding was to take place."

Martina looked up at Rod, shocked that a bride would do such a terrible thing, and caught him trying to keep a straight face. Realizing that she was being teased, Martina started laughing at his silliness. By the time they joined Freebird and Julie in the living room, Martina's jitters were gone.

Rod gave Freebird a look of relief and then said, "Okay! It's photo time, and then we've got to hit the road." Suddenly remembering the wrist corsages for the girls that had been delivered by the florist that morning, Rod exclaimed, "Hold it! I've forgot something." Running to the kitchen, he snatched the two boxes containing the white orchid corsages out of the fridge, and ran back into the living room. Handing one of the boxes to Freebird, he said, "This one's is for Julie." Rod opened his box and gingerly removed the large delicate white orchid. Taking hold of Martina's arm, he slid the corsage onto her wrist and closely examined the exotic flower for a moment. "It's almost as beautiful as you are," he told Martina, his tone quite serious. Bringing her hand to his lips, he locked his eyes onto hers and hoped she read the intensity of the love he felt for her.

Staring deep into Rod's eyes, Martina was stirred to her soul by the passion she saw radiating from him. Measure for measure, she returned with her own steady gaze the love and desire that had grown in her own heart for him. Any doubts she may have had earlier about getting married at such a young age to a man whom she had not known all that long were now completely erased. Everything about being with Rod felt so right.

When the camera's flash suddenly broadcast a burst of light into the room, Rod and Martina looked up, surprised. For the past few moments they had drifted into a time warp, aware only of each other. Julie had taken a photo of them, gazing intently into each other's eyes.

"That's going to be a great picture," Freebird predicted.

"C'mon, you two," Julie called out to Martina and Rod.

"You can do all that love stuff later. Let's get everyone's photos taken, so we can get going."

Between Rod, Freebird, and the automatic timer on the camera, every possible photo combination of the four celebrants was taken, and then they finally headed out the back door.

"Hey!" Julie exclaimed. "What are we going to ride in? The only cars here are the Corvette and the Jag and both are only two seaters."

"We're going on our bikes," said Rod, with all seriousness.

Julie's mouth dropped open. "We can't ride bikes to Clanton in these dresses. We'll be all windblown."

"Don't be silly, Julie," Rod said, still carrying on with his serious act. "We have side cars with glass domes to attach to each of our bikes for just such an occasion."

Julie looked at Rod and then Freebird, not knowing what to believe. But the two men were playing it so straight faced that she was taken in by their act.

Rod threw a set of keys to Freebird, and said, "Let's get the sidecars out." Freebird grabbed the keys out of the air and took off running before Julie could see the grin on his face.

"Sidecars?" Martina asked. "Are we really riding in sidecars?" She looked at Rod's face and saw the glint of amusement in his eyes. "Don't listen to those guys, Julie. They're just trying to put one over on us again."

"Okay," Rod said, still keeping his face deadpan. "You'll see."

"I'm not riding to my wedding in a sidecar with a glass bubble," Julie said, folding her arms across her chest for emphasis.

Weighing in, Martina said, "Me neither."

Rod was having a hard time controlling his urge to laugh.

Freebird had by then disappeared around the back of the garage building, where, unbeknownst to the girls, there were two wider stalls where the larger vehicles were kept. Presently, a white four door Cadillac convertible, its canvas top appropriately in place, appeared from behind the building and drew up next to where Rod and the girls were standing. The door opened and Freebird climbed out, laughing at the amazed expressions on the girls' faces. Rod took Martina's arm and escorted her into the back seat and then he went around and climbed in on the other side, while Freebird helped Julie onto the front passenger seat.

"Sidecars!" Muttered Martina, as they headed down the driveway on their journey to Clanton. And then they all started laughing.

21.

Justice of the Peace J. Winslow Torpy, who was a portly man with white hair and a kind face, conducted a surprisingly meaningful ceremony for the two couples, considering he was used to people rushing in and out of his makeshift chapel for weddings on the fly. Justice Torpy could see by the way these young folks were dressed that they would want his extra special nuptial service, and Mrs. Torpy even produced a gold plated candelabra and lit the candles for the occasion.

After the service, there was a lot of hand shaking, back slapping, embracing, and tears. Justice Torpy wished each beaming couple all of the happiness and prosperity that righteous souls living together in the sanctified state of marriage could reasonably expect from the "Great Savior on High", and even gave them a pep talk on the proper way for a husband and wife to treat each other if they wanted to enjoy a long, blissful marriage, such as he and Mrs. Torpy had for the last forty years.

"Yessir," proclaimed Justice Torpy, "always treat each other with the utmost respect and kindness and your marriage will endure." The two newly joined couples thought that was good advice and nodded their agreement.

As he affixed his bold, ostentatious signature to the couples' nuptial certificates, J. Winslow took great pains to caution Martina and Julie about the evils of high-minded and independent women, and the importance of being loyal and obedient wives, and read to them a brief passage from the Bible about cleaving from the ways of their parents and conforming to the ways of their husbands, and being a good example to their future children, although he hoped they wouldn't have children right away, seeing as how they were so young themselves.

Rod kept an eye on Martina's facial expressions during Justice Torpy's instructions concerning her wifely duties. He had to bite his lip a couple of times to keep from snickering.

Sneaking a sideways glance to check Martina's expression, he could tell that she wasn't buying the Justice's rhetoric denouncing "high minded and independent" women. The bit about "obedience" didn't seem to sit well with her, either. Rod wasn't sure exactly what kind of a wife he'd be getting with Martina, but he was willing to bet she would not fall within the definition proffered by the well-intentioned J. Winslow. And, frankly, Rod was concerned that if the JP didn't wind it up real soon, Martina might feel inclined to set the old boy straight about her staunch views on equal rights for women.

For most of their ride back to Millborough there was not much conversation. In the front seat, Julie was snuggled against Freebird and giggled intermittently. In the back, Rod had his arm around Martina and held her close. It seemed as though the four young people were mulling over the gravity of the commitments they had just made.

After nearly a half-hour of pensive quiet, Rod whispered in Martina's ear, "So...my beautiful bride...how does it feel being Mrs. Roderick J. McDonough?"

Looking up at Rod's beaming smile, Martina did not have the heart to tell him she was worried about Martino's reaction whenever he found out what she had done. Instead, she gave him a heavy-lidded, suggestive smile, and said, "I'll let you know after the marriage has been consummated...Mr. McDonough."

"Whoa! Listen to you!" Rod said, with a surprised laugh. Sliding his hand under the slit in her dress, he caressed the length of her thigh while he held his gaze steady on hers. His voice was heavy with passion when he said, "I hope you won't be disappointed."

Placing her hand on his muscled chest, Martina slowly massaged his body, moving her hand downward until it rested on his thigh. "I'm not expecting to be disappointed," she whispered.

Reacting to her touch, Rod moaned and brought his lips down on hers. He found the soft fullness of her lips so sensual and inviting that it seemed he could not look at them without feeling the strong desire to kiss them. He was so taken with the exotic beauty of his young wife that he did not notice how adroit she was with her hands. Perhaps, subconsciously, he did not want to notice. For, then, he would have to wonder how she acquired her experience.

Reaching the outskirts of Millborough, Freebird called back to Rod, "Where's that restaurant where we have the dinner reservations?"

"La Trianon! It's over on Riverside," Rod answered.

"You have good taste, Rod," commented Martina, assuming Rod had made the arrangements, since Freebird was unfamiliar with the restaurant's name. "They have the best French food in town."

"Have you been there before?" asked Rod, thinking how little he knew about her life.

"My parents ate there frequently," she said,

Rod picked up her left hand and fingered the delicately carved gold band he had placed on her third finger during their wedding ceremony.

130

The ring had been his Grandmother's. "Do you like your ring?" he asked.

"It's beautiful, Rod. I wish I had one to give you...but everything happened so fast and there was no time to get to a jewelry store." She sounded as though she had committed an unpardonable social blunder.

"Don't worry about it," Rod assured, "we'll go get us a matching set of bands before we leave for our honeymoon."

Surprised, Martina looked up at his face with a quick movement of her head. "Honeymoon?" A sudden rush of panic flooded her body. "I...I can't go on a honeymoon. I have to go to school Monday and Martino would be furious if—"

Having heard Martino's name mentioned once too many times in the course of the past several hours, Rod cut her off, "Martina! Remember what the preacher said about cleaving from your family? Your relationship with your father no longer takes precedence in your life, and he can get as furious as he wants. You are my wife now and we are going to have a righteous honeymoon." Wisely, Rod made no reference to Martina about what the preacher had said concerning a wife's duty to be obedient to her husband. But he was annoyed that, once again, Martino Fiasconi had managed to overshadow what should be a happy occasion for them.

Martina bit her lip. She sensed Rod's annoyance and knew her response was childish and stupid. "I'm sorry," she said, tears of embarrassment stinging her eyes. "I guess I have to get used to being married."

Rod pulled her closer and nuzzled the side of her head. "It's okay, Baby. We'll both have a lot to get used to. You're just going to have to trust me to take care of things. We're not going to have your father in bed with us."

Martina stiffened at Rod's last comment. She wondered if it was simply a figure of speech or did he know or suspect anything about her relationship with her father. Rod felt her body go momentarily rigid and wondered why.

In the front seat, Freebird had overheard the conversation between Rod and Martina and squeezed Julie's hand as if to say, "Uh-Oh! Here it comes!" In his mind, Freebird likened Martina to a high-spirited filly that Rod was going to have to break in, using a gentle but firm approach. Rod sure has his work cut out for him with breaking in Martina, thought Freebird, suddenly feeling a chill ripple across his shoulders. Looking in the rearview mirror at Rod's shadowy form in the back seat, he was overcome with a dark sense of foreboding. Of course, Freebird could say nothing about it to his friend at the moment.

22.

The Provence inspired atmosphere of La Trianon and the delicious food did wonders to enliven the spirits and conversation of the four newlyweds. The episode which had occurred earlier in the car, where Rod diplomatically asserted his now dominant position over Martina's father, seemed a minor territorial issue that was now permanently settled. But it was not, nor could it be so simply dealt with. Rod was, at the moment, blissfully unaware of the calamitous situation that he would soon be sucked into. In the meantime, in lieu of a wedding cake, he and Martina shared a cream filled pastry covered with brandied cherries, after their full course filet mignon dinner. Now, they were full and happy and eager to go home.

When the valet parking attendant brought the Cadillac up under the *porte cochère*, Rod took the wheel for the drive home, since Freebird wanted to sit in the back with Julie and smoke a joint. When the Cadillac finally turned the corner onto Scenic Drive, Rod could feel his heart wildly pounding in his chest. He glanced quickly at Martina and saw she was staring straight ahead. He had a feeling she was going through some heavy changes over that cleaving business the justice of the peace had spoken about. Rod reminded himself that despite her seeming maturity she was, after all, still only seventeen and he would need to be patient and understanding with her. Reaching over toward her, he affectionately rubbed her arm.

"Are you tired of me already?" Rod asked Martina.

At first, she responded with a curious look, then she asked, "What do you mean by that?"

"Well…you're sitting way over there looking all grim faced."

When she scooted across the seat and leaned up against him, he felt his heart surge with the pleasure of her nearness. "That's more like it," he told her. "I always want you close by my side."

Nosing the wide body sedan between the two stone pylons demarcating the driveway entrance to the McDonough estate, Rod slowly navigated the curves as though he were taking a ship into its home port. "Here we are folks," Rod called out.

"Home at last!"

For a few seconds it was totally quiet in the car and then Freebird said to Rod and Martina, "See you guys sometime tomorrow…let's go, Julie." In a flash, Freebird was out of the car and pulling Julie out after him.

Rod switched off the engine and looked at Martina. "Welcome to your new home, Mrs. McDonough," he said, taking her into his arms and kissing her gently, almost chastely, on her intriguing lips. He could have easily ravaged her right then and there in the front seat of his father's prized Cadillac, his aching to have her was so strong, but Rod knew he would have to take it slow and easy with his new wife. If he was reading her body language correctly, she looked as though she was mentally wrestling with a monstrous dilemma: unable to choose between two unsatisfactory alternatives. And Rod didn't want to be the losing one of the two.

He studied her face for a moment, hoping for a smile in response to his attempts to dispel her nervousness, but in the dimness of the light reflected from Freebird's apartment window above the garage, he saw only a look of worry in her eyes. Always direct in his approach to life, Rod asked her, "Do you want me to take you home?"

Martina let out a heavy sigh and shook her head. "No! It isn't that," she quickly answered, her voice sounding thin.

"What is it, then?" Rod took a soft, undemanding approach, while all the time gently rubbing her back and brushing his lips, like the light strokes of a feather, along her worry-crinkled forehead. He heard her release another deep, ragged sigh and felt her shoulders sag.

"You need to know something...about me," she said, with a resigned tone in her voice.

Rod thought she was going to finally tell him what he already suspected about Martino was true and braced himself. He sensed that if he lost it and became enraged over the confidences she shared with him now, she would never again entrust him with her secrets or innermost feelings. He couldn't stand for there to be any kind of a barrier between them. He continued stroking her sagging shoulders. "Tell me what it is," he encouraged.

"I... I'm sorry, Rod...but I'm not a virgin."

Rod tightened his embrace and pulled her closer against him. Into her ear he whispered, "Neither am I, Baby." He felt the tenseness of her body immediately loosen and dissipate.

She turned her head to look at his face. "I love you so much, Rod." Her declaration sounded like it came from a sudden realization.

"And I love you, too, Martina...so very much."

Rod didn't realize how tense he was until he suddenly felt his own body relax upon hearing her heartfelt declaration of love for him. He had needed to hear that more than he realized.

Looking deep into each other's eyes, wordlessly reaffirming their love for each other, they established in that moment the all important connection between them. Neither could turn away from the other now; they were truly joined as husband and wife. But there would be many tests of that connection in the days ahead.

When the moment of affirmation had passed, Rod opened the car door and stepped out. Extending a hand to Martina, he said, "C'mon, Baby. Let's go do some of that consummating you were talking about earlier." Martina smiled and took his hand.

23.

Rod fumbled with the tricky braided cord frogs that fastened together the top flaps of Martina's Oriental dress. Not having had any previous experience with the annoying contrivances, Rod would have preferred to tear them apart than to come off like an incompetent idiot on his wedding night. But his ingrained sense of decorum overruled his baser, more reactionary, instincts. Nor did he want to frighten the hell out of his already skittish bride by tearing off her clothes. Besides, the dress looked so beautiful on Martina and he did want to see her wearing it again. So, he fumbled patiently with the frogs.

When they first entered the house, over an hour ago, Rod noticed that Martina suddenly seemed nervous and unsure. So, instead of rushing her upstairs to the bedroom, which was what he really wanted to do, he took her into the living room and poured a couple of drinks: she a club soda and he a light bourbon and water. He tried to behave like taking her to bed was the last thing on his mind but, with the lateness of the hour, it became inevitable that it was time to go upstairs.

Taking Martina's hand in his, he led her up to the bedroom. There were no more words to be spoken at this tender moment of expectation. Over the last months and the last hours, they had talked and kissed and caressed each other to the point where they were both hungering for a deeper, more intimate connection. They climbed the stairs slowly, but their hearts raced. Hers from nervousness. His with anticipation.

The lace canopied bed never seemed more appropriate to the occasion, its ambiance heightened by the sensual aroma from the several vases of fresh cut gardenias that had been selectively placed around the room. There were two smaller vases of the gardenias, one on each of the nightstands that stood on either side of the bed, that were positioned to perfume the air under the canopy with their seductive scent. Martina knew that Rod had decorated the room with the flowers to commemorate their wedding night and was touched by his thoughtfulness. And as if by some magic, a full moon was now suspended just beyond the open French doors, illuminating the balcony and the bedroom with a soft, phosphorescent glow. It was the most beautiful setting Martina could have ever imagined for their first night together.

Martina tried to control her nervousness when Rod drew her close, to begin the ritual of undressing her. She felt his fingers fumbling with the braided frogs that fastened the top of her dress. Instinctively, she knew better than to interfere and attempt to show Rod how to undo the frogs; she didn't want to insult his intelligence at such a seminal moment on their wedding night. So she held her hands in check and hoped he would not lose patience and rip them loose, especially since the dress had been her mother's and Martina had always loved the way Jacqui had looked in it.

But after several frustrating attempts to open them, Rod was close to tearing the confounding fasteners off of Martina's wedding dress. The only thing stopping him was that it would be an unpardonable offense. He knew that women had a sentimental thing about their wedding dresses and kept them in plastic bags in their closets for as long as they lived. Even if they never wore the dress again they never got rid of it. And the last thing he wanted was for Martina to get pissed off at him for being an insensitive oaf on their wedding night. But those damn things she called frogs were making him feel like an inept schoolboy, as well as holding up a long-awaited moment. Talk about Chinese puzzles! And putting on a light in order to better see them was out of the question. A bright light would totally ruin the atmosphere he had worked so hard to create. So he would have to use some old-fashioned stealth to figure them out. He was not about to be outfoxed by the frogs.

Finally, by feeling the apparatus with his fingers, he was able to determine it was nothing more than a cleverly disguised hook and eye and when he crunched the two pieces together in his hand, they popped apart. Silently, he rejoiced at his conquering of the frogs. Martina exhaled a quiet sigh of relief.

Peeling away the top of the dress, he saw she was wearing a lacey blue bra and decided not to take it off just yet. It looked so sexy against her smooth caramel skin. Slowly, he pulled her dress downward until her slender arms hung free, and the dress slid down over her narrow hips, revealing blue lace bikini panties. Helping her to step out of the dress, he picked it up from the floor and draped it across a nearby lounge chair as carefully as he could, given the rising excitement of the moment. Then Rod turned his attention to removing the carved Abalone combs from her hair, letting it fall loose to cover her shoulders and back like a long shawl. It was the first time he had ever seen her with so little clothing on, so he curiously studied her lithe body, admiring her flawlessly smooth skin and running his fingertips over her as though she were an object of art. Martina did not feel self-conscious or violated by his staring or touching; she understood his need to see her every curve and beauty mark, and she was looking forward to undressing and seeing all of him.

When Rod guided her hands to the buttons on his shirt, she deftly opened and removed it, laying it next to her dress on the upholstered lounge. Placing the palms of her hands on his well developed chest, she slowly massaged his nipples for a few moments, causing him to close his eyes and simply feel the ecstasy of the wonderful sensations she aroused in his body.

Downward, over the curly dark hair on his chest, her soft, loving hands roamed until they confronted his belt, which she seamlessly unfastened. Having thoughtfully prepared for this moment beforehand Rod wore no underwear. Taking advantage of his nakedness, Martina purposely allowed the back of her hand to brush against his hardness as she removed his pants.

Physically, he was everything she had imagined, and more. Feeling the delicate touch of her hand against his sensitive skin, Rod suppressed an urge to groan. Now was not the time to destroy his cool, masculine image by turning into a mass of quivering flesh from the mere touch of her hand. Now was the time for overt, masculine action.

With sudden, effortless motion, Rod whisked Martina up into his arms and lowered her ever so gently onto the moonlit bed, his eyes locked upon hers with such a burning intensity of passion her body visibly trembled with desire. Lithesome as a jungle cat, Rod positioned himself astride her hips and began slowly trailing kisses from her lips downward over her body, removing her last lacy bits of clothing as if by sleight of hand.

By the time Martina realized she was now completely nude, she was beyond being embarrassed by her moonlit nakedness. In many respects, she was as innocent as a virgin to the ways of making love, and just how much so she would soon find out.

She had never been kissed or fondled or ever really been made love to as Rod was now doing. She had never known such excitement and passion, nor had she ever been kissed in such a sensually probing manner. Never before had she moaned, cried out, thrashed, and begged as she found herself doing while Rod stroked, massaged, and rubbed, or teased her with his tongue.

When she felt her insides pulsating, she had no idea what was happening to her, only that it felt like she was free-falling through space and every nerve ending in her body was on fire with an intensity of passion she did not know was humanly possible to experience.

Rod had never seen a woman so sexually aroused, and Martina, in turn, excited him beyond his wildest imaginings. Their foreplay had gone on for well over an hour and even though he had been close to orgasm several times he was able to hold himself in check. He owed his impressive endurance, in large part, to Freebird. It seemed his friend possessed a vast array of indigenous pharmacopoeia and a cure for every ailment known to mankind. As Rod's luck would have it, while they were in the men's room at the La Trianon earlier that evening, Freebird slipped him a few wilted leaves, with only the laconic instruction that he should "chew before laying down with the woman." Following Freebird's prescription to the letter, Rod chewed the wickedly bitter leaves just before ushering Martina upstairs to their nuptial chamber. But, now, the mysterious herb had run its course and he was ready to consummate their marriage. And he could tell from Martina's body language that she, too, was more than ready.

Surprisingly, the moment he entered the moist warmth of her body he felt a brief resistance, and there was no mistaking Martina's cry of pain for what it was. Rod immediately withdrew and rolled onto his side, his chest heaving and his breath too ragged to speak. Even if he could huff out an intelligible sentence he was too confused for words. Nor did the timing lend itself to any clinical discussion of what constituted virginity. As he lie there panting, his excitement ebbing away, he had to restrain himself from bellowing like an injured animal.

Martina quickly realized the gravity of the situation. After all of Rod's thoughtfulness and consideration for her feelings and her pleasure she had allowed her ignorance to ruin their wedding night, and maybe even damage their future life together as well. Her heart sank in a flood of guilt as she watched this wonderful man, whom she truly loved and wanted to please in every way, lie panting and miserable with frustration beside her. Silently, she berated herself for being so stupid and ignorant about her own body that she did not even know that she was still a virgin. Had she been truthful with Rod from the outset about her relationship with Martino this embarrassing scene could have been averted. But this was no time to beat herself up over past mistakes; she had to make it up to him somehow and salvage what had been up until that moment a magical night of lovemaking. She could not allow her childish stupidity to mar the happiness of their wedding night or, worse yet, compromise the future of their relationship.

Ignoring her own searing discomfort Martina moved quickly to recapture the intensity of their passion before it completely evaporated, and with one fluid movement she was suddenly cloaking him with her musky warmth. Immediately, she set to work with her hands, her tongue, the movement of hips, and even the mounds of her breasts to revive his excitement, making note of the techniques that yielded the most groans of pleasure from him. It did not take long before her ministrations were generously rewarded. Whatever raw passion was lost by the momentary interruption in their lovemaking was now being doubly reclaimed as Martina poured her heart and soul into pleasuring the man she knew she would love for the rest of her life. She wanted him to remember this night for as long as he lived and to know how deeply, how viscerally, she loved him.

No one could have been more surprised than the beleaguered Rod when Martina swiftly took control of the situation and his body. He wondered, but only briefly, where and how she could have learned such an amazing repertoire of pleasure enhancing techniques, but his curiosity was soon overshadowed by the powerful sensations elicited by the caressing touch of her tongue and the artful stroking of her hands. Not only was their earlier momentum regained but it was swiftly surpassed as they responded to each other's desires with the intensity of lovers who had long known each other's every erogenous pleasure. For hours, they explored each other's body before finally succumbing to a satiated exhaustion.

Unable to let loose of each other even after their extended lovemaking, they slept entwined in each other's limbs. But even more important than her salvaging the splendor of their wedding night, her act of reclamation sealed the deeper, more emotionally sensitive bonds of their union: those of loyalty, trust, and unselfish caring for the needs of the other.

The following morning Rod came awake in the crosshairs of excitement and a sobering realization: the woman curled up next to him was not a one-night-stand or passing affair; she was now his wife, his gladly-accepted responsibility, and she would be sleeping beside him for as long as he dared to hope. He knew that nothing in life was permanent, but he wanted their togetherness to be as permanent as life would allow. For a long time he lay still and watched her in the act of sleep, an intimate aspect of her he had never seen before, and marveled at the smoothness of her caramel skin, her hair, all wild and tangled, and the delicateness of her eyelashes. There was more to this woman of flesh and bone and feelings than her extraordinary beauty. He thought about how nervous she was last night when he brought her home. That she should work herself up into a bundle of nerves over such a stupid issue as virginity seemed a cruel and senseless guilt trip. But Rod couldn't help wondering whom she had been with and what they could have possibly done to make her think she had lost her virginity when, in fact, she obviously had not. He was puzzled that she could be so unaware of such a thing and yet so adept at sexual pleasure. There was much he needed to learn and understand about his young wife.

While Martina slept, Rod slipped down to the kitchen to fix a breakfast tray to bring up to her. Unsure of what she might like, Rod prepared an assortment of traditional morning foods: orange juice, melon slices, hard-boiled eggs and croissants with fruit preserves. On the way back to the bedroom he spied a peacock feather in a hallway flower arrangement and plucked it as he passed by. Quietly placing the breakfast tray on the dresser, Rod used the feather to awaken Martina. Gently lifting the rumpled sheet, he ran the feather lightly down the length of her back and over the curve of her well-formed posterior. When she stirred and opened her sea green eyes, her smile was at once both sensuous and innocent. Rod knelt on the bed and lifted her into his arms. Their first kiss of the day was tender and sweet, showing nothing of the wild sensuality they had aroused in each other only hours before.

"How are you feeling this morning?" Rod said, gently massaging her stomach. "I'm so sorry—" His concerned expression alluded to the surprise discovery of her virginity. He decided not to pursue the matter just at that moment; it didn't seem to be the right time for such a discussion, despite his curiosity.

"I'm okay." She smiled, somewhat embarrassed that he brought up last night's *faux pas*. He pulled her close and brushed her cheek with his lips. "I've brought you breakfast, so let's get you comfortable…"

Shifting his position, Rod stacked the pillows behind Martina and helped her lean back against them. He brought the breakfast tray to the bed and carefully set it across her lap.

"Mmmm. Everything looks so good. Thank you, Rod," she said, beaming an appreciative smile. Then added, "But I should be making breakfast for you."

"Says who? Is that one of the Ten Commandments? Thou shalt serve your husband breakfast every morning."

"Well…it is the traditional role of the wife to do the cooking," she countered.

"Not in this house and not in our marriage. We make our own traditions. Okay?" he said, taking her hand and kissing it.

"Okay." she answered, loving his boyish grin.

"That's the spirit. For a minute I thought maybe you had been brainwashed by the Justice of the Peace and all his talk about being an obedient servant of your husband."

Martina laughed and pinched his arm playfully. "I know he meant well, Rod, but that was such a crock of horse manure. What was that he said about high minded women?"

"Oh— Yeah! I saw you grinding your jaw when ole J. Winslow started talking about that," he said, chuckling.

"Well…let's never mind about his sermon. The service was very nice. And I appreciate your making breakfast," she told him.

"I was the first one up and I wanted to bring you breakfast in bed on your first morning as my wife. After you have had an opportunity to explore the kitchen and see where everything is at, then I'll chain you to the stove. But since this is your first day on the job," he joked, "I thought I'd cut you some slack."

She laughed at his silliness. "My thoughtful husband." She said, patting his cheek. "I actually like to cook and I'm pretty good at it too."

Rod sat down on the edge of the bed and handed her a glass of juice. "Here's to our long, happy marriage, where we make our own traditions," he said, tapping his glass of orange juice against hers. Martina curled her arm around his and they drank their juice in the manner of a matrimonial champagne toast. Their positioning was awkward but they managed to do it without spilling a drop.

Martina set her glass down on the tray and looked at the array of food. "I didn't realize I was so hungry until I saw this food," Spreading the preserves on a croissant, she took a large bite.

Rod smiled sheepishly. "After last night you should be as hungry as a bear in the springtime." She blushed and he patted her leg affectionately. He was now sitting next to her, sharing the pillows, and peeling a hard-boiled egg.

"You are a fine one to talk," she said, playfully defending herself. "I didn't hear you call for any time-outs."

"*Touché*, my sweet." He handed her the peeled egg.

When they finished breakfast, Rod set the tray on the floor outside the bedroom door, as they would do if they were staying at a hotel. He then went to open the French doors to the balcony. Martina reflexively pulled the sheet up over her breasts. Rod noted her modesty and went back to lie beside her on the bed. "No one will see those two beauties

142

up here, except me and possibly a squirrel or two," he said, lowering the sheet again.

After a few moments of kissing and fondling, Rod sat up and announced, "I know just the thing to clear the cobwebs and soothe the aching limbs."

When he didn't attempt to make love to her again, she asked, almost timidly, "My husband is tired of me already?"

"Is that what you think? Believe me…your husband would love nothing more than to make love to you all day but I'm trying not to be an insensitive oaf and wear out my welcome."

He took her hand in his and kissed it with obvious reverence.

His voice was soft and serious when he added, "I know what you did last night after—" She placed her index finger across his lips, wanting to avoid any conversation that would lead to questions she was not prepared to answer about her past.

"I love that you are sensitive and caring," she said, her voice quavering with emotion. "That's what attracted me to you right away. I don't want you to ever change. I love everything about you and you'll never wear out your welcome with me."

Rod wiped away the tears that had spilled from the corners of her eyes with the edge of the sheet. He could sense that she did not want to talk about what led her to believe she was not a virgin, and he certainly did not want to force the issue, but he felt the need to apologize for hurting her in such a way.

"Martina— (He paused to take a deep breath and make sure he had her full attention.) When I realized I was head over heels in love with you and wanted you to be my wife, it is the wonderful person you are that I fell in love with. I didn't base my feelings on anything other than how you and I got along together. I just knew right away you were a good fit. I know you're very young, but you are also very intelligent and mature. The fact is…I've never met anyone as sweet and lovable and exciting as you and that's the simple truth of it. When I took you into my heart, my only concern was that I do everything possible to take care of you…to keep you safe and happy. I've not asked you for any information about who you've kissed or held hands with or anything else. All that is important to me is that you want to kiss and hold hands with me and lay up against me at night…that you want to share your life with me. I'm just sorry that I wasn't more careful last night…and we won't talk about it anymore unless you want to."

For several moments, Martina could say nothing. It wasn't just what he said but the heartfelt way he said it. Looking into his eyes she saw his naked, raw emotions and felt so undeserving of his love. How could she possibly deserve such a loving man, she wondered? Finally, her mouth opened and out tumbled, "Oh— Rod." It was all she could say.

Seeing she was overcome with emotion, he decided to lighten up the moment. "I pour my heart out to you and all you can say is 'Oh Rod'," he gently teased.

Emitting a heavy sigh, she then said, "I'm kind of blown away. All I can say is that I feel the same way about you and I just hope I can live up to your love."

"There's no such thing as having to live up to someone's love. I don't expect you to be anything other than who you are."

* * * * *

On the other side of Millborough, Martino Fiasconi was pacing in his study and conjuring up graphic thoughts of what he intended to do with his wayward daughter when she finally returned home. Wearing the same stained, rumpled polo shirt and khaki trousers he had been wearing for the last two days, Martino Fiasconi blended into the early morning darkness of his paneled study, sipping a breakfast of straight Scotch and seething with anger. Feeling very much cuckolded, he wondered what a fitting punishment would be to teach Martina a lasting lesson. While most parents would be alarmed and call the police if their child had vanished from their house on a Friday afternoon and had still not turned up by Saturday morning, Martino had none of the normal reactions of most parents. He knew exactly where Martina had gone when she left the house on Friday, taking the Jaguar without his permission—she was with that despicable biker, Rod McDonough. And when she returned home, as he knew she eventually would, he would render the appropriate punishment for her transgressions. In the twisted reasoning of his demented mind Martino Fiasconi had come to believe that Martina was his exclusive possession, and it was unforgivable of her to give herself to another man. As for Rod McDonough, Martino had already decided what his fate would be.

24.

"So what would you like to do on your first day as Mrs. Rod McDonough? I'm open to all suggestions that are lawful and pleasurable." Rod had just returned from bringing the breakfast tray downstairs to the kitchen, and had come back with a cup of tea for Martina, who was still lolling in bed.

"There's a beautiful, sunny day waiting outside for us."

"I'm up for anything you are," she said, not sure she even wanted to leave the house.

"But we agreed that this is your day, and I am here to serve your every whim." He bowed playfully, and his loosely cinched cotton robe fell open provocatively, as if on cue.

Martina cocked an eyebrow, amused. "I don't remember agreeing to any such thing but it sounds like an offer full of intriguing possibilities. Let me think about it." She studied the lace canopy for a moment. "Well— the first thing I'd like to do is take a nice, hot bubble bath."

"A bubble bath, eh?" Rod grinned lecherously. "One bubble bath, coming right up."

A giant cloud of iridescent suds awaited a surprised Martina when Rod escorted her into the bathroom. "Where's the tub?" She asked, astounded by the mountain of froth.

Grabbing a towel, Rod swatted at the suds until they had disbursed enough for her to vaguely make out the porcelain boundaries of the extra large, free standing tub. "There you are, my dear." He held his hand out to her. "Hop in."

The just-right hot water felt heavenly as it enveloped her body and she moaned with delight. She attempted to lie back, but the bubbles would have completely covered her, so she hugged her knees to her chest and let the heat of the water soothe her taut, aching muscles. Rod, she saw, was rummaging in a well-stocked linen closet that was hidden behind two full-length sliding mirror panels and came away with several thick Turkish towels. Then, to Martina's surprise, he threw off his robe and climbed into the tub, facing her.

At first, they splashed and tickled each other like playful children, but it was inevitable their play would settle down to more serious touching. Beckoning to Rod with her index finger, Martina said, "What was that you said earlier about serving my every whim?"

"I thought you'd never ask, my Princess."

Nearly an hour later, Rod was patting Martina's back with a thick Turkish towel, when he said, "I think we should start every day of our married life this way."

Martina turned slowly and slid her slender, caramel arms around his neck. "It's a wonderful way to start off the day, Rod," she said, her voice soft and sensual, "but would we ever get past the bedroom door?"

Rod smiled and kissed the tip of her nose. "Would it be such a bad thing if we didn't?"

"I have no objections but I don't know how practical it would be," she said, tickling him under the chin. "We should probably do something unique on our first day of married life together."

"We can do just about anything you desire. We can fly to the Bahamas and spend some time on my parents' boat. Or we can go see a Broadway play in New York City. How about surfing in Oahu?"

"Be serious, Rod. I have to go to school on Monday."

Playfully snatching the towel from his gesturing hand, she wrapped it around her torso and disappeared into the dressing room-closet.

"I am being serious," Rod called after her, pulling on a pair of black Levis. "You asked what shall we do and I'm just trying to give you some ideas." From a dresser drawer he plucked out a neatly folded black Harley-Davidson T-shirt and slipped it over his head.

Martina, now wearing the same white tank top she wore the day before and lacey red bikinis, peaked through the closet doorway to check Rod's face for a telltale smile. But she saw he was dead serious. "Are you saying that we can really fly to the Bahamas or Hawaii if we wanted to?"

"Yep. That's what I'm saying…and don't forget New York."

"Can we afford to do those things?" It was the first time Martina thought to consider their finances. Obviously, she had no income to contribute to the marriage, at least not until she turned eighteen and became eligible to receive a monthly income from the trust fund her mother left in her name. And she knew very little about how Rod made his living, other than his family owned a construction company, where he worked as a project supervisor.

Seeing Martina's confused expression, Rod went to her and cupped her face between his palms. "I would not have asked you to marry me if I was unable to give you a good life, Martina. I do have a job in the family business." He paused to kiss her tantalizing lips, and then, with a less serious tone, he added, "Even though I have been goofing off a lot since I met you. But that's going to be changing soon. My brother,

Travis, has been getting on my case about it…and I can't say I blame him."

"So you are blaming me for your goofing off." She pretended to be outraged.

Dropping to one knee, Rod grabbed Martina's hand and pressed it to his cheek. "Who else can I blame for all those days I was AWOL from the office because I was trying to win your affections? I couldn't help myself. I was smitten from the moment I first saw you. So I had to pull out all the stops to make you mine." His plea was basically a statement of truth delivered in his innate playful manner.

Martina giggled at his melodramatics, but she knew there was some truth mixed in with his theatrics. "Well— Now that you have won my affections don't think you can stop trying," she joked back, but Rod heard the kernel of truth in her words as well.

"I shall never stop pursuing your affections," he said, with great seriousness. Then, he again asked, "So what shall we do today?"

"How about just staying home and spending a quiet day getting to know each other," she answered.

"That sounds perfect to me," he said, beaming with happiness. Spending an entire day with Martina, without having to think about taking her home, was exactly what Rod had been looking forward to for months. He was ecstatic. His life was now complete.

After drying and brushing out her long honey brown hair, Martina stepped into her red gypsy skirt and adjusted the waist drawstring. She wished she had brought more clothes with her, but she had been in such a hurry to get out of the house yesterday afternoon, before Martino returned and stopped her from leaving, that she had no time to pick and choose the clothing she wanted to take with her. Plus, Martino would get suspicious if he saw that her closet was half empty. So great was her haste she had even forgotten to take her school books with her.

Thinking about what she had done last night - sneaking over to Clanton County and getting married in a double ceremony with Julie and Freebird -she could hardly believe it really happened, or that she even had the courage to go through with it. She was now Mrs. Martina McDonough, Rod's wife. Just thinking about it made her heart pound with nervous excitement. Although she had no regrets about marrying Rod, she knew that Martino would absolutely freak out if he ever found out about it. She would have to be extremely careful that he didn't. At least, not until after she turned eighteen in October, in only five months.

But there was still the tricky matter of her living arrangements. She knew Rod expected her to now live with him. Martino was certainly not going to agree to that. In fact, she had no doubt that he was probably flipping out right now because she sneaked out of the house and didn't come home all night. Martina knew there would be hell to pay when she returned home, but she could not let thoughts of possible mayhem ruin her weekend with Rod. Somehow, she would find a way to pacify Martino. Checking her hair and make-up in the mirror one last time, she rushed out of the bedroom.

Downstairs, Rod had put an Eagles' record on the stereo turntable, and the words "...*take it easy, take it easy, don't let the sound of your own wheels drive you crazy....*" wafted up the stairwell to greet Martina. Indeed, she couldn't think of a more apt song for the moment. With each step downward, she felt her own load loosen, and when Rod took her hand at the bottom of the stairs, she was smiling happily, as he twirled her into his arms.

"Pick out some tunes, Babe." Rod encouraged, gesturing to several shelves in the huge entertainment center that were lined with LPs.

"Do you have any Zeppelin?" Martina asked.

"That's my girl!" Rod beamed, and whisked out *Kaleidescope*, *Houses of the Holy*, and *Physical Graffiti*.

Martina took the *Physical Graffiti* album from Rod's hand. "This one," she said, sliding the inside sleeve up and down to maneuver the pictures in the window cut-outs. Rod smiled at her, amused.

"I'm really glad you wanted to stay home today," he told her. "We've never had a chance to just kick back like this."

Taking the album from her hands, he stood it on the shelf next to the stereo, and took her into his arms, gently kissing the fullness of her taunting lips and caressing her body. Swaying to the music of *Desperado*. How strange, it suddenly struck Rod, that this woman was now his wife but he knew so very little about the music she liked or any of the innumerable bits and pieces that made up this person who had the power to make him dizzy with love. He wondered if he would ever learn all that he wanted to know about Martina, as she kept so much of her life to herself; she was hardly an open book and difficult to read, in any event. Holding her tight against him, he could only hope that in time she would open up to him, let him read her secrets. Just then, she threw her head back and twirled out of his arms and he caught the glint of happiness in her phosphorescent eyes, which seemed greener and more mysterious to him than ever.

It was close to noon when Freebird and Julie sauntered through the back door, their hair wet from a recent shower and their faces aglow with matching, dreamy smiles. "Hey Bro!"

Freebird called out from the kitchen. "Are you guys decent in there?"

"C'mon in and join the party," Rod shouted back from the living room.

After several rounds of hugs and conspiratorial smiles between the couples, Freebird announced, "Hey, Bro…and Sis (acknowledging Martina as his sister), it's a beautiful day for a ride out to the country."

Rod immediately jumped up, ready to take off, but then suddenly remembered that he was no longer a single entity, with only himself to consider. He looked at Martina to see if she was receptive to the idea.

Martina would have been just as happy to hang out at home all day, listening to music and doing whatever else might come naturally, but she knew how much Rod loved riding his motorcycle. "Guess I'm going to have to get me some proper riding gear," she said.

Rod's face erupted into an appreciative smile. "Right on, Sister Sookie!" He said, chucking Martina under her chin. "Maybe we can stop by the bike shop and look at some leathers for you ladies," he suggested to Martina and Julie.

Julie squealed with delight. "Ooh! I've always wanted a black leather jacket. They are soooo tough."

Luckily, Martina had thought to bring a pair of jeans with her, just in case Rod wanted to take her riding on his bike, and her boots were in the Jaguar, so all she had to do was change out of the red skirt and white top she had thrown on after her bath.

"You girls go get ready," Rod said, as he and Freebird headed for the back door. "We're going to dust off the bikes and we'll be waiting for you out in our den of iniquity." He effected a sepulchral tone to emphasize the words "den of iniquity", to poke fun at the girls' for their earlier comments about their "little boys' macho hangout".

"C'mon, Julie," Martina said, grabbing her friend's arm, "Keep me company while I change."

As they climbed the stairs, Julie whispered to her friend, "After boffing all night, I don't know if I can even sit on a motorcycle."

Martina had not heard the expression "boffing" before but quickly surmised its meaning. "Now that you mention it— that might be a problem."

Laughing, the two friends locked arms and headed down the hallway to Martina's new bedroom.

"Yeh, but it was sure worth it," said Julie, playfully walking pigeon-toed and smiling blissfully. "No wonder my mother is out prowling around all hours of the night, wanting another husband."

Martina laughed at her friend's silliness, but refrained from any comment about Julie's mother. Truth be told, Martina did not approve of Mrs. Owens's prowling the local bars every night, when she should have been spending her time with Julie.

Then, switching to a more serious tone, she told Julie, "I think I'm the luckiest person on earth. Rod is just so wonderful to me. I really don't deserve him."

Julie stopped in mid-stride and gave Martina a puzzled look. "That's a crazy darn thing for you to say, Marty. Why would you not deserve him?"

Martina shrugged nervously and averted her eyes from Julie's penetrating gaze. "I just don't," she said, and continued walking toward the bedroom.

Following her friend into the bedroom, Julie said, "Don't ever let me hear you say such a thing again, Martina. You do so deserve Rod and you deserve to be happy."

Martina said nothing and went into the closet, where Rod had hung up the few clothes she had brought with her. Removing her jeans from a hanger, she brought them over to the lounge chair.

Julie gaped at the double-sized canopy bed, which was so amply tented with white lace that its yardage billowed out from the four posts like boat sails whenever a breeze drifted into the room through the open balcony doors. Shaking her head, she remarked, "I can't believe a big, muscular biker guy like Rod sleeps in such a frilly bed. You must have felt like a princess last night."

"Rod's mother decorated the room and he doesn't dare change it," Martina said, stepping out of her red skirt.

"He's still afraid of his mother, too?" asked Julie, incredulous.

"Let's just say that he respects her authority," Martina said, noting the precise way Rod had made up the bed that morning after he changed the sheets.

Julie laughed at something that had just come into to her mind. "Freebird said he was going to hang our sheet from a window, you know the way they used to do in olden days to prove to the whole village that the bride was a virgin." She looked over at Martina, who was wiggling into her jeans, and hissed. "I told him that hanging out a sheet doesn't prove a thing. Someone could put ketchup on the sheet and pretend it's the real deal."

"Julie!" Martina laughed, truly amused. She snapped the fly of her jeans closed. "You can think of the weirdest things."

"Yah. Like going to North Hampton to pick up guys," Julie said, giggling.

Removing her white tank top, Martina was about to pull on a red scoop neck top with cap sleeves, when Julie stopped her.

"No! Martina! You can't wear that."

"My red top? Why not?" asked Martina.

"No, silly. I don't mean your red top. I mean your bra,"
Julie admonished. "Biker chicks don't wear bras."

"How do you know that?" Martina asked, giving Julie a quizzical look.

"Freebird told me. He told me that now that I'm his wife he doesn't ever want to see me wearing a bra again. In fact, when he took my strapless bra off last night he threw it out the bedroom window and now it's down there in the bushes behind the garage."

Hearing that, Martina fell onto the lounge chair laughing hysterically. "Stop it, Julie! You're killin' me with your crazy stories."

Just then, Rod yelled up from the yard, "What's keeping you ole ladies? We're ready to go."

Martina stood up and gave Julie an impish grin. Taking off her bra and then pulling on her red top, she walked out onto the balcony and dropped the bra over the railing. They heard Rod shout, "What the heck? Martina! What's going on up there?"

Then they heard Freebird laughing.

"Okay!" Martina confirmed to Julie. "We braless biker babes are ready to roll."

"Sounds like a good title for one of those funky B movies."
Julie said, laughing, as they left the bedroom.

Rod was waiting for Martina just outside the back porch door when she came out of the house. He held up the white silk bra she had dropped off the balcony, and said, "I know this must be some kind of a statement, but what exactly are you trying to say?"

Gently rubbing his muscled chest, she smiled up at him with the wickedest grin she could muster, and repeated Julie's admonition, "Biker chicks don't wear bras." Then she sauntered off barefoot toward the red Jaguar to retrieve her boots. Rod watched the swing and sway of Martina's curvy butt as she walked off, and let out a long, low whistle. Shrugging, he went back to the garage, clutching the discarded bra in his hand.

Freebird, who was kneeling beside his bike, and fussing with something or another to do with the engine, looked up in time to see Rod hang the bra from a vacant nail sticking out of a wall stud.

Giving Rod a strange look, he asked, "What's up, Bro?"

"Hell if I know. Martina just threw her bra at me," Rod shrugged, his expression was both confused and bemused. "She told me that biker chicks don't wear bras. I wonder where the hell she heard that crap? Now I have to worry about other guys checking out her tits. Jesus! What's next?"

Freebird could hardly keep a straight face while he listened to his friend's fretting. "Lighten up, man," he kidded Rod. "You've been married less than twenty-four hours and you're already acting like a jealous husband." Standing up, Freebird swung a leg over his bike and dropped his butt into the saddle. Reaching down, he pulled out the kick pedal. "Let's get into the wind, Bro, and you'll enjoy the hell outta those braless tits bouncing against your back."

25.

It had been a perfect weekend until Sunday morning, when Rod woke up and found that Martina was gone from his bed and the red Jaguar was gone from the driveway. Distraught, he pulled on his Levi's and headed over to Freebird's apartment.

Even before opening the door to let Rod in, Freebird knew the reason why his friend was there pounding on his door.

"I heard the car start up real early this morning," Freebird said without prompting, as he motioned his friend to come in. "I thought you two were taking off someplace for the day."

Julie had brought each of them a steaming mug of coffee, but it was undrinkable. She had not quite perfected the grounds to water ratio, so her coffee was more like a bitter syrup. But they thanked her, and she returned to the kitchen, downhearted about her missing friend, while the two men discussed Martina's disappearance in the living room.

"Didn't she say anything to you about where she was going?" Freebird asked.

Rod, who sat hunched forward, with his head in his hands and his elbows jabbed into his thighs, shook his head.

"Nothing," he said, his voice barely audible.

"Where d'ya think she went?" Freebird asked.

"I'm sure she went back to him," Rod said, with disgust.

Freebird knew Rod was referring to Martina's father, and shook his head in disbelief, "Why would she go back there?"

"Because she's got this stupid idea that it's her job to take care of him since her mother died." Rod answered with a grimace, as though the words were as distasteful as their meaning. Then he jumped up and started pacing around the living room, obviously upset. Freebird had never seen Rod in such an emotional state.

"What do you want to do? Go get her?"

Stopping in front of the large picture window that overlooked the driveway, Rod looked out at the empty spot in the driveway where the Jaguar had been parked. He suddenly felt lonely. Turning to look at Freebird, he said, "Yes. I have to go get her."

"Let me do it, Rod," said Julie, rushing back into the room from the kitchen, where she had been listening to their conversation. "If you go over there, her father might call the police. But if I go, he'll think I just dropped by to visit. Let me at least talk to her first. Then I can tell you what's going on."

Rod looked at the young girl, hating to admit to himself that she was probably right, then he looked at Freebird. "She's probably right, Bro, but you have to approve. She's your ole lady."

Freebird looked from Rod to Julie and then nodded his assent to Julie's plan.

"Okay, Julie," Rod said, but we'll will be waiting right outside, so if anything weird gets to happening in that house we can jump right in…but I sure as hell hate to use you as the Trojan horse."

Julie gave him a quizzical look. "Trojan horse? What d'ya mean?"

"It's a long story…from the Greeks. I'll tell you about it some other time. Right now, I can't even think straight," said Rod, sounding pathetic.

Julie ran over to Rod and gave him a hug. "I'm sorry, Rod," she said, her eyes overflowing with tears. "I know Martina loves you. She even told me yesterday that you were wonderful to her, but that she didn't deserve you—"

"Doesn't deserve me?" Rod cut in. "Why would she even think that?"

"I don't know why, Rod. That's just what she told me…like you were too good for her."

Rod resumed his pacing, now more upset.

Freebird said to Julie, "Hey, Sweetie! How about going in the bedroom and finding me some clean clothes to put on."

When the girl left the room, Freebird went over to Rod and put his hand on Rod's shoulder. "Sorry, man. She's just trying to be helpful."

Rod nodded and flashed Freebird a weak smile. "I know. She's cool, Bro. Don't worry about it."

"I'm going to wash up and get dressed, so we can take off," said Freebird, "Try to relax. No sense going off the deep end until we find out what's going on."

Giving his friend a quick nod, Rod said, "I'll be down in the garage."

* * * * *

As silently and methodically as two men suiting up for a covert mission, Rod and Freebird donned their black leather chaps and jackets, and rolled their bikes out of the garage, onto the driveway cement. Rod looked up at the overcast sky, which seemed to aptly reflect his somber mood, and pulled on his black leather gloves. "Pissy day...all the way around," he commented to Freebird, and then climbed onto his bike.

"Maybe not," Freebird answered, with an enigmatic tone, and then said. "I'd better go upstairs and see what's holding up Julie." But just as Freebird was about to run up the steps, he saw Julie coming out of the front door to their apartment, somewhat suited up herself, wearing the new black leather motorcycle jacket and the chaps that Freebird had bought her yesterday, when they stopped by the Harley shop.

"Whoa! Julie! You can't wear leathers when you go to Martina's house...her father might get suspicious," Freebird observed.

"I know, Lover Boy. I'm just wearing them on the ride and I'll take them off before I go into Martina's house."

Freebird nodded in agreement, thinking that he sometimes did not give Julie enough credit for having the smarts to think of such things. He saw that as a shortcoming he would have to work on. When Julie got to the bottom step, Freebird grabbed her and gave her a hug.

"Hey, Rod!" Julie called out, pulling a school text book out from under her leather jacket, and waving it at him. Rod gave her a puzzled look. "I'm going to use this book as the reason why I need to see Martina when I get to her house. I've got a story all worked out."

Rod looked at Julie in her new leather jacket and chaps and smiled for the first time that morning. "Well...will you look at Mattel's new Biker Barbie," he kidded her. But that would be the extent of Rod's levity that day. After that one brief smile, Rod reset his jaw into a grim cast and stuck with that mean expression while they rode across town, toward Martina's house.

Rod led Freebird into a neighborhood of tree lined streets and stately homes in the College Park section of Millborough, where young men wearing black leather jackets and riding on thunderous motorcycles would be considered intruders and, thus, suspect. After a series of left and right turns, Rod switched off his engine and coasted to a stop at the end of a narrow lane that intersected with a slightly wider road, and signaled to Freebird to do likewise. There, across the street from where they stopped was the back section of the high white wall that surrounded the two story Georgian house where Martina lived. The house occupied a full block, which was probably close to an acre of land.

The two men sat on their bikes and grimly stared at the enormous walled estate as though it was some hated obstacle.

After a moment Freebird wryly observed, "That dude Martino could use a landscaper. It looks like a monster of a jungle has already swallowed up the house and now it's creeping over the walls looking for more land to devour."

"I drove all around the block the first time I brought Martina home from a date and the place is like a fortress. There's only one way in and one way out...and that's through the driveway with a wrought iron security gate...probably electronically controlled. And that's located way down there, at the other end of the block." Rod pointed to his right, down the wide road known as Kittredge Avenue.

Julie slid off of Freebird's bike and started removing her leathers. "Un-uh!" She interjected. "There's a door in the outer wall if you know where to look. It's hard to see, 'cause it's painted the same white color as the wall and it's practically covered with hanging vines. That's the way I go in and out."

Rod gave Julie a considered look. "You're going to have to show me where that is."

"Just watch where I go in. It's just this side of the driveway." Then, with her school book tucked under her arm, she gave Freebird a kiss on the lips and took off across the street toward a grassy footpath, between the wall and the road, which served as a sidewalk.

Rod called after her, "Be careful, Julie." She turned and waved back at them. "Damn! That girl's got a lot of heart," Rod commented to Freebird, keeping his eye on Julie as she walked. He didn't want to miss her signal, when she arrived at the front gate. Rod heard Freebird counting Julie's footsteps and said nothing further, so as not to screw up the count. Just as Freebird recited "two hundred and fifty-one," Julie raised her arm and pointed, to indicate where the gate in the wall was located and they watched her disappear from the footpath.

Freebird commented with a sigh, "I hope she doesn't stay in there too long."

Rod merely folded his arms across his chest and sat staring straight ahead, grim-faced, at the overgrown wall. He wondered if life with Martina would always be full of complications, recalling the way she smiled up at him yesterday morning, when they were dancing after their bath. Her eyes gave no hint of her intention to abandon him today.

Although it seemed much longer to Rod, only about ten minutes had passed when he heard Freebird utter, "Oh shit, Rod! Here comes the red Jaguar."

Rod immediately turned to look up the road and saw the red car, with its top down, nosing out of the driveway of Martina's house and onto the street, turning in their direction. Hopeful that it was Martina and Julie, Rod sat up straight and squinted into the distance, trying to see who was in the car. He could only make out one person, who appeared to be a man. Quickly, Rod put on his sunglasses. "I think it's her ole man," Rod muttered under his breath.

The Jaguar slowed down to a crawl as it approached the intersection and the man who was driving, a distinguished looking type with longish salt and pepper hair and dark goatee, gave Rod and Freebird a hard, suspicious look before continuing slowly down the street.

"I think he made us," said Rod, his eyes trailing after the red car. "If so, he might turn around and come right back. He won't want to leave Martina alone in the house if he knows who we are."

"Shit!" Freebird exclaimed. "If he goes back to the house I'm goin' in there and getting' Julie out right away. An' I don't care if he does call the cops. I don't like the looks of that dude and I don't want my Julie in there with him."

Continuing to look at the rear of the Jaguar as it traveled further down the road, Rod assured his concerned friend, "Don't worry, man. If that's Martino…he looks like a good stiff breeze would blow him over. We won't have any problem getting her out of there."

Freebird nodded, but not in agreement with Rod's simplistic assessment of retrieving Julie. He knew that guys like Martino could be pretty dangerous when they were pushed into a corner. If the vibes he picked up when Martino drove past them were any indication, that dude was one squirrelly bastard.

* * * * *

Just before going through the door in the wall that encircled Martina's house, Julie turned and waved her hand at Freebird and Rod, so they could see where the hidden portal was located. She thought it was funny the way the two guys carried on before leaving to ride over to Martina's. They thought Mr. Fiasconi was some kind of an ogre, but Julie downplayed their criticisms. She had told them that Martino may be a strange bird but he was certainly no axe murderer. Julie had never so much as heard Martina's father raise his sophisticated voice.

But Julie had not been around the Fiasconi house for a long while and was unaware of the professor's further descent into obsession, jealousy and fear of losing Martina. She was completely unaware her best friend's father was teetering on a razor's edge of mental derangement. So, when Martino opened the front door and looked somewhat wild-eyed, Julie merely assumed he was upset because Martina had been absent without leave for two nights and a whole day.

"Hi, Professor Fiasconi! Is Martina home?" Julie bubbled. Holding up her textbook, she explained how she had been sick last Friday and missed school. And, now, with a big test coming up, she needed to find out from Martina what chapters were covered in class, so she would know what to study. Julie assumed Martino believed her story because he invited her to come right in.

"Martina's in the sitting room," he told Julie, his voice stiff and formal. "We're having a bit of a disagreement just at the moment, but you may go in and speak with her. I need to go out and run an errand anyway, so you may visit with her until I return." He ushered Julie to the sitting room, where Martina was huddled in an armchair, wearing a long pink satin lounging tunic that Julie recognized as having belonged to Jacqui. Julie noticed right away that Martina's eyes were red and swollen from crying and one of her cheeks was emblazoned with what appeared to be a red handprint. Seeing Martina in that condition was Julie's first inkling that something even weirder than usual was going on at Martina's house. Then, when Martino pointed at Martina and said, with a stern tone she had never heard him use before, "You are not to leave this house for any reason. And we will resume our discussion when I return and your friend leaves."

Then, Julie knew for sure that the calm, permissive Martino had undergone a radical change.

After Julie made certain Martino had left the house, she ran to her friend and knelt on the floor in front of the chair. "What happened, Martina? Ohmygod! Your face! Did he hit you?"

Martina nodded and burst into tears. Julie grabbed Martina's knee. "That bastard!" She exclaimed. "He can't hit you. You're a married woman. Rod will really be pissed off when he finds out."

Martina stiffened. "No! Julie. You can't tell Rod anything. I don't want Martino to know anything about Rod and us getting married. Please! You can't say anything."

Julie stood up and took her friend's arm. "C'mon Martina. Let's get outta here. You've got to go back to Rod. He's your husband and he's really upset and missin' you." Tugging Martina's arm, Julie pressed

"C'mon! We've got to get outta here before Martino comes back. Rod and Freebird are waiting down the street for us."

Martina looked up at Julie, a light of hope flashing in her eyes for a second and then rapidly dying out. "I can't leave right now, Julie. You don't understand. Martino is too upset."

Julie looked at her friend, confused. "What about Rod, Martina? He's pretty darn upset, too. You just bugged out this morning and didn't tell him anything. We all woke up and you were gone. Poor Rod. He didn't know what to do." Once again, Julie tugged her crying friend's arm. "Please! Martina! We've got to go…now! Rod really needs you."

Martina shook her head and waved off Julie. "I can't. Tell Rod I'll come back as soon as I can…but I can't leave Martino like this. He needs time to get used to things."

"That's just plain crazy, Martina. You're his daughter, not his mother." Unable to make any headway with Martina, Julie threw her hands up with frustration. "Okay! Fine! I'm leaving, Martina. If you want to stay around here in this depressing overgrown jungle and be slapped around by someone who doesn't want you to have a life, that's up to you. But you should at least go talk to Rod. You owe him that much."

Wiping the tears off her face, Martina said, "Okay, Julie. I'll talk to Rod. But he's got to understand I can't go with him today."

"That's between you and Rod. I only volunteered to come in here and be the Trojan Horse."

Martina looked up at Julie, surprised. "What? What do you mean? Be a Trojan Horse?"

"I don't have time to explain right now. We'd better go outside, so you can talk to Rod before Martino comes back and gets pissed again." That said, Julie turned and started to leave the room.

Languidly, Martina rose from her chair and followed Julie outside, into the overgrown, leaf strewn brick courtyard in front of the house. The gate to the road was hanging open and she saw Julie standing out on the footpath, waving an arm back and forth, presumably signaling Rod and Freebird. Martina felt her heart grow heavy with trepidation when she heard their motorcycle engines rev to life somewhere down the end of the block; she dreaded facing Rod. She knew he would not understand the difficult situation she was embroiled in with Martino, one that only she could resolve, nor could she even explain to Rod just at the moment what that situation was about. She had mired herself in a terrible mess, all of her own creation, and the worst thing about it was there seemed no way out at the moment. And, now, she had two men pulling at her from opposite directions.

The motorcycles were now idling just on the other side of the wall from where Martina stood. Steeling herself for an upsetting confrontation, she walked through the gate and came face to face with Rod. Seeing the expression of deep hurt in his eyes, Martina was overcome with shame and lowered her head.

Rod switched off the engine of his bike and kicked out its stand. Dismounting, he shouted to Freebird, "I'll see you back at the house."

Freebird nodded, waiting only long enough for Julie to put on her leather jacket and hop back on his bike, and then he roared off down the road.

The first thing that disturbed Rod was the weird pink dress, or whatever it was, Martina was wearing. It looked like something a two-bit brothel whore would wear and he could see just enough through the delicate material to know she had nothing on underneath it. It struck him as very odd that she would be dressed like that in the first place, let alone in the middle of the day.

Looking up and down the street, to make sure the red Jaguar was not in sight, he took hold of her arm and guided her back through the open door in the wall, into the overgrown courtyard. When she looked up at him, Rod saw her eyes were red and puffy from crying and wondered why one of her cheeks looked so inflamed. Alarm bells were going off in his head as he looked her over, and his hands shook with anger and uncertainty. He wanted to throw her over his shoulder and carry her away. He wished he had brought his car instead of the bike. Obviously, she was not dressed for riding on the bike and it might be too late for her to change. Martino could return at any moment and Rod wanted to avoid any contact with him, mainly because he wanted to punch out the perverted bastard. His heart was pounding so hard he could feel it in his head. He waited for her to say something, to give him some explanation of why she abandoned his bed, but she only stared at him with her sorrowful eyes, that seemed to have taken on the grayish cast of the sky.

Rod felt himself loosing the battle with his emotions. Forgetting all about his earlier resolve to be firm and unequivocal when this moment arrived, he now only wanted Martina to leave with him and how he accomplished that result no longer mattered. He felt the urge to throw himself on the ground and beg her to come home with him. Somehow, even in his anger and hurt, he knew that she did not need a heavy-handed approach from him right now. The sad, tense expression on her face softened his heart.

With a soft and gentle voice, he asked, "Tell me what's going on here, Martina? It's not a good thing to wake up and find my wife has left me…and just a day after we were married."

Then, placing his hands lightly on her shoulders, he added, "I need to know what's going on with you, Baby. Are you my wife…or what?" He gestured toward the forbidding looking house.

Dropping her head to avoid the naked intensity of his gaze, Martina wiped away the resurgence of tears that spilled from her eyes. When she was finally able to speak, her voice quivered from the tightness of her constricted throat. "I love you more than anything, Rod. I didn't leave you. I came back here to get my clothes and stuff for school…but when I went into the house Martino was right there waiting. He was upset and worried that something terrible had happened to me…at first. Then he got really mad and wouldn't let me leave. When I tried to call you he pulled the phone out of my hand—" Her words were suddenly choked off by sobs.

Envisioning the entire scenario between her and her father as she related what had happened, Rod felt his rage building.

"That sonofabitch!" He grabbed her by the arm and pulled her toward the front door. "Go get a jacket on. You're coming home with me."

Martina pulled her arm free, and stepped back. In an instant, her expression changed from misery to alarm and then to defiance. "No! Rod! I can't go with you right now. You don't understand—"

Rod cut in, "Make me understand, Martina! Because right now I am at a loss to understand what's going on in your head." His tone was strained as he attempted to control his frustration with her and the craziness of the situation she had put him in.

"It's not his fault. I can't tell you anymore than that right now," she cried, putting her hands up in a gesture that warned him not to pursue his questioning any further.

It was then Rod noticed she was not wearing the wedding ring he had placed on her finger when they were married only two nights ago. He reached out and took hold of her left hand and pointedly stared at it. "Where's your wedding ring," he asked, upset.

"I had to take it off before Martino saw it and asked any questions," she explained, sounding a bit defensive.

Rod nodded his head, clearly unhappy. "So, that must mean that you didn't tell him we got married."

"How could I, Rod? He's never even met you."

"And that's a very good point, Martina," Rod said, trying to maintain his patience. "Just exactly why is it that you have never brought me home to meet your father?" She could only gasp at his statement and lower her head, embarrassed by its truth. Struggling to keep his temper from flaring, which would only send her running into the house, he tried to reason with her. "What am I supposed to think? You tell me you love me. Then you run out on me in the middle of the night…take off your wedding ring…and now you're telling me you won't come home with me. Sounds to me like it's over between us."

Throwing herself against him, Marina burst into pitiful sobs. Burrowing her head into his chest, she tried to tell him he was wrong, but the words would not come out. She knew she had made matters worse than they were, and now she was in danger of losing the one man she truly loved. Surely, Rod must know how much she loved him. But, instead of holding and comforting her, she felt Rod push her away from his body.

Holding her at arms' length, he simply said, "If you are not going to be my wife and wear my ring, then give me the ring back right now and I'll leave. I guess our marriage means nothing to you."

His words shocked her out of her emotional stupor, but just as she opened her mouth to tell him she had every intention of being his wife, the red Jaguar entered the driveway and stopped just long enough for Rod and her father to exchange the kind of hateful, challenging glances that promised a certain future confrontation between the two men. Then the car sped off down the long, straight driveway leading to the back of the house and a detached garage. Rod looked back at Martina and saw a look of fear in her eyes that caused him to wonder if she was afraid of Martino. Or was she afraid what Rod might do to Martino?

Suddenly, her words poured out in an excited string of pleas. "Please…Rod! I do love you. You must know that I do?

I am your wife and I do want to be with you. But you've got to give me some time to get things straightened out with Martino."

With his peripheral vision, Rod kept an eye on the front door of the house while, at the same time, trying to look at Martina's face and listen to her words. He knew there would be trouble if he stayed there much longer. Listening to her words only frustrated him more. And she, too, was nervously looking over her shoulder, to check the door, as though she was expecting Martino to come bursting through it at any moment, brandishing a gun.

"Then come with me now, Martina." He urged her.

"Please, Rod. Just give me tonight to talk to Martino and I promise to go home with you tomorrow."

The sincerity of her plea overshadowed Rod's sense of logic. He loved Martina too much to be objective, so he did not bother to ask her how one more night could possibly make any difference in Martino's attitude. Especially now, after Martino had glimpsed the obviously older man his young daughter is keeping company with and displaying his utter contempt for her choice. To keep Martina in his life, Rod agreed to give her the one more night she begged him for.

"Alright, Martina. You have one more night...but that is it!" His tone was adamant. "When I pick you up after school tomorrow you better be prepared to come live with me from there on out...and don't even worry about bringing your clothes if it'll make your move any easier and faster. If you don't come home with me tomorrow." Rod didn't finish the sentence but the drift of his intention was unmistakable. He was clearly unhappy with being put off.

"I will go home with you tomorrow, no matter what," she promised, then turned to run back inside the house.

Rod grabbed her arm and spun her around to face him. "Can I at least have a kiss before you run off?" He asked. He saw her expression grow fearful again, and when she did not make a move to kiss him, he encircled her with his arms and pulled her to him, kissing her roughly on the mouth. She tried to pull away but he would not let her. When he finally let her go, he said, "I'm not fooling around, Martina. This is real."

"But— Martino." She weakly protested.

"You're not married to Martino," he reminded her. Then, brushing a stray lock of hair behind her ear, he said softly, "I love you, Baby."

"And I love you," she answered, tears brimming in her eyes.

After giving her one last, serious look, Rod turned and left, pissed off to the high heavens but determined not to make a scene.

As if on auto-pilot, Rod slowly navigated his bike up and down random side streets, rehashing in his mind the scene he just went through with Martina that had left him with a chaffing uneasiness. Several times he circled back toward the walled mansion, stopping within visual distance of the imposing white wall. *What the hell is going on in there?* He wondered. Bits and pieces of Martina's words replayed. Snapshots of her reddened eyes, nervous and pleading, and that ridiculous dress she was wearing filtered into his mind's eye. It was all too bizarre and unsettling. Why didn't he drag Martina out of there when he had the chance? But that was just it - he had no authority to drag her anywhere. That asshole father of hers was holding all of the cards in this dangerous game. Rod knew that if he lost his cool and did anything stupid, he would be the big loser.

Someway, somehow, Rod told himself, I have to draw up on Fiasconi.

Taking one last look at the Fiasconi house, he whispered, "See you tomorrow, my love," Then he turned his bike around and finally headed home.

26.

Martino was waiting just inside the front door when Martina went into the house. He grabbed her by the arm and yanked her toward him, so that his angry, distorted face was only millimeters from hers. "So…is that who you spent the last two nights with?" He ridiculed. "I would have given you more credit than to take up with that kind of trash. I should have him arrested for corrupting a minor."

The crazed look on his face frightened Martina. She had never seen him in such a violent state before, but without thinking, she said, "He's not trash. If you would only get to know him you would see that he's not what you think." It was the wrong thing to say to a man who was beyond the pale of rational thinking. Martina did not realize that her father had indeed drifted into a dangerous gray area. In his mind this young girl, who belonged to him by virtue of their blood relationship, had been unfaithful and she needed to be taught a harsh lesson. Shoving Martina toward the stairs, he ordered, "Go upstairs to your room. You have defiled yourself beyond redemption."

Martina thought he merely intended to make her feel guilty by making such an ugly statement and then restrict her to her room for a few days. She figured it best to just go along with him. She could see there was no sense in trying to reason with him at the moment, as he was much too agitated. It almost seemed like he was on some sort of drug that caused him to act wild and bizarre. To get away from him, Martina quite willingly rushed up to her bedroom and locked the door.

It had always been a sacrosanct rule in the Fiasconi house to never enter another person's room when their door was closed. Thus, Martina felt she was safe from intrusion. Unfortunately, Martino Fiasconi was also now beyond respecting the closed door policy. She was sitting on the edge of her bed, wishing she had gone home with Rod, when Martino crashed through the bedroom door. The crazed look in his eyes was horrifying. She was caught completely off guard by his intrusion and realized that it was too late now to escape from what was about to happen.

27.

Rod waited for nearly an hour in his usual parking space, a block away from Martina's school. When she did not show up as promised, he cruised the streets around the school, thinking she might have been detained for some reason, but she was nowhere in sight. As he drove slowly past the main entrance of the school one last time, he tried to recall every nuance of Martina's conversation with him yesterday, while they stood in the front yard of her father's house, and the sincerity of her voice when she told him she would go home with him after school today. Rod refused to believe she would lie to him. At the end of the block he saw there was an open parking space in front of a delivery truck and he nosed the Corvette into the vacant spot. He needed a moment to think.

In a deserted classroom on the second floor of the Millborough High School, Martina stood by a window watching the street below. Her heart quickened when she saw Rod's Corvette cruise slowly past the front of the school, and then her heart began to ache. Clear as a bell, she could hear in her head Martino's threatening words from last night, when he warned her he would turn Rod into the police for statutory rape, and how Rod would spend the rest of his days in jail if she ever attempted to see him again. And as if the thought of Rod going to jail did not terrorize her enough, Martino shockingly reminded her that he knew people who would be happy to take care of Rod for a price. Then, out of his own sense of impotence and fear of losing her to another man, Martino removed his belt and whipped her with the buckle end of it until she promised to never see or communicate with that low class biker trash again. Martina's first fifteen minutes of defiance, when she refused to give in to Martino's crazed demands and promise never to see Rod again had cost her dearly. When he had finally broken her will, he made her repeat the words, "I will never see that low class biker trash again," over and over like a demented mantra until, mercifully, she passed out

The following morning she saw in her wardrobe mirror that she was covered with bloody welts, which were mostly on her back, buttocks, and upper thighs; they were so swollen and painful she could hardly move around to get ready for school. There was other soreness, too, but she attributed that to lovemaking with Rod. Yet, Martina could not be sure. She had passed out last night during Martino's beating, leaving herself vulnerable to whatever punishment he fancied. After seeing the brutality he was capable of, she could no longer put anything past him.

Moving slowly, she attempted to dress herself for school. There was no way she could wear a bra over her painful welts, so she slipped on a T-shirt and the long red broom skirt she wore home yesterday. Even raising her arms to brush her hair was excruciating. She didn't even bother with make up. Two or three times, the battered young woman almost passed out from dizziness. When she finally made it down to the kitchen, Martino was waiting for her. He was not the least bit contrite about what he had done. In fact, he acted as though nothing out of the ordinary had happened.

When she complained to Martino about her pain, he minimized the extent of the injuries he had inflicted and insisted she go to school anyway. He even drove her to the school to make sure that she did indeed go. With great difficulty, she sat through class after class, trying to keep her full weight off of the welts, but it was next to impossible since she had to sit directly on them. Luckily, she did not have any classes with Julie on Mondays, as Julie would have certainly noticed her discomfort and the peculiar way she was walking.

When the last bell sounded, dismissing all classes for the day, Martina found an empty classroom that overlooked the street in front of the school, so she could watch for Rod's car. She thought about calling Rod and telling him that Martino was threatening to turn him in to the police for keeping her at his house overnight, and it would be best if they did not see each other until things cooled down, but she knew Rod would only flip out and go after Martino. And Martino would surely be on the lookout for any excuse to have Rod thrown into jail. She decided that the only thing she could do to protect Rod from Martino's revenge was to make it appear as though she had stood him up by not meeting him after school this afternoon. Rod had made it pretty clear to her yesterday that if she did not go home with him today, their relationship would be over. And even if it were her intention to defy her father and move in with Rod, she could not go through with it now. If Rod ever saw the belt marks all over her back he'd be hell-bent to kill Martino for laying a hand on her. She had to protect Rod at all costs, even if it meant she could never see, touch, or feel him again. She could only blame herself for the awful mess she was in and she would have to live with her mistakes.

As Martina stood at the classroom window and watched Rod's car disappear from view, she braced herself for the pain of walking to the bus stop, and then the lurching bus ride home. Gathering up her purse and books, she sighed and tearfully shuffled out of the room. Luckily, there was no one in the hall to witness her misery and ask questions. Descending the two flights of stairs from the second floor was torture. Martina had to lean heavily on the banister with her one free hand and her progress was slow. Each step she took was like receiving another crack of the belt and brought tears to her eyes. Reaching the first floor, she breathed a sigh of relief and stood motionless for a moment. Then she painfully pushed open the heavy front door and stood looking down at another flight of at least twenty cement steps leading to the sidewalk.

While Martina teetered slowly down the school's front steps, she could not see that Rod's Corvette was parked only several spaces away, in front of a wide box truck. All of her concentration and flagging energy was focused on making it down the steps without collapsing from the searing pain that was shooting down her back and legs, and the awful dizziness and nausea that accompanied it.

Sitting in his Corvette, unaware of Martina's nearby plight, Rod had his eyes closed and was trying to work through the knot in his stomach. Martina's no-show was completely unexpected. He felt certain she had been sincere when she said she would come home with him today. Recalling the fear on her face last night, just before she ran back into that house, Rod had no doubt that her father was somehow preventing her from meeting him. What if he had her locked in her room? Or hurt her? Bristling at the thought of Martino mistreating his wife, Rod decided it was time for him to go on the offensive with Fiasconi and have it out with the man. Tired of the passive role he had been playing, it was now time to go get his wife and bring her home. Otherwise, what kind of a man would he be?

With his course of action now determined, Rod sat up and shifted into first gear. Out of habit, before pulling away from the curb he checked all of his mirrors and that was when he noticed in the miniature frame of his right side view mirror the familiar red skirt, shapely legs, and red satin slippers coming unsteadily down the sidewalk, toward his car. Shifting into "Park," Rod threw open his door and sprung out of the car. He walked quickly along the street side of the box truck, sneaking around to the rear of the truck and up onto the sidewalk, to surprise Martina. Hearing footsteps behind her, Martina half turned her head, but could not move fast enough. Rod noted the stiffness of her movement and the halting way she was walking.

"Martina?" He called out to her, worried. "What's wrong?"

Hearing Rod's voice, Martina cried out with surprise, and her purse and books fell to the sidewalk with a clatter. Despite Martino's threats and beating she was happy to see him. "Rod! You scared me," she said, clutching her hands to her chest.

Rod picked up her purse and books and held onto them. "What's happened to you? Did you fall or something? Why are you walking like that?" he asked, suddenly concerned.

"I'm okay," she said.

"When you didn't meet me after class I thought maybe you had been locked up in your room. I was just about to drive over to your house."

Martina was getting nervous about standing around on the sidewalk with Rod. She looked around, worried that Martino might be parked nearby and watching them; she knew he had a class at this time on Mondays, but he could have canceled it just to spy on her.

Rod put his arm around her shoulders and she jumped, gasping in pain. "Jesus! Martina. What's wrong with you?"

"It's nothing," she told him, struggling to act and sound like she was really okay. "I slipped and fell in the gym this morning," she lied, "I'll be okay." Then, with a tone of urgency in her voice, she said, "Rod, we need to go someplace and talk."

He gave her a strange look. "And I know just the place," he said. Opening the door to the low-slung car, he attempted to help her in.

"No! Don't help me!" Martina cried out when Rod placed his hand on her back.. "Let me just take my time getting in by myself."

"Jeez! You must have really hurt yourself. Maybe I should take you to the Emergency Room?"

"No!" She said, sounding even more panicky. She knew that if a doctor saw those welts on her body the police would be called in a heartbeat, and she being a minor would be taken away to some facility for abused kids. They might even think Rod was the one who beat her, and Martino would be only too happy to let the police think Rod was responsible.

"Please...just let me get in the car by myself."

"But it's hurting me to watch you," he winced sympathetically.

"Just don't drive too fast," she said between pain-clenched teeth.

Taking her straight to his house, it took another few painful minutes for Martina to extricate herself from the car. This time, she held onto Rod's hands to pull herself out. When she finally stood up in the driveway she looked as though she might pass out. Rod put his arms around her, to keep her from falling, and she let out an ear piercing scream and collapsed in a faint.

Catching her as she went limp, Rod picked her up and started to carry her to the house. Just at that moment, Julie came running out of the apartment, to see what had happened. "Julie!" Rod called up to her. "I need your help. Come open the doors for me."

"What happened?" Julie asked, seeing Martina passed out in Rod's arms and hurrying down the steps.

"She said she fell at school," Rod told Julie, but he was beginning to have his doubts.

Carrying Martina straight up to the bedroom, Rod placed her on the bed. "Help me get her undressed," he said, lifting Martina's hand and attempting to feel her pulse.

"Undressed?" Julie asked, unsure. "You mean like naked?"

"No, Julie. I mean like her skirt and blouse…so I can see where she hurt herself. For her to pass out she must be hurt pretty bad. We have to check her out. Let's unbutton her blouse and when I hold her up you can slip it off." When Rod unbuttoned her blouse he was surprised to see she was wearing a man's white T-shirt underneath, instead of a bra or something more feminine. It struck him as odd, but he didn't have time to waste thinking about it. He immediately turned to Julie, and instructed, "I'll lift her up and you slip off the T-shirt."

The second Julie lifted the bottom of the T-shirt she saw the raw welts on Martina's back. "Ohmygod! Rod!" she exclaimed, horrified.

"What? What is it?" It was difficult for him to see what Julie was freaking out about due to his positioning.

"It looks like she's been beaten with a stick. Ohmygod! We'd better leave the T-shirt on and roll her over, off of her back. The T-shirt is kind of stuck to her in places," said Julie, now getting hysterical.

Rod carefully rolled Martina onto her stomach and then lifted up her T-shirt to see what had Julie so freaked. When he caught a glimpse of the swollen, bloody welts on her lower back, his stomach churned with nausea and a slow burning rage began to fill his senses. But he had no time to be sick or blinded with rage. He needed to focus on taking care of Martina's wounds right away. "Let's get her skirt off. It looks like the welts go all the way down. Jesus! What kind of sick fuck would do a thing like that?" Rod immediately envisioned Martino's smirking face, and his rage boiled over anew. "I'm going to kill that miserable bastard!" He said, trying to put a lid on his rage. If it were not for Martina needing his immediate attention he would have gone straight over to the Fiasconi house and beat up on her father with a stick until he was turned into a bloody pulp. There would be time for that later, Rod told himself.

Fighting back his anger, Rod gently untied the drawstring in the waistband of Martina's skirt, and with Julie's help, they managed to slide it down and off. Then they saw the full extent of her injuries. Rod bit down hard on his lip. "Stay with her, Julie. I'm going to get some water to wash these wounds."

Julie nodded, overwhelmed by the number of bloody welts covering Martina's body. Looking up at Rod, she said, "I should have never left her yesterday. She was so upset."

"Don't blame yourself, Julie. How were you to know he would do such a thing? He must be crazy." Rod patted the crying girl on the shoulder. "If anything...I'm the one who should not have left her with that sonofabitch. I should have dragged her home with me last night. But she begged me to let her have one more night with that—" Choking off the rest of his words, he went to get a washcloth and a bowl of warm water.

Rod called upon the deep breathing and focus techniques he learned in his martial arts training to quell the rage that was pounding in his head. Now was not the time to give vent to his fury. He had to concentrate on taking care of Martina. Right now, that was the most important thing. There would be time later to take care of Martino Fiasconi, and he vowed that Fiasconi would pay for what he did to Martina.

28.

It took nearly two hours for Rod to gently sponge Martina's wounds with warm water and then dab each welt with an antibiotic ointment.

But first, he had to saturate the bloody fabric of the T-shirt with warm water infused with hydrogen peroxide and carefully peel it away from the areas where it was stuck to the broken, congealing skin. Once she calmed herself down and restored her wits, Julie was a big help with carefully peeling away the cotton fabric while Rod concentrated on cutting it with a scissors. It was a painstaking process, and they had to be careful not to poke the welts with the point of the scissors or tear away loose skin. They also had to cut off Martina's underwear, so as not to re-injure the welts on her buttocks and the back of her thighs by trying to pull the tight elastic bandings down over her cuts.

Despite their efforts to be as gentle as possible, Martina cried out in pain several times, which unnerved Rod and Julie. They did their best to comfort Martina as they worked, but there were a few occasions when Rod doubted the wisdom of his decision to not take her to the hospital. If he thought for one minute her injuries were life threatening there would be no question about bringing her to the Emergency Room at Millborough General, but he was pretty sure that once they were able to fully cut away the T-shirt and apply the antibiotic ointment to the broken skin that she would be okay. And it didn't help that Rod had to keep his anger at bay while he reassured his mutilated wife that she was going to be okay.

"I wish Freebird was home," Julie said. "I know he would have some herb that would dull the pain."

"Knowing Freebird he's probably got some miracle cure he could whip up," said Rod, attempting to inject a bit of levity into an otherwise stressful situation. He stood up and walked into the adjoining bathroom.

Julie heard a cabinet door open and shut.

Rod returned to the room with a small plastic pill vial in his hand. "Ordinarily, I'm against the use of prescription pain pills but I think this situation merits at least a half of a Percodan." Opening the container he fished out a pill with his finger. Julie watched as he wiped the blade of the scissors with an alcohol swab and then used the blade like a knife to chop the pill in half. With some effort Martina was able to swallow the half pill by sipping water through a straw.

"That should take the edge off the pain for her," he told Julie. "Let's give it a few minutes to get into her system."

Martina soon fell asleep and Rod resumed dressing her wounds. When he was done, he covered her with a sheet.

"Well..." he said to Julie, "nothing to do now but to let nature take its course and hope she doesn't get an infection." Then he smiled at her and added, "You'd make a great nurse, Julie. I don't know what I would have done without your help...you were fantastic."

Rod could see from the wide-eyed expression on Julie's face that she was still somewhat freaked out from seeing her friend so badly injured. He pulled her into his arms and gave her a heartfelt hug. "You're a cool sister," he told her, "Thank you for helping."

Julie nodded and emitted a deep sigh. "I'm glad I was here to help, Rod." Looking over at her sleeping friend, she said, "Gosh, Rod...I never thought Martino would do such an awful thing like that." Tears filled her eyes.

"He's a coward and an animal," Rod said with a matter of fact tone that belied his absolute hatred for the man.

*	*	*	*	*

Over the next several days, while Martina was bedridden with her stiffness and pain, able only to lie spread-eagled on her stomach, he straw fed her potent broths and pureed foods containing various herbs that Freebird gave to him. Anticipating the difficulty she would have getting out of bed to use the bathroom, he even prevailed upon the wife of one of his biker brothers, who worked at a local hospital, to supply him with a bedpan. But Martina insisted on getting up to use the bathroom. It was painful and cumbersome but with Rod's help, and sometimes Julie's, she was able to do it.

Faithfully, Rod performed the ritual of the sponging and dressing Martina's abrasions with ointment several times a day, refusing to leave her bedside. If she woke during the night with pain, Rod wanted to be certain that he was there to immediately give her medication to relieve any discomfort, so he moved the lounge chair closer to the bed and maintained his sleepless vigil. During the day, Freebird and Julie took turns coming over when they were able, so that Rod could take a shower, go to his office for meetings he could not put off, or run errands. Freebird even took time off work to be of more help. On the fourth morning of his vigil, Rod's efforts were rewarded when he saw the swelling and redness of Martina's cuts were starting to abate. He considered it a miracle that she did not get an infection, but proudly attributed that to the good care she was getting from not only him, but also from Julie and Freebird.

On the afternoon of the fourth day, Freebird appeared with a huge, foul smelling bowl of paste he claimed to have made from mashed aloe plants, ground comfrey leaves, and some other mysterious ingredients he refused to divulge. He told Rod that it was imperative that the paste be put on her wounds as soon as they scabbed over in order to prevent scarring. When Rod attempted to take the bowl of medicinal paste from Freebird, the young man told him that he would need to inspect all of Martina's wounds to make certain they were at the proper stage of healing before the paste could be applied. He said it had something to do with the Comfrey leaves. Rod could see that Freebird was very serious, but the rollicking nature of their friendship would not permit the younger man's request to go unchallenged.

"Yah! Right!" Rod exclaimed with mock suspicion. "You just want to check out my ole lady's sweet little ass."

Freebird looked at Rod with his enigmatic smile, and said, "If that were the case I'd wait until it was healed. But if you want to see it heal up as good as new, I need to look at it now."

"Okay, Bro. But it's going to cost you," Rod kidded, as he carefully lifted the sheet that covered Martina, who was barely awake but could hear the two men talking.

Up until now, Freebird had only seen the beating marks on Martina's back, which were bad enough, but the full view of her injuries shocked and upset him. He set down the bowl of paste on the night table and bent over Martina's body, minutely inspecting each and every welt to make certain there were no open sores, and then he gently draped the sheet over Martina's buttocks until he was ready to work on that area. Sitting on the edge of the bed, Freebird grabbed the bowl and began slathering the awful smelling concoction all over the welts on the young woman's back with a spatula like implement he had carved from a soft wood of some sort. Martina was embarrassed that Freebird should see her in that condition, but the soothing effects of the paste made her soon forget her nakedness.

Closing her eyes, she drifted off into a comfortable sleep, while the young Shaman quietly and efficiently completed his task. When he was finished, he cautioned Rod to leave the paste on for two days, and then hurriedly left the room.

Julie later told Rod, "Poor Freebird...he's really upset to see Martina beaten up like that. He practically cried like a baby."

Rod sighed and said, "I'm still trying to figure out how she made it through a whole day of school in that condition. She should have called me to go over to the school and pick her up."

29.

The pungent odor of Freebird's paste seemed to permeate the entire house, giving Rod pause to wonder how anything so nasty smelling could possibly do any good. But early in the morning, after the second full day of its application, Freebird came over to supervise the removal of the paste. Martina was awake at the time and seemed to be more responsive. Freebird told her it would be best if she stood in the shower, as it would take a lot of warm water to remove the paste. Martina was afraid to move, but Freebird assured her that it was time for her to start walking around and using her muscles. Loosely wrapping her in a sheet, Rod and Freebird helped her out of the bed and down the hall to another bathroom, where there was a tiled shower stall, then Freebird left. Rod took off his clothes and climbed into the shower with her to make certain she did not fall. It was the first time he felt her body up against his in over a week, and although he could not embrace her, he was happy just to see she was able to stand up again. And Martina was amazed at how much better she felt. By the time Rod soaped down the front of her body and helped her shampoo her long hair, Freebird's miracle paste had all but washed away, and Rod was astonished to see how well she had healed. There was actually very little evidence left of the awful beating she had received.

Wrapping her wet hair in a towel and helping her out of he shower, Rod had her stand with her back to a full length mirror on the bathroom door, and then he held up a hand mirror so she could see how beautifully her injuries had healed. She was delighted to see there were no scars on her back, her buttocks, or thighs. There was, she saw, still some residual bruising of various shades and she was still somewhat sore, but now, especially after a wonderful shower with Rod, she felt relatively terrific compared to a few days ago.

"Do you want to try walking around a bit?" Rod asked solicitously.

"Like this" She said, looking down at her nakedness.

Rod thought she looked absolutely beautiful in her natural glory. But with all she had just been through, still being weak and barely able to move, he was not even of a mind to pursue the thought. He was too exhausted and still shaken himself by the ordeal. Instead, he diverted his thoughts to his Mother's Hawaiian muumuus.

"Well…I don't know whether you'll like them or not but I found a couple of my mother's muumuus. You can wear those until we get you something more of your style."

Martina smiled up at him. "I'll be happy to wear your mother's muumuus. I doubt if I'd be comfortable in anything else right now."

With Rod's help, Martina lowered herself gingerly onto he bed to see if she could sit. Her last recollection of sitting was extremely unpleasant. Testing her butt, she happily remarked, "I think I can sit now."

"Good! Because I've gone to your school and picked up your books and Julie has been collecting your class assignments…so while you finish recuperating you can catch up on your schoolwork. There are only a few more weeks of school before your graduation. I've talked with your teachers and Principal Becker and they've all told me that if you catch up on what you've missed and pass your finals you'll graduate with your class." Seeing her scrunch up her face at the mention of schoolwork, Rod smiled and bent down to kiss her on the nose. "And…," he added, "your graduation present is a honeymoon in the Bahamas, where you will meet your new in-laws."

Martina, who had been drying her hair with the towel, looked up at him with an expression of surprise and alarm.

"Meet your parents?" She asked, sounding uncertain about the prospect.

"Yes. And they are looking forward to meeting you. My mother will be so happy to finally have a daughter," Rod said, as he disappeared into the large bedroom closet. Coming out with a pair of jeans for himself and a blue muumuu with splashy white flowers for Martina, he handed her the muumuu.

"Let's see how beautiful you look in this?"

Martina slowly stood up and attempted to put on the shift. Wincing, she said, "It still hurts to raise my arms." Rod took the dress from her and lowered it over her head, helping her get her arms through the short sleeves. "You look fabulous," he told her

"It feels fabulous," she said, happy to be standing upright again.

"There's a bit of sun out on the balcony this time of day," he told her. "How about if I take you out there and see if you can handle getting into a lounge chair?"

"Mmmm. Sitting in the sun would feel good," she said dreamily.

It took a bit of patient engineering but Rod finally got Martina settled onto the soft cushion of a lounge chair and rolled it into the dappled sunlight. "There!" He told her. "Sunshine and fresh air are good for what ails you."

She weakly reached up to touch his face, "I don't know how to thank you for everything you've done, Rod."

Taking her hand and kissing her long, slender fingers, he said, "I am your husband, Martina. I am supposed to take care of you...I want to take care of you." Then, dropping to one knee, his expression grew serious. "I just don't understand why you didn't call me to come and get you from school last Monday? When I think of how you must have suffered all day, it really upsets me. Why didn't you call me, Baby?" His tone was inflected with hurt and frustration.

Martina really did not want to think about the horror of that torturous Monday or the night before when Martino burst into her bedroom and beat her with his belt. It was painful to even think of it. But Rod was her husband and he had just suffered through a terrible nightmare with her. Without his loving care over the past week she might very well be dead. Certainly, she owed him an explanation. But she would not tell him all of the details of Martino's sadistic brutality. She was thankful she had passed out in the middle of his crazed frenzy. There was no sense in inflaming Rod any further; she was already worried that he might go after Martino for revenge. Rod was the one thing in her life that made living worthwhile and she did not want to lose him for any reason, especially not to a prison cell for maiming, or possibly even killing, Martino. Choosing her words carefully, she told him, "I was afraid Martino would hurt you. He told me I could not see you any more and made all kinds of threats."

Rod waited for Martina to tell him the rest of the story but she seemed to retreat within herself. Probably, he thought, she would just like to forget about it. And, really, he didn't want to hear the ugly details anyway. He saw all of the injuries, even the ones that were not as obvious as the ugly welts on her skin.

Rod was sure that Martino had mutilated her to get back at him. So, in a very large and personal sense, Martino had hurt him by hurting the woman he loved. And Rod had already made up his mind that the psycho bastard was going to pay for what he did to Martina. As far as Rod was concerned, the man was a sick and perverted son of a bitch and didn't deserve to live.

Rod continued to hold Martina's hand, gently rubbing it between his palms. "Let's just forget about...him," Rod said, finding Martino's name so distasteful he would not even say it. Looking directly into her eyes, he told her, "There's only you and me and our life together from now on. I hope you realize who you belong with now."

Martina's heart quickened with the tremendous love she felt for this wonderful man who had taken such good care of her. His words were the real balm that healed the awful hurt and anguish she had suffered. From now on, she told herself, her only focus would be on making sure she made Rod happy in every way. He was all that mattered to her now.

She now realized how foolish she had been to be so concerned with Martino's feelings when he obviously didn't care about her. She had seen the pure evil in his eyes when he had crashed through her bedroom door and came at her swinging a belt: it was like looking into the eyes of Satan. She shivered to think that he was actually the man who fathered her. But now, she had finally cut Martino loose; he was no longer her concern and she wanted nothing more to do with him.

"Yes," she agreed with Rod, "I never want to hear his name mentioned again."

If only, Rod thought, it was that simple to obliterate Martino Fiasconi from their lives.

30.

With Martina now on the mend and busy studying for her final exams at school, Rod decided it was now time to deal with Martino Fiasconi. Rod would have no problem snuffing him out like a bug. He wouldn't even have to get his own hands dirty squashing the asshole. Some of his Viking brothers would be happy to do the job. But then Rod had an epiphany. He wanted Martino neutralized in the sense that he wanted the man to suffer for the rest of his days with the misery of never seeing his daughter again. And he wanted Martino to suffer with the knowledge that Martina was alive and well and sleeping in Rod McDonough's bed every night. And he wanted Martino tied up in a nice little legal package.

So, Rod called the attorney who handled all of McDonough Construction Company, Inc.'s corporate affairs, J. Bradford Crenshaw, a former NFL linebacker, and invited him to lunch. Crenshaw was the sort who looked like he'd sooner kick an adversary in the groin than shake their hand, so Rod knew he'd be the perfect man for the job of neutralizing Martino Fiasconi. And when Rod met JB, as Crenshaw liked his friends to call him, for lunch he brought with him the dozen or so Polaroid snaps he had taken of Martina's injuries, when she was out of her mind with pain.

JB shook his head with a combination of disbelief and revulsion as he examined each of the photos. "Her own father actually did this to her?" he said.

"Yes," Rod confirmed, "and then sent her off to school." Rod related the entire story to JB how he had found Martina after school in a state of near collapse and how he and his friends took care of her round the clock.

JB set the photos upside down on the table and picked up his beer mug. He took a long draught and then sat thoughtful for a few seconds. "You say this dude Fiasconi is a professor of philosophy at Wingate?" Again, JB's tone reflected his disbelief.

Rod simply nodded.

JB cleared his throat and looked at Rod with a serious expression. "Well...I don't ordinarily do these kinds of cases anymore, but you are a good buddy and a valuable client so I'll be happy to take it on just for the pleasure of taking that Fiasconi dude out of commission. He shouldn't be allowed to walk the streets much less teach philosophy."

Rod emitted a sigh of relief; he thought for a minute that JB was going to tell him he wouldn't take his case against Fiasconi.

* * * * *

Within a week, Rod and JB were sitting across the table from a very pasty looking Martino Fiasconi and his attorney Vittorio Travante.

JB actually liked Travante, they served on some of the same Bar Association committees and belonged to some of the same social clubs. But JB took an instant dislike to Professor Fiasconi and, for that, Travante would earn his $300.00 per hour.

"So…Vito!" JB said slyly, opening the dialog across the conference table, "I'm encouraged to see you sitting here today.

Your client must be worried if he's retained a heavy hitter such as yourself."

Vito eyed JB suspiciously. He knew JB wasn't one for idle chatter or compliments. There was an ill wind blowing across the table in his direction, and Vito knew it wasn't empty hot air.

Vito was a card sharp and an observer of nuance. He knew that a guy like JB didn't make cocky statements unless he had some sort of an ace in the hole. But Vito was being paid to represent a client, so he responded, "Doctor Fiasconi has no need to be worried. He is an esteemed scholar and a solid citizen of this community."

JB gave Fiasconi a dismissive once-over. JB would have liked nothing more than a good verbal sparring with his old buddy Vito Travante and to drag it out as long as he could just to run up his slime ball client's bill. But that would mean he would have to spend needless time in the same room with the slime ball and that did not appeal to JB in the least. So, he said, "Let me edify you Vito as to how esteemed and solid your client is." JB reached into the inside breast pocket of his suit jacket and fished out the color photo's Rod had taken of Martina's injuries and placed them down on the table in front of Vito as though they were a full house.

The allegedly esteemed professor took one look at the array of photos and his pasty face blanched even whiter. Vito took his time looking at the gut-wrenching photographs of the badly beaten girl. Finally, Vito emitted a heavy sigh, and said, "What is it your client would like from my client?"

"First of all, these injuries were inflicted on my client's wife." JB paused to let his statement soak into the atmosphere and when he saw

Fiasconi's face turn purple and contort with disbelief, he went on with his diatribe. "Mr. McDonough and Ms. Fiasconi were married just two days before Doctor Fiasconi committed these heinous actions upon his daughter on a Sunday night in her bedroom and then sent her off to school on a Monday morning like nothing out of the ordinary happened to her. He had to have seen the injuries he inflicted. My client's wife will testify that Doctor Fiasconi inflicted these merciless injuries and Mr. McDonough will testify that he found his wife wandering outside of her school in the state of near collapse.

"In my opinion, I believe Doctor Fiasconi should be prosecuted for assault, battery, and a host of other serious criminal charges, if not attempted homicide. But my client feels that his wife has been through enough suffering without dragging her through the public spectacle of a notorious trial, as you can imagine this matter would surely turn into, and he merely wants your client to never communicate in any form or fashion with his wife (he paused for effect) ever again."

"I see," Vito commented when JB concluded his statement. "But my client will neither admit verbally to inflicting these injuries, nor will he stipulate in writing to having inflicted the injuries. Furthermore, since we are talking about a father and daughter here, we may want to leave the door open for a future reconciliation."

JB snorted at such a preposterous idea and looked at Rod, to see his reaction to Vito's proposal.

Rod shook his head and said, "Absolutely not. Either he (Rod pointed to Fiasconi) agrees in writing to stay away from my wife or I will press charges against him. I'd like nothing more than to see his ass in jail for what he did—" Feeling his temper surging, Rod abruptly stopped talking. He felt JB pat his arm sympathetically.

Taking up where Rod left off, JB ruminated, "Of course, my client could apply for a restraining order prohibiting Doctor Fiasconi from contacting or going within a hundred feet of Mrs. McDonough, in which case I would have to prepare a motion outlining all of the reasons why such a restraining order is necessary, and then there would be a hearing on the issue. Then all these photos would be entered into evidence…and once the District Attorneys office got involved in the matter things could really heat up for your client. And there is the possibility of the press getting wind of the matter, which could negatively affect the Professor's job and his standing in the community. There's a lot to be considered here."

Vito Travante was nodding attentively now, having caught JB's drift. He knew that his client was boxed in and wished his client realized it also. Unfortunately, his client was determined to press the issue.

Suddenly erupting with anger, Martino Fiasconi yelled, "What is this talk about my daughter being this man's wife? I don't see how my daughter can legally be this man's wife? She is a minor and I am her legal guardian. I did not give my consent for him to marry my daughter."

JB came right back with, "My client has a legally sufficient Certificate of Marriage signed by a bona fide Justice of the Peace in Clanton County. Martina McDonough did not need Professor Fiasconi's permission, and the marriage is quite legal."

"I'd like to see a copy of that Marriage Certificate," said Vito Travante.

Rod was starting to feel threatened by the sudden turn of the conversation. His standing as Martina's legitimate husband was being called into question and now he was getting pissed off.

He wanted to tell Vito Travante and his perverted client to go fuck themselves, but somehow he found the presence of mind to heed JB's advice and keep his cool. Instead, he drilled Fiasconi with an ominous glare and left it up to JB to tell them to go fuck themselves in more polished legalese.

Vito Travante flicked a tiny piece of lint off the sleeve his blue suit jacket while JB concluded his statement detailing his client's right to privacy. Travante was a man who obviously didn't miss too many meals. He wasn't obese, but he could have benefited from the consumption of less pasta and more exercise. With his slicked back, dark wavy hair, he could have easily been mistaken for a Mafioso; he had that heavy-lidded, rough, no-nonsense look about him.

When JB stopped talking, Travante nodded with seeming agreement to JB's proclamation. After a moment of sincere consideration, he said, "Well...then, JB...if your client's marriage certificate is legally sufficient then Mr. McDonough should not mind letting us review it and make that determination of ourselves. After all...my client's daughter is in fact a minor under the law."

Rod jumped up so fast his chair fell over backwards and crashed to the floor. Against his lawyer's advice, he had lost his cool. "This is bullshit! Your so-called client nearly beat his daughter...my wife...to death and then dropped her off at school, bleeding and in such pain she passed out in my arms. She was laid up for over a week and nearly missed her high school graduation. Who the hell is he to make any demands?"

Rod looked like he was about to lunge across the highly-polished conference table and tear off Fiasconi's head and shit in his lungs. Fiasconi's hands were on the arms of his chair and he was positioned to spring from his seat. He eyed Rod McDonough warily. JB stood up and grabbed Rod's arm. "Cool it, Rod! It's no big deal if they want to look at a legal document."

Rod didn't see the production of his Marriage Certificate in quite the same light as JB. In Rod's mind, that was how scavengers, like Travante, worked – they chipped away at their adversaries, one concession at a time, until they had everything they wanted.

"They can kiss my ass!" Rod exploded and stormed from the room.

Travante watched Rod's angry departure with a bemused expression. "That's one hot-headed young man," he remarked to JB.

"Can you blame him, Vito? You saw the photos of what your client did to his wife...so you can hardly expect him to be in a bargaining mood." JB picked up the photographs, his legal pad, and pen and tossed them into his briefcase. "I guess this meeting is over," he said and strode toward the door in pursuit of his client.

31.

It was shaping up to be another bad day. Ever since the meeting with Fiasconi and his greaser attorney two days ago, Rod felt his mood descend into darkness and nothing seemed to be going right ever since. All morning he had been on the phone with sub-contractors and vendors and was hit with one stumbling block after another. After just slamming down the phone in frustration, he looked around his cluttered office at McDonough Construction and wondered how his father had been able to build such a successful business when the industry was so full of morons. Maybe things were easier when his father was getting started, he wondered. But they sure as hell weren't now.

Just as Rod was about to get up and go look for his brother Travis, the intercom line on his telephone buzzed. Sighing with annoyance, Rod picked up the receiver. "Run it, Janis," he said to the receptionist in his usual bikerspeak.

"JB's on the line four for you," Janis informed in her sweet Southern drawl.

A sudden burst of anxiousness rattled his already taut nerves. "Thanks," he said, and pressed the lighted button for line four. "Hey, Bro! What's up?" Rod affected a more upbeat tone in an effort to mask his anxiousness.

"The only thing that's up today, my man, is the sky," JB responded, sounding annoyed.

"I freakin' hear ya!" Rod groaned, now knowing JB's call couldn't be good news either.

"Just wanted to give you a heads up, Rod. Travante's filed some sort of emergency complaint for injunctive relief on behalf of his client. He's asking that Fiasconi's minor child be returned to his custody, and is claiming your marriage is not legal…since Martina is a minor and not old enough to give her consent. I fully expected Travante would do something like that. What the hell…he can bill his client $300 an hour. He knows it's a lost cause but that client of his is pushing the issue."

There was a lot more to Travante's complaint but JB didn't want to go into all of the details with Rod over the phone. After witnessing how easily Rod's temper ignited at the meeting with Travante and Fiasconi two days ago, JB figured he'd better keep his commentary to a minimum. He didn't want to incite Rod to go looking for Fiasconi or Travante, for that matter. But JB had underestimated Rod's flash point.

"Are you shittin' me?" said Rod, becoming incensed.

"Where the hell do they get their balls?"

"Ours are a hell of a lot bigger, my man," JB reassured his fired up client. "I've filed an immediate response in opposition and included as an exhibit a montage of the graphic photos showing the horrendous injuries inflicted on Martina by Fiasconi. When the judge cocks a gander at those photos, Fiasconi will never get custody of Martina."

Rod felt somewhat relieved by JB's words, but he still did not trust the legal system to do the right thing. Certainly, he told himself, any decent judge who saw those photos would likely order Fiasconi to undergo psychiatric testing or, better yet, throw his ass in jail for a long, long time. Thinking out loud, Rod commented, "Good thing I took those photos."

"Indeed," agreed his lawyer, "Those photos will go a long way to dissuade the judge from giving any credence to Travante's complaint."

Hearing that, Rod's relief was short-lived. "What?" He exclaimed with outrage. "You don't mean to say that Travante's complaint has any juice at all?"

"Well...now, Rod. Let's not jump the gun on this. I make it a practice to never predict outcomes...but there is a hearing scheduled this Friday...at three in the afternoon. I'll swing by your office at noon on Friday and take you to lunch. That way I can run down the questions I'll be asking you if I find it necessary to call you to testify. Okay, buddy?"

No, Rod thought, it was not at all okay. When he hung up the phone he felt as though a three hundred pound boa constrictor had coiled itself around his midsection and was squeezing the breath out of him. Staring out his office window at the sunny spring day and his gleaming Harley parked outside, his mood darkened. "I should have killed that asshole," he muttered to himself.

"Killed what asshole?" Someone asked from behind him.

Rod turned, surprised, and saw his brother Travis standing in the doorway. Rod hadn't even heard him walk up. "Just some personal shit about Martina," Rod told his older brother.

"Don't tell me there're comin' after you for robbing the cradle?" Travis joked.

"Not funny, Travis," said Rod, looking grim. "Actually, yeah. Her psycho father is comin' after me."

Travis took a seat opposite his brother's desk and Rod told him about Fiasconi's bid to reclaim Martina through the court. When Rod finished his account several minutes later, Travis let out his breath with a loud whooshing sound.

"Man…that sucks," Travis commented, feeling upset for his brother. Then, breaking into one of his big smiles, Travis assured, "But you've got JB as your first line of defense…so you're in good shape." Underneath his everything's going to be alright countenance, Travis had some serious misgivings about his brother's involvement with Martina, and not just because she was so much younger than Rod. It seemed to Travis that the girl was surrounded by a cloud of constant drama, and he worried that his brother was being pulled into it.

It was understandable to Travis why Rod was drawn to Martina, she was personable, obviously intelligent, and so very beautiful. She reminded Travis of an orchid, beautiful and fragile. He, too, was drawn by her exotic, sea-green eyes, but he had caught glimpses of the troubled currents that lie just below their surface calm.

It was shortly after Rod met Martina that he had brought her to the lake house, the McDonough's summer home where Travis now lived most of the time, and introduced her to his bachelor brother. It had been a beautiful spring day, so Travis took Rod and Martina out in his boat for a ride around the large, pristine lake the house overlooked. The water was still much too cold for swimming, which Travis thought was unfortunate, as he would have liked to see what his brother's new girlfriend looked like in a bathing suit. She certainly did wonders for the jeans and T-shirt she was wearing. As it was, with her long, thick honey-colored hair and her tanned, exotic appearance, Travis thought Martina looked like an elegant Egyptian princess he was ferrying down the Nile River. And from her demure comportment he would have never guessed she was all of seventeen; she seemed to have the presence of an older person. Travis could easily see that Rod was much too elated from his newfound love to see anything other than what he wanted to see. As Travis piloted the boat around the lake, his eyes kept returning to the young woman, so gracefully composed, and wondered how she had acquired the sophistication she exuded.

Now, seeing the strain on his brother's face, Travis's misgivings were fortified, but he wasn't sure what he could do about it. Rod was too committed to Martina to walk away from her at this point. After listening to his brother's faunching and bellowing like a wounded water buffalo for almost twenty minutes, Travis summarily ended the bitch session. "Here's what you need to do…" said Travis, with a no-nonsense tone.

Rod looked up, a hopeful expression on his face. Travis stood up and pointed to the doorway of Rod's office, "You need to get your whining ass outta here right now and go to lunch with me…it's my treat," he said.

"We're going to lunch." Travis informed the receptionist, as the two brothers passed by her desk on their way to the front door.

At first glance, the McDonough brothers looked as though they might have come from different parents. Where Rod was dark haired and brawny, Travis was blonde and wiry, but they shared a similar height and both had the same boyish faces, framed with curly hair. Only fifteen months apart, they were as close as twins and seemed to read each other's minds. Travis, the oldest, had inherited his father's acumen for the construction trade and was really the brains and muscle of McDonough Construction. Travis kept the wheels of the business turning and the machine of its operation humming smoothly. While Rod enjoyed the building supervision side of the business and excelled at finessing the sub-contractors and ground crews, he lacked Travis' patience and became easily frustrated when things did not go according to schedule. Insofar as running the day-to-day operations of McDonough Construction since their father's retirement, the brothers complemented each other fairly well. But it could be said of Rod that he'd rather be riding his Harley, and did so at every opportunity.

32.

Martina wasn't sure what was wrong with Rod. He had come home early from work that Wednesday afternoon, and she thought he seemed restless and distracted. It was the same day that JB had telephoned Rod with the news of Travante's Complaint, but Martina was completely unaware of the legal posturing going on behind the scenes regarding her custody. And Rod did not want to upset her by telling her about it. She wasn't even aware of the meeting Rod had with her father and Vittorio Travante two days ago, on Monday. She had been occupied with studying for her final exams but was not so completely immersed as to not notice Rod ranging around the house, haunting the place like an unhappy ghost.

From her position on the balcony she could see Rod as he wandered in and out of the bedroom, and to and from the garage. He seemed not to want to be anywhere in particular, just always on the move. Finally, around four in the afternoon he came to her on the balcony and announced he would take her out to dinner that night. She noticed there was none of the usual playfulness about him. Looking up at his serious face, Martina asked, "Is there something wrong, Rod?" She was worried that he might now be having regrets about marrying her and taking on her difficulties. Thinking about it made her suddenly feel insecure. Rod picked up on the troubled look in her eyes and lightly brushed her arm with his hand.

"Just the usual craziness at work," he reassured her. "Nothing seemed to go right today." Then, changing the subject, he asked, "How's the studying going? Will you be ready for your tests next week?" He was thinking about getting away to the Bahamas once she was finished with school. Smiling, Martina gave him the thumbs up sign. "I'm as ready as I'll ever be," she said, closing the thick text book she had been reading.

At dinner, Rod tried to make an effort to relax and be more talkative, but his attempts fell far short of his usual banter. Other than to complement his young wife on how pretty she looked in her new emerald green sheath dress he couldn't seem to generate much else to say after that. Martina noticed the lack of conversation as well but said nothing about it.

Later, as they slipped into bed together, Rod took her into his arms and held her close. "I'm sorry I've not been good company tonight, Baby," he told her, sighing deeply. Martina merely cuddled more closely against him and enjoyed the feel of his hand stroking her back, hoping that he would make love to her tonight. "Are you feeling better today?" He asked. It had become his nightly question since he was able to join her in bed again, now that her injuries had pretty much healed.

"I'm feeling lot's better…thanks to you," she answered, nuzzling her face against his warm, muscular chest and inhaling his wonderful masculine scent.

Rod ached to make love to her and awaited some signal from her to let him know it would be okay. And Martina wanted him, too, but she was hesitant to make any overtures given his anxious mood. So, the two eventually fell asleep, unaware of each other's desires.

33.

When Martina was finally able to return to school Rod insisted she drive his Corvette. At first, she rejected the idea out of fear she might cause damage to his prized car. But after he assured her over and over that it was more important to him that she have convenient transportation, she finally agreed. For good measure, Rod took her to a deserted parking lot one afternoon to let her drive around and get used to the feel of the car. Since Martina already had the experience of driving her mother's Jaguar, which was also a stick shift, she did not have much trouble getting used to the Corvette.

As it turned out, it was Thursday, the day before her own custody hearing, that Martina finally returned to school. Thankfully, she had no idea that her father was trying to use the court system to effectuate her return to his control, or she might not have left the safety of her new home with Rod. If anything was gained from the beating she suffered at her father's hands, Martina now understood that her father was an extreme danger to her. Had she known what Martino was up to and what Rod was up against, she would have fully understood her husband's strange mood, and she would have been quite depressed about it herself.

Julie was still half asleep when she lowered herself onto the passenger seat of Rod's Corvette. She dropped her book bag onto the floor between her feet and immediately adjusted the seat to a reclining position. Martina glanced over at her drowsy friend and shook her head as she started the car. Julie looked as though she had just rolled out of bed and threw on whatever rumpled clothes she found lying nearby on the floor, "Did you even brush your hair or teeth this morning?" Martina chided, assessing her friend's haggard, rumpled condition with concern.

"Barely," the girl dreamily responded.

"I think you need to go to bed earlier or something…you look really awful."

"Thanks for the compliment, Martina, but I did go to bed early. The problem is Freebird…he's at me all night long."

"Can't you tell him you need to sleep…I mean…he knows you have to get up early for school."

Starting to come to life, Julie giggled lasciviously and then said, "But I'm just as bad as he is…I want him all the time, too."

The familiar, impish grin on Julie's face made Martina smile in spite of her own niggling anxieties. She wished things between her and Rod in the bedroom were going as well; their sex life was nonexistent at the moment and the closeness they once shared seemed to have dissipated. Ever since Rod brought her home, since the time of her beating, his attitude toward her had changed. Now, whenever she was with him he was distant and so obviously preoccupied that Martina was certain he was having second thoughts about having married her; he hadn't even attempted to touch her intimately in weeks. When Rod did embrace her there was no longer any passion in his body. She didn't know what to think of Rod's confusing behavior. He had so tenderly nursed her while she recovered from Martino's beating and, now, it seemed as though he had erected a barrier between them.

It was all so evident the other night when he took her to dinner, when he appeared to be forcing himself to talk to her or even to smile. It was not in Martina's emotional make-up to live in an atmosphere of uncertainty; she had become nervous and edgy from it. She knew she had to say or do something to get Rod to talk to her about what was going on with him, because she could not stand the present situation between them much longer.

Julie was quick to notice the troubled look on Martina's face and thought perhaps she was nervous about today being her first day back to school. "It'll be okay," Julie said in a comforting tone.

Martina turned and looked at Julie with surprise, wondering if Julie knew what was bothering her. She commented, "I don't know that it will ever be okay again, Julie."

"Don't worry about the other kids, Martina. I spread the word around that you were in a bad automobile accident...and you'll be graduating next week anyway." Julie reached over to touch Martina's arm reassuringly and saw the tears in Martina's eyes.

"It's not school I'm worried about, Julie...it's Rod. I don't think he wants me anymore—" Sobs choked off her words.

Julie gasped. "That's not true," she said, jumping to Rod's defense. "Rod loves you."

Trying to stifle her sobs, Martina's words were heavy with sadness when she responded, "Then why doesn't he touch me anymore?"

"Gosh, Martina! Maybe he's afraid he'll hurt you...you did have some serious injuries," Julie reminded, as she rubbed Martina's shoulder. Then she added, "You've got to give him time to get his head back to normal...he was really spazzed out about what happened to you."

What Julie said did make some sense to Martina but it did not explain Rod's distant, distracted behavior. Wiping the tears off her face with her hands, she remarked, "I can understand he was *spazzed*, but ever since then he's been like in another world. He hardly talks to me...he doesn't laugh anymore...it's not like it was before between us. There's no passion anymore."

Martina could see that Julie was seriously considering what she had told her and was searching her mind for a satisfactory answer. After a few moments, Julie responded, "I know Rod loves you...I've heard him tell Freebird over and over." Then she gave Martina a sly, wicked smile and suggested, "Maybe what you need to do is stoke his fire a little bit."

"What do you mean?" asked Martina, who was halfway curious but looking at Julie with mild trepidation. She knew all too well about the wild side of Julie's nature.

"Oh...I'm thinking about you in a sexy red dress and a candlelight dinner...and some wine and music. That might be just the thing to kick start Rod."

For the first time in over a week Martina felt a sense of lightness replace the dull ache in her heart. Perhaps Julie was right. What Rod needed was for her to remind him she was his wife and lover, not his patient. She reached across the console separating the front seats and hugged her friend. "That's a great idea, Julie. We'll go the mall after school and look for just the right dress."

Infused with a new hope, Martina eased in the clutch, put the car in first gear, and started slowly down the winding driveway toward their school.

* * * * *

Martina took great pains to make sure the dinner was perfectly timed with Rod's arrival home. He had called her a few minutes earlier, around five o'clock, and said he would be home in an hour. Luckily, she had plenty of experience planning and cooking meals; after her mother died she had taken on the added role of Martino's personal chef. Now, she was thankful for that experience, as she looked around the stone kitchen to make sure everything was in order. The breakfast room table had been set for two, using Rod's mother's best China and an

Irish linen table cloth with matching napkins. She had even decorated the table with two ornate candlesticks and a small vase of fresh cut flowers. Martina had to admit that the table setting looked very romantic. Before going up to the bedroom to shower and dress, she put the Chianti on the table and double checked the scalloped potatoes, which were baking in the oven and the tossed salad that was chilling in the refrigerator. For dessert, she had stopped by Rod's favorite bakery and picked up a cherry cheesecake. Now, all that had to be done to complete the meal was to broil the thick cut sirloin steaks she had taken out of the freezer to thaw when she first got home. After she had assured herself that everything was in order, she ran upstairs to take a quick shower.

The red thong was the perfect accessory to wear under her new fitted red crepe dress that Julie picked out and insisted she buy for the occasion. Ordinarily, Martina would not have chosen such a revealing dress—it had a plunging neckline that was probably not street legal, but Julie whined and carried on until Martina had to buy it just to shut her up. But, now, as Martina examined the way the dress looked on her in the full length mirror, she was glad Julie forced her to buy it. The crepe material clung to her body like a second skin. Studying her image in the mirror, both front and back, she noted the way the clingy material accented the rounded curves of her hips and *derriere*. The final touches were a pair of dangling, red beaded earrings and backless red sandals with low heels. Confident that her dress would have the desired effect on Rod, Martina gave her long hair a final brushing, and then ran downstairs to check on the potatoes once again. With everything in the kitchen under control, she went into the living room to turn the music on low and take up her calculated position on the sofa to await Rod's arrival.

It was almost six o'clock on the dot when Martina heard the engine of Rod's Harley tearing up the hill on Scenic Drive. She felt her heart begin to pound with excitement, knowing that he would be coming through the back door in just a few moments. Unable to sit any longer, Martina stood up and walked to the center of the dimly lit living room. Her stance was both tentative and defiant. She was determined to get her lover back, although a sliver of her consciousness feared he might possibly reject her overtures.

34.

Coasting into the garage with the engine off, Rod braked the bike, kicked out the stand with the toe of his boot, and leaned the machine over onto it. He continued to sit on the bike for a few moments, thinking about the absurdity of his life at the moment. Tomorrow he would have to appear in court for what, essentially, would be a custody hearing to determine if he had the right to be married to his wife. And to think that this custody hearing was called up by none other than his wife's father, the same person who had beat her nearly senseless and did God only knows what else to her. If the court wanted to protect Martina from a harmful situation, the judge should ensure that her father was not ever again allowed to have any contact with her. Yet, it was conceivable the judge might rule Rod had taken advantage of her youth and enticed her to marry him without first obtaining her father's permission.

As much as Rod hated to admit it to himself, he was scared about which way the judge would rule. And just a few hours ago, when he met with JB, for the second time, to discuss his testimony at the hearing JB could offer no assurance of any kind as to how it would all play out. Ever since Wednesday, when Rod first found out about the hearing, he had been stewing and worrying. Now, on the eve of the hearing, with no words of encouragement from JB, Rod was really starting to freak out. What if the judge ruled his marriage to Martina was invalid? At just the thought of it, Rod broke into a cold sweat.

He knew he had to get a grip on himself and come off cool and sensible at tomorrow's hearing. Rod also knew that he had better start paying some attention to Martina; he had been so preoccupied since that meeting with her father and his attorney last Monday there was no telling what she might be thinking about what was going on with him. Maybe when this custody nonsense was over with he would tell her all about it but, for now, he didn't want to trouble her with it. Even though it was Rod's sole intention to spare Martina from unnecessary worrying by not telling her of her father's legal maneuvering to get her back, it was a decision borne of ignorance and one that would eventually backfire on him.

As Rod swung his leg over the saddle of his bike he noticed Martina's discarded bra hanging from the nail on the garage wall, where he had hung it the day after their wedding. It seemed like many months had passed since Martina had playfully dropped her bra over the side of the balcony but, actually, it had only been a few weeks. The sudden realization of how intense the interaction between him and Martina had become in such a brief space of time hit him hard. It then occurred to Rod that Martino Fiasconi had succeeded in surreptitiously inserting himself into their marriage. Bristling at the thought, Rod headed for the back door, vowing to reclaim his marriage and his wife from the insidious intrusion of that rotten son of a bitch.

The aroma of food cooking was a pleasant greeting when Rod stepped into the back porch. Entering the kitchen he noticed the table had been set for an intended romantic dinner for two, complete with cut flowers and his grandmother's favorite candlesticks. Stopping in front of the wall oven, Rod peered through the glass window and saw scalloped potatoes bubbling in a Pyrex casserole dish. Smiling to himself, because he had once told Martina that scalloped potatoes were his all-time favorite side dish and she had remembered, he continued on toward the arched stone entrance to the living room. Just inside the doorway to the living room, Rod stopped abruptly.

The jaw-dropping sight of Martina standing in the middle of the living room, wearing an incredibly sexy red mini-dress brought him to a complete standstill. Her transformation from a pretty schoolgirl to an exotic beauty caught him by complete surprise. He couldn't help but notice how the low cut dress revealed the tanned mounds of her breasts, barely concealing her nipples, and the way its shimmering crepe material hugged her tiny waist and accented the curve of her narrow hips, making her appear more fragile to him. Rod knew why she was wearing such an eye-popping dress and he felt ashamed of himself. That his wife of barely a month should have to even think about putting on a provocative dress to get his attention spoke poorly of him as a husband and a man. And so, instead of being fully turned on by the sight of Martina in the sexy dress, he was overcome with a mixture of remorse and guilt that she should have to sell herself to him, because he had been a neglectful lover.

Despite the elegance of her lithe body in the shimmering red dress and the appeal of her long, shapely legs, Rod was more captivated by her sea green eyes, in which he saw a turbulent undercurrent of hurt, worry, and defiance. He was reminded of the defiant look she had flashed at him that day he first saw her in the alley in North Hampton. It was that look of defiance that caught his interest then and stirred him now.

Continuing to keep his eyes locked onto hers, Rod crossed the room and pulled Martina into his arms, squeezing her tightly against his body.

"I'm so sorry, Baby," he apologized, stroking her silky hair.

"What are you sorry for?" Martina asked, truly perplexed by his reaction. Then she felt his body tremble as he released a deep sigh.

"I'm sorry that I've not been a better husband to you."

Martina said nothing and continued to hold him, enjoying the feel of his body against hers after such a long lapse in their intimacy. She supposed the red dress did have the desired effect, although, while getting dressed, she had entertained visions of him tearing it off of her and making love to her on the living room floor. But, now, as he held her tightly in his arms, she was ecstatic with his simple apology. It was enough that he had received her message.

Oddly enough, however, it was the oven and not the red dress that orchestrated the next move. Suddenly aware of the baking potatoes, Martina panicked. "I'd better go check the potatoes...I don't want our first home cooked dinner together to be burned," she said.

Rod released his hold on her just enough to place an unhurried, tender kiss on her lips. When he broke away, he said, "You look very beautiful tonight...but you always look beautiful to me." He gave her a long, sincere look. Then he added, "I'd better go shower and get ready for dinner. But before I go upstairs, do you need my help with anything?"

Martina smiled up at him. "No. Everything is under control. Go take your shower and by the time you are done, dinner will be on the table."

Rod took her hands in his and brushed kisses across her fingers, all the while staring at her with great feeling, and then told her, "I hope you know how much I love you, Martina. I know that lately I've not been very attentive and haven't been in the best of moods...but it's not because I don't care about you."

Martina looked up into his eyes and saw he was speaking directly from his heart. His words were just what she needed to hear to dispel the heaviness that had been accumulating in her own heart from thinking he no longer cared for her. She smiled up at him, relieved, and affirmed, "I love you, too, Rod...and I always will."

Rod lowered his head and gently rested his forehead against hers. It should have been a tender moment between them, but thoughts of tomorrow's hearing plagued him, resulting in a chilling effect on his sexual energies. This, too, worried Rod and exacerbated the problem.

Ever tuned in to Rod's body language, it did not escape Martina's notice that in this intimate moment between them, he showed none of his former passion or eagerness to make love. And for Rod to take a shower and not even attempt to coax her into joining him seemed unusual to Martina as well. She instinctively knew that something was on his mind, continuing to distract him, and she intended to find out what it was. But in the back of her mind she felt certain that whatever was troubling Rod must have something to do with Martino, and when the time was right she would talk to Rod about it.

35.

The steaks were sizzling in the broiler when Rod playfully strolled into the kitchen, fresh from his shower. He was wearing his black dress pants and a long sleeved red silk shirt, unbuttoned just enough to allow a glimpse his hairy, muscular chest. His hair, still damp, was starting to pull up into loose curls.

"You look like a sexy gypsy," Martina said, liking that he matched the color of his shirt with her dress.

"I don't look as sexy in red silk as you do." He proclaimed, affecting a dry expression. "But that's okay with me," he crooned and encircled her waist with his arms. "There's only room in this house for one sexpot and I'd just as soon that you do the honors."

"You're too kind, Mister McDonough."

Gesturing toward the oven, Rod asked, "What've you got sizzling in there?"

Martina brandished her long handled barbecue fork, warning him away from the oven. "It's a surprise for you, Rod, so don't try to peak in there."

"Well, I want to do something to help you...what can I do?"

"You can open the wine," she told him, pointing with the fork to the bottle on the table, as she stood guard at the oven.

Rod looked over at the table and saw that the long, tapered candles had been lit. "The table looks very nice," he complimented her, as he walked over to the table to open the wine. Teasing her, he asked, "Are you old enough to drink?"

"I am tonight," she quickly responded, as she turned the steaks over for a few minutes more of broiling. Behind her, Martina heard Rod's lecherous laugh and turned to look him.

She noticed that he was barefoot and smiled at his silliness, and how she had missed that playfulness about him in the last few weeks. "Okay, Rod!" She called out. "I want you to sit down and close your eyes."

"Where do you want me to sit?"

"In a chair...pick anyone. Just sit!"

One by one, she brought the crystal bowl containing the salad, the casserole dish of scalloped potatoes, and the platter of steaks to the table, setting them around Rod's plate.

"Okay... now you can open your eyes," she said, proudly surveying the food she prepared for him.

Opening his eyes, Rod felt a wave of complete happiness. He jumped up from his chair and pulled her into his arms. "You are quite the cook," he complimented her between kisses. "Everything looks so wonderful. Thank you, Baby." It was the first meal that any woman, aside from his mother, had ever cooked for him. So, he was truly pleased with her efforts, and Martina was warmed by his effusive response. He ushered her to her chair and held the chair while she seated herself. After adjusting her chair, he poured them each a small glass of wine, and raising his glass, he said, "To my beautiful wife and the wonderful dinner she has cooked. I hope we have many good meals together as husband and wife." Tapping their wine glasses together, they each took a sip of the mellow Chianti.

Beaming happily, Martina watched Rod eat the last of the scalloped potatoes. He had already eaten the two steaks she broiled for him, a huge helping of salad, and several pieces of French bread. When Rod finished the potatoes he sat back in his chair and sighed contentedly. "And I thought my Mother was the only one who could cook like that," he commented, giving Martina an appreciative look. "That was fantastic, Baby."

Martina felt a swell of pride. The best compliment he could have given her was the way he gobbled everything up. Then she remembered the cheesecake. "I hope you saved room for dessert?" She asked.

"Dessert! There's always room for the kind of dessert I have in mind." Saying that, Rod stood up and casually walked over to her. Before Martina realized what he was going to do, he had slid her chair away from the table, scooped her up in his arms, and threw her over his shoulder.

"Rod! Put me down!" Martina squealed unconvincingly, as he carried her out of the kitchen.

Once upstairs, Rod's playful mood escalated. After weeks of captivity, his wild and silly persona needed to be released. Enough with the intense bullshit, he told himself. Lowering Martina gently onto the bed, he then went into his best imitation of a male stripper. Slowly, slowly unbuttoning his red silk shirt, giving Martina little peeks at his amazing chest. A flash of one nipple, the other, and then holding the front tails of the shirt away from his body to bare it all—his brawny pecs and taut abs. The audience was small but obviously enthusiastic: Martina smiled and eyed all of his movements appreciatively as her private dancer slowly, sensually swayed his hips, turning by degrees and letting the silky fabric of the shirt slide down his back and onto the floor. Hips still gyrating to some jungle-drum rhythm that played in his head, he turned to face Martina, who was by now ready to leap from the bed and speed up the process but didn't want to spoil the tantalizing fun. Now, it was time for the big reveal. His fingertips toyed with the tab of his zipper, pulling it down just enough to peak her interest, then slowly back up. The ziptease, as Martina called Rod's finale, was her favorite part of his private dance. Things started happening between them when he got down to the zipper. Excitement was building. He slid it down further and further until there he was in all his maleness and ready to rock and roll.

Martina gasped, surprised. "That's cheating," she said with a seductive giggle. "You're not wearing any underwear."

Tossing his head to one side, he affected a heavy-lidded expression and Bogart-like tone. "You're not the only one who can dress for success around here, Baby."

Hours later, after they had exhausted every ounce of their pent-up desires and energies and Martina had fallen into a deep, contented sleep, Rod continued to hold her close and stroke her back, which was now completely healed and bore only one tiny scar to mark the incident of her beating. Although no one would have even noticed the small linear mark under her left shoulder blade, every time Rod's fingertips passed over it he was reminded of his unfinished business with Martino Fiasconi.

And now, lying next to his sleeping wife, feeling the softness of her body nestled against his side, it burned him that thoughts of her father should invade their most private space and time.

Tomorrow's hearing would be upon him soon enough, when he would have to once again be in the same room with the evil bastard. Clutching Martina more tightly to his side, Rod tried to wipe from his mind the ominous feelings that assailed him and kept him from falling asleep. But he couldn't help but wonder if tonight would be the last night for a long time that he would be able to hold her in his arms. It was a difficult balancing act to keep thinking positively while preparing himself for the worst. There would be no sleep for Rod tonight.

36.

JB could see that Rod was nervous and uneasy as they took their seats at one of the two counsel tables positioned before Judge Reginald Gridley's dais. Earlier, at lunch, JB had hammered on his testy client about the importance of not showing any anger in the courtroom. "Look interested, but don't let your emotions rule your brain." JB could only hope that Rod would control his temper and not piss off the Judge. Reminding Rod, "When I tell you that Judge Gridley doesn't stand for any bullshit in his courtroom, I kid you not."

Looking around the dark paneled room, with its ornately framed paintings of stern-faced jurists he did not recognize, Rod was glad that Fiasconi and his lawyer had not yet come into the courtroom. They were at the moment, he knew, huddled out in the hallway, talking in hushed tones, and doubtlessly plotting their conspiracy to take Martina away from him. Closing his eyes and taking a deep breath, Rod called upon his martial arts training to focus and steel his nerves.

JB clicked open his briefcase and took out a sturdy, dark brown file folder and a legal pad and placed them on the table before him. Rod looked at the multi-indexed file folder, with its typed label identifying it as "***McDonough Advs. Fiasconi***", and shuddered. The legal folder seemed to emphasize the serious nature of the adversarial proceeding that would take place in less than fifteen minutes. Rod's stomach churned as he watched JB flip through several pages of his legal pad, on which he had written copious notes.

When Attorney Travante did finally enter the courtroom, with an ashen and grimfaced Martino Fiasconi trailing behind, Rod glowered at the two opponents and subconsciously clenched his fists. Suddenly, the Bailiff announced that court was in session and Rod caught his first glimpse of Judge Gridley, who entered the room through a door behind the dais.

The lawyers and their clients jumped to their feet while the Honorable Reginald Gridley settled himself in his seat at the elevated bench. Even discounting his elevated position in the courtroom and the black robe, the Judge was an imposing man. He had a shock of white hair and deep set dark penetrating eyes that first raked over Martino Fiasconi and then studied Rod. It was an easy assumption, without being forewarned by one's attorney, that Judge Gridley did not brook any nonsense from anyone in his courtroom, attorneys and clients alike, and stuck to a rigid procedure.

Since Attorney Travante was the motioning party, he presented the facts of his client's Motion for Injunctive Relief to the Judge first. The Judge merely sat back in his oversized chair and stared, thoughtfully at the ceiling while Travante explained why his client was demanding the return of his minor daughter to his custody.

When it was JB's turn to present his rebuttal arguments to the Judge he started by referring to the photographs of Martina's beating injuries, which had already been placed into evidence when he filed his Response to Travante's Complaint.

Travante attempted to object to the photographs, citing their lack of validity, time taken, and authenticity, but he was soundly overruled. The Judge indicated that he had already spent considerable time reviewing each photograph prior to the hearing and he would make certain their validity was determined, stating for the record, "I would certainly not expect Attorney Crenshaw to file false or misleading evidence with the court."

"Your Honor," JB began, "My client is lawfully married to Martina Fiasconi, now known as Martina McDonough. He has just spent weeks nursing her through those horrendous injuries you saw in those photographs. My client loves Martina and has pledged to take care of her for the rest of her life. She is happy and thriving with my client and has no desire to return to the home of Martino Fiasconi. Although she is seventeen years old, Your Honor, she has been raised in a very liberal, if not Bohemian atmosphere, where she was not even allowed to call her parents "Mom" or "Dad," but encouraged to use their first names. And she is not your average seventeen year old girl, Your Honor. She is a very mature, self-sufficient young woman and is currently preparing to take her college entrance exams. To return Martina to the custody of (JB turned and gestured with great distaste toward Martino Fiasconi) … this man…would not only be injurious to her well being but would disrupt a very compatible and happy marriage—"

Judge Gridley raised his hands in a silencing gesture. He had heard enough. JB ceased talking immediately.

"I've thoroughly read the pleadings submitted by both parties to this action and I have reviewed the evidence introduced…I'm going to order that since Ms. Fiasconi…uh…McDonough is still a minor in the eyes of the law (saying that, the Judge inclined his head toward Rod) I am going to appoint a Guardian *ad Litem* to protect her interests while this matter is pending before the court, and that she be interviewed and evaluated by her Guardian within the next week. Further, I am going to request that Home Study Evaluations be conducted by the Department of Family Services on both Mr. McDonough and Mr. Fiasconi, and until I receive the reports from both the Guardian and Family Services, I am going to order that this minor be made a ward of this court for the term of the case. But since the minor is only a week away from graduating high school, in order to avoid any disruption to her school studies and final tests, which I understand are scheduled for Friday, June thirteenth, I am going to allow her to remain in the home of Mr. McDonough until after her school tests are completed.

However, on the Monday following the minor's final exams…that would be on June sixteenth…I am ordering that Ms. McDonough shall be moved to a protective residence, where she will stay until after I have had the full opportunity to review the reports of the Guardian and Family Services and make my final ruling."

Then, specifically addressing Rod, Judge Gridley advised, "Mr. McDonough, just so there will not be any question about it, you are to bring Ms. McDonough to the office of her Guardian *ad Litem*, on Monday, June sixteenth, at or before two o'clock in the afternoon. Make sure she brings enough clothing and personal effects to last her three or four weeks." Seeing the shocked expression on Rod's face, the Judge added, "I am being very lenient with you concerning this matter and I hope you realize that. Normally, I would have arranged to have her picked up this afternoon." The Judge stared at Rod, who found himself nodding in agreement, although he was not at all in agreement with Judge Gridley's ruling.

Continuing with his ruling, Judge Gridley then looked at JB and said, "I have appointed Attorney Dalena Linton as Ms. McDonough's Guardian. I want your client to make certain he delivers Ms. McDonough to Ms. Linton's office on June sixteenth, on or before two in the afternoon, no ifs, ands, or buts. Understand?"

JB nodded affirmatively to Judge Gridley, as he made some quick notes of the Judge's ruling. "One thing, Your Honor," JB interjected when the Judge had paused, "will my client be allowed visitation with his wife during the period of time she is separated from him?"

Leaning back heavily in his chair and staring up at the ceiling, Judge Gridley knitted his brows and pursed his lips, as he pondered JB's question for a few moments. "What are we talking about here, Mr. Crenshaw?" asked the Judge, who was still looking up at the ceiling as he spoke. "Do you mean like taking her to lunch or dinner or spending the entire day together?"

JB saw his opening in the Judge's broad question. "Well...both, Your Honor. Ms. McDonough will be out of school for the summer after her final exams on June thirteenth...they had a lot of things planned for the next couple of months...including a trip to the Bahamas to visit with Mr. McDonough's parents, who live there most of the year."

Judge Gridley nodded soberly, considering the implications of JB's statement. After a few moments he looked down, first at JB and then at Rod. "I am going to allow Mr. McDonough three visitations per week, starting at ten o'clock in the morning and ending at nine o'clock at night. He may choose which days of the week he wants to schedule his visitations, but the time is not negotiable. He must coordinate his visitations with the administrator of the residence where Ms. McDonough will be staying...so the schedule over there will not be disrupted. But I will not allow Ms. McDonough to be taken out of the country while she is under the jurisdiction of this court...and I'm telling your client right now that if I hear of any abuse of his visitation privileges (the Judge paused to wag a finger of caution) I will immediately rescind his right to visitation. Is that clear?"

JB and Rod nodded in unison.

Then Judge Gridley turned his attention to Vito Travante. "Mr. Travante...my ruling here this afternoon should not be construed in any way to be prejudicial to your client's interests in the minor. My only objective is to protect the rights of his daughter, whom Mr. McDonough also alleges is his wife. I have to be mindful of the fact that she is both a minor and a wife. So, at this time, I am not going to order any visitation for your client...especially in view of the evidence submitted. Once all of the reports are submitted for my review you may submit a motion for visitation but, as of this moment, your client is not to have any contact...and I do mean none whatsoever (the judge emphasized the words "none whatsoever" with a stern voice, raised eyebrows, and a wagging finger) with Ms. McDonough."

Although Vito Travante obediently nodded his understanding to the Judge, he was visibly perturbed. Even more so perturbed was his client, Martino Fiasconi, who had assumed the Judge would forthwith return Martina to his custody. Nor did he like the way the Judge kept referring to Martina as "Ms. McDonough."

Everyone stood while Judge Gridley exited the courtroom.

Travante hastily gathered up his files, muttered a few words to Fiasconi, and both men rushed from the courtroom.

JB looked at Rod and gave him a beaming smile. "I do believe the Judge is in your corner," he announced to Rod.

Unfamiliar with courtroom procedure and legal nuances, Rod only comprehended that Martina was to be taken away from him. He was stunned. "I have to take my wife to live with strangers?" He asked, incredulous.

"Rod! The Judge gave you a very favorable ruling. He could have demanded you turn her over this afternoon. He really cut you some slack," JB assured. "Trust me, Rod. I know Gridley and he really gave you serious deference. I'm surprised he granted you visitation. I'm sure those photos had a big influence on him."

JB's words did nothing to assuage Rod. He was bereft and didn't know how he would ever be able to tell Martina about any of it. "Oh, Jesus! What am I going to do. Martina is going to freak out."

"She doesn't know about any of this?" JB asked, incredulous.

"No. I haven't told her anything. I didn't want to worry her."

"Do you want me to have a talk with her?" JB offered.

Rod looked at him with a wary expression. "I think I should talk to her first," he said, sounding defeated. Standing up, he added, "I'll call you if I run into a problem."

JB shook his head and put the file and legal pad in his brief case. "I know you don't believe it, Rod, but we did very well."

Rod didn't believe it and felt as though he had just gotten a swift kick in the ass. But, he thought, there was no point in belaboring it. He just wanted to go home and spend what little time he had left with his so-called alleged wife.

"Thanks, JB," Rod said, shaking his lawyer's hand and trying to sound upbeat. "I'm sure it'll all iron out once the investigation is done. If not, Martina will be turning eighteen in a few months and then her father will have no legal standing to control her life anymore."

"When's her birthday?" JB asked, interested from a legal perspective.

"In October," answered Rod.

"I'll note that on my office calendar. If this case is still ongoing at that time I'll file a motion for termination based on her reaching her majority." Snapping his briefcase shut, JB looked at Rod with a serious expression, and said, "I know you think this case is a lot of bullshit but I can assure you that it is not...especially as far as Judge Gridley is concerned. My best advice to you at this time is to play the game, stick to the terms of the Judge's Order, and you'll come out smelling like a rose. I know you're not happy about Martina being made a ward of the court but the Judge had no alternative in order to keep her father away from her. It all works to your benefit in the end."

The two men walked out of the courthouse together, going their separate ways on the sidewalk in front of the granite structure. Rod crossed the street to the private parking lot where he had parked his bike. Maybe JB is right about the Judge being on his side, Rod told himself, at least that asshole father of hers can't get near her.

Arriving home about twenty minutes later, Rod found Martina at the sink in the kitchen, getting ready to peel several potatoes. She was wearing a bright pink tank top with the tiniest denim mini skirt he had ever seen. The skirt barely covered her buttocks and show-cased her fabulous tanned legs.

She looked over at Rod and flashed him a wide smile.

"You're home early tonight," Martina said, happy to see him. She had been thinking about him all day and their incredible lovemaking the night before. She put the peeler down on the counter and turned to face him, her entire body vibrating with the love she felt for him.

Wasting no time, Rod went over to her and removed her pink tank top. Studying for a moment the magnificence of her caramel breasts, with their dark ruby tips, he then took them in his hands and began gently massaging the pliant mounds. The erotic effect on Martina was instant; she closed her eyes and emitted a low moan. The soft, fullness of her lips caught Rod's attention and he had a sudden desire to taste them. Pressing his lips to hers, his tongue probed the sweet moistness of her mouth, all the while his hands continued kneading her breasts. Before long, the two were hot and sweaty from their excitement for each other.

Reluctantly, Rod withdrew his lips from hers and whispered in her ear, "Let's take all this passion upstairs and play around in the bathtub." Martina smiled up at him, knowing how much he loved to play with her in a tub full of warm, bubbly water. Sometimes they would just soak and talk. Other times, it was a prelude to their later lovemaking. Tonight, she thought, was probably going to be a prelude night, since he was already tearing her clothes off. Nodding her assent to his proposition, he took her by the hand and led her upstairs to the bathroom.

37.

Martina awoke early the next morning, Saturday, contented to simply lie next to Rod and wait for him to wake up. They had fallen asleep in the early morning hours, satiated and entwined, and one of Rod's arms was still stretched across her body. She thought about how lucky she was to have met such a wonderfully considerate, loving man, who was both strong and masculine, yet so delightfully playful at times. Tears of emotion welled in her eyes and spilled down the sides of her face. She wiped them away with her hands but more fell in their place. Feeling her movement, Rod opened his eyes. Ever since the morning she had disappeared from his bed, on the weekend of their marriage, he always tried to keep one of his arms or legs in contact with her body, as sort of an alarm system to monitor her movement. Seeing her wiping the tears from her eyes he raised himself up on an elbow, and placed the palm of his free hand on the side of her face in a comforting gesture.

"What's wrong, Baby?" He asked, concerned that she was upset about something. When he saw her smile he was relieved.

"I'm just happy, Rod…happier than I've ever been in my life. You are so wonderful to me," she told him, her voice was barely above a whisper and quavered with emotion. Rod leaned over and kissed her lips, overwhelmed by her sensual beauty. "Why would I not be wonderful to you? You are my wife and I love you," he said.

Martina wrapped her arms around his neck and pulled him close against her body. "I love you, Rod, and I love being your wife."

The way the tears in her sea green eyes sparkled when they caught the early morning light at just the right angle made her appear more mystical to Rod. Her long, dark hair was pulled to one side and clipped at the nape of her neck, where its thickness covered her shoulder and breast. Rod brushed the hair aside so he could suck and tongue her ruby nipple. Martina gasped from the sheer pleasure of his touch, encouraging Rod to continue with seductive movements of her body, but his desire for her had already passed the point of self control, so he needed little encouragement. Rod was keenly aware that she wanted him to make love to her. Breakfast would have to wait until they first had their fill of each other's passion.

Martina had on one of Rod's long tailed Chambray shirts when she joined him in the kitchen later that morning. She snuggled up behind him, wrapping her arms around his waist, while he monitored the pancakes he was cooking for their late breakfast. There were also bacon and eggs sizzling slowly in their frying pans on the other burners.

"These are about done," Rod said, motioning to the thick, golden brown pancakes with a spatula. With his free hand he rubbed the soft skin of her hands, which were clasped at his stomach.

"Smells so good...and I'm starving," she said dreamily, still under the spell of his lovemaking.

"Then let me loose, so I can get the plates and then we can eat," he said, laughing and trying to break out of her hold.

"I'll get them," she yawned, padding barefoot across the floor to the cabinet, where the dishes were kept.

As they ate breakfast, Rod asked, "What would you like to do today? Anything special?"

Martina glanced out the window and appraised the overcast sky. "It looks like it might rain. How about if we just hang out here and listen to music...it's been a while since we've been able to do that."

"Whatever you want, Baby," said Rod, trying to sound casual. "Hangin' out here sounds fine to me."

He thought about how he would soon have to tell his unsuspecting young wife about her father's attempt to wrest her away and Judge Gridley's ruling. Rod didn't look forward to admitting he had been withholding from her the legal jousting which, of course, seriously impacted her life. He hoped she would not be angry with him, for it had been no great joy for him to carry the weight of it all on his shoulders. In some respects, it would be a relief to finally be able to share the burden. He feared what her reaction would be when he told her she would have to go live at a juvenile residential facility until the case was resolved. Just thinking about it made his stomach sour. And his time was running out. He couldn't very well spring it on her an hour before he had to turn her over to that Guardian *ad litem* the judge had appointed.

"**Rod!**" Martina said loudly to get his attention. "I've been talking to you and you haven't heard a thing I've said."

Snapping back into the moment, he reached over and stroked her arm apologetically. "I'm sorry, Babe...I was thinking about one of our construction jobs," he lied. "What did you say?"

"I said...maybe we could ask Julie and Freebird to come over for dinner tonight."

At first, Rod thought of flat out nixing that idea, but then he saw it as an easy out to his dilemma. Freebird and Julie were their closest friends; actually, the couple was like family to them. Especially after all of their help when Martina was recovering from her injuries. If it were not for Freebird's secret concoction of herbs, nasty smelling as it was, there was no telling how scarred Martina would have been left. And with Freebird and Julie there when he broke the news to Martina about the court case, they would be able to help him calm her down. Suddenly, a smile came over his face, and he responded, "Great idea, Babe. I'll get some steaks out of the freezer. I'll run over there now and catch them before they go out."

Martina jumped up and started clearing the breakfast dishes from the table. "While you do that, I'll clean up the kitchen." Looking up at Rod, she exclaimed, "This will be our first dinner party as a couple, so it will be very special. Can we use the dining room and your Mom's good China?"

It was good to see her so happy and excited, but Rod hadn't given any thought to the special aspect of the dinner. Only a woman would attach a higher significance to something as mundane as friends coming over to eat. How could he possibly say anything to her now and ruin their first dinner party. With his plan of using Freebird and Julie as a buffer no longer feasible, Rod was back to putting up a front until he could find the proper time to approach her. So, for the moment, Rod joined in her excitement. "Of course we can use the dining room...and the china, the gold plated flatware, the Irish linen tablecloth, and anything else that's in there," he told her, "that's what it's there for."

"Oh, Rod! Thank you. The table is going to look so beautiful tonight."

Rod looked at Martina with great pride. It wasn't just her exotic beauty that bowled him over. She had such an unexpected creative, homey nature that he found really endearing, like the way she enjoyed planning dinners, cooking his favorite foods, and decorating the table. He watched her rinse off the dishes and stack them on the counter. It occurred to Rod that the reason Martina was so adept with domestic duties was because she had been coerced or manipulated by her father to do his cooking, cleaning, and laundering; he wanted to keep her so busy doing household chores that she would have no time for a social life of her own. Especially, no time to date.

Rod suddenly felt an overwhelming sadness for this young woman who was now his wife. While her friends were out having a good time, Martina was made to feel obligated that she should be at home, taking care of her father's needs. And despite all of her efforts to please him he had beat her so horribly.

Rod suspected Martino Fiasconi had an attraction for his own daughter that went beyond the realm of fatherhood, and he couldn't help but wonder if that attraction was responsible for Martina's thinking she was not a virgin. What would she say if he asked her point blank about it, he wondered? Would Martina tell him the truth or would she protect her victimizer, as most victims do? In any event, he could not possibly ask her about any of that now, not with Judge Gridley's order hanging over his head. Perhaps it will all come out in the course of the upcoming investigation for the present court case brought by Fiasconi. It would be sweet justice if Fiasconi was thrown under the bus by his own hands, Rod thought.

"Are you going to keep standing there looking weird or are you going to go over and invite Freebird and Julie to dinner?" Martina asked, wondering about Rod's peculiar expression.

With just a few strides Rod was across the kitchen and encircling her within his muscular arms, pulling her tight against his body. It seemed as though he had suddenly become possessed. Martina attributed his quixotic behavior to his passionate nature, unaware he was actually moved by a heavy feeling of sadness that momentarily captured him.

"I love you so much Babe" he whispered, exhaling his words with a rush of sudden emotion and squeezing her so tightly that she could hardly breathe. "My feelings for you are so strong…there just aren't the words to tell you the way I feel inside." And then, for emphasis, he squeezed her even tighter, as if he were trying to meld their two bodies into one, so that no one could ever separate them. Martina almost cried out from the pain of his squeeze but stifled it in her throat. After the recent drought of passion between them, she surely did not want to do anything to dispel his passionate mood by complaining he was hugging her too tight.

Although, Martina could not help but be puzzled by Rod's sudden intensity and the seeming sound of desperation in his voice. And why was he holding her as if he were afraid someone was about to tear her away from him? It was then that Martina began to wonder and worry that something was not right—there was something going on that Rod was not telling her about. In Martina's mind, that could only mean whatever was troubling Rod was serious and she needed to know what it was. So, she asked him point blank. "Don't I deserve to know what's going on, Rod?"

Stunned by the accuracy of her perception, Rod took a step back to read her face and saw her look of determination. Taking a deep breath and exhaling slowly, Rod considered her question for a moment and decided that now was the time to tell her all about what was weighing so heavily on his mind. "Let's go sit down in the living room," he said, his shoulders visibly sagging with his burden. Taking her hand in his, he led her out of the kitchen. "It's going to be a long story."

There would be no special dinner that evening ... or ever again.

38.

Thinking about those magical days when she and Rod were together always left Martina in a deep melancholy. Looking around her beautifully decorated apartment, carved out of what was once a huge Victorian mansion in the affluent Pacific Heights area of San Francisco, it still seemed a stark contrast to the fabulous stone mansion on Scenic Drive, where she had briefly lived with Rod and briefly knew the fullness of his love.

Maybe he would be still alive and with her right now if she had agreed to run away with him to the Bahamas, as he had begged her to do after telling her about the court battle with Martino. Instead, she insisted they stay in Millborough and follow the Judge's ruling to the letter, which left Rod open and vulnerable to Martino's vengeance.

The memory of that awful day when Rod finally confessed to what was really behind his recent bout of anxiety played crystal clear in her mind. She recalled how she had insisted on not going to the Bahamas, where they could have hidden out forever, because she was just trying to show Rod that she was not mad at him for leaving her out of the loop. He felt guilty and miserable. They were supposed to have invited Julie and Freebird to dinner that night. Instead, they spent that night hanging onto each other, as though they expected the Millborough Police to break down the front door at any minute and haul her away. As it turned out, it was more of a relief to Martina when she did check into the group home. At least then the unknown became known, and she did get to see Rod almost as much as before and he wasn't so gloomy anymore.

Forcing the thoughts of the past from her mind, she reminded herself that what's done is done, and the main thing she needed to concentrate on is being the best mother that she could possibly be to her little son. While Martina was at that moment doubling down on her determination to focus on being the model of motherhood to Roddy to make up for his not having a father, she would have been chagrined to know that on the other side of the country, back in her hometown of Millborough, Rod McDonough had taken up residence with a woman named Carol Bennett, and that one day this Carol Bennett would pose a terrible threat to both her life and that of her son's.

39.

In August of 1975, Nurse Carol Bennett had just been dumped by the fifth or sixth boyfriend she had taken up with after her third divorce when she cast her covetous eye upon a handsome patient named Rod McDonough. She was making her rounds in the orthopedics ward at Millborough General Hospital and came upon the dour-faced young man who was recovering from a gun shot wound and broken bones he received in a motorcycle accident. After taking a few moments to read his chart she entered his room with a big smile that belied her exceedingly poor social skills.

Carol was an attractive enough package to get a man's attention: her figure was trim, yet she was curvaceous on a five-foot five-inch frame; she wore her black wavy hair in a modish shag cut that framed an oval face with blue eyes; and although her legs were a bit too long for her torso, it wasn't her proportional imbalances that men found objectionable.

Carol was what some might call a "pig in a poke". Underneath her attractive veneer there was nothing of any substance. She possessed the temperament of a pit viper and completely lacked the ability to nurture long term relationships. After a while, even her voracious sexual appetite was not enough to keep men interested in coming back for more. Not only was she self-centered, arrogant, needy and demanding, her vicious temper could be triggered by the least perceived slight. Although she was careful not to go off on her hospital co-workers, those who spent any time at all around her picked up on the imperious attitude that lurked just below the surface of her personality. Most of her co-workers just automatically chose not to spend any more time in her presence than they had to.

Initially, Rod showed no interest whatsoever in Carol. He simply accepted her presence as just another aspect of the hell he was living in since his accident. And Carol couldn't seem to break through the wall of indifference he had built up around himself. But Carol was resourceful and tenacious; she circled Rod's wall every time she was on duty, looking for a weak spot in its construction. She found the weakness on the day Rod was told he would probably be a cripple for the rest of his life. He was so shaken by the prospect of spending the rest of his life in a wheelchair he actually responded to Carol's conversation for the first time since he landed in the orthopedics ward.

"I've heard that Doctor Telvie told you not to be hopeful of walking again," Carol spoke as she was adjusting the position of Rod's bed. With his broken right leg in traction he was constantly being raised and lowered and his butt being shimmied from side to side and propped with pillows. And, of course, there were also the ordeals with the bedpan and the urine bottle and the daily sheet changing disturbances. There was no shortage of opportunity for her to chisel at his wall of silence, so when he responded to her comment with mere grunt she saw that as progress and continued her conversation. "I wouldn't accept Doctor Telvie's opinion as law. I've seen people with worse cases than yours get up and walk again." She paused to see if she had his attention. Although he was looking straight ahead she could tell he was listening, so she went on. "If you'd like another opinion you might want to contact Doctor Paul Larkin…he's also an orthopedist who is on the staff here. You'll be in for a lot of therapy but he'll have you walking again if you are willing to do the work."

Rod turned and looked at Carol. "I'd like to talk to him," he said, and then added, "Thanks."

When Rod began his therapy under the direction of Doctor Larkin, Carol became his cheer leader and then, eventually, his coach. And over time it was natural that Rod would open up to her. She brought him magazines and made sure his pain medication was increased to the maximum dosage that could be prescribed. Rod told her about how he came to be shot and his motorcycle crash. It took him a while to finally bring up the subject of Martina, but when that floodgate of emotion opened up he poured out his heart. And Carol listened to it all, feigning sincere sympathy, and all the time wondering how she could turn Rod's shattered life to her advantage.

It would probably take a team of psychiatrists to decipher Carol's motivations and her need to "collect" men; it was not as though she were capable of loving any of them. Rod McDonough was just another warm body to take the place of the last one who passed through her revolving door of transient relationships. Nor could it be certain if Carol felt a real sexual attraction to any of the men she became involved with or did she just use them for her own gratification?

Love and sex were inconsequential to Rod at this point; his physical and mental pain was so great that he could not think of either. He saw Carol only as a sympathetic friend. So wrapped up in his day-to-day struggle to cope with the loss of Martina and the dysfunction of his battered body, Rod was vulnerable to Carol's guile. He could not see beyond his own bitterness.

When Rod turned down the offers of his parents, his brother Travis, and Freebird and Julie to live with them when he left the rehabilitation facility in early January of 1976, and announced that he would be moving in with his nurse, Carol Bennett, they were all dismayed at his decision. Freebird was the most vocal about his disapproval.

"What do you know about this Carol, Bro?" Freebird reasoned with his best friend. Of course, he had to be careful not to alienate Rod while trying to talk some sense into him. "We are your family and we want you to come live with us."

Rod appreciated their offers but he felt he needed a clean break from all ties to Martina, and Freebird and Julie were the closest of all ties. He responded by saying, "It's not like I am moving out of the country. I'll only be across town. We'll keep in touch."

To Freebird, Rod's words sounded like a kiss-off and he was saddened. He wished Rod could see the evil inside of Carol that he saw. There was no point in telling Rod what he knew about the woman, Rod would not believe him.

Julie, who had been listening quietly to Rod's and Freebird's conversation, finally spoke up for the one person who seemed to be totally left out of the equation, "What about Martina, Rod? Don't you think you owe it to yourself and to her to talk to her?"

Rod recoiled with obvious distaste at the mention of Martina's name. "Isn't it pretty obvious by now that she's left me. It's been over six months and no one has heard a word from her…so much for love and marriage."

Not about to give up on Martina, Julie added, "But we won't know anything for sure unless you talk to her, Rod. I was the last one to see her and she was sick with worry about you. She only left town because her crazy father wanted her to get rid of your baby."

Rod gave Julie a look of disgust. "My baby! If it was my baby she would not have run away."

"That's not fair, Rod!" said Julie, bursting into tears and leaving the room.

"You have my telephone number, Bro," Freebird said with a note of disappointment. "Call me if you need me." The he, too, turned and left the room.

As soon as Freebird and Julie were gone Carol Bennett appeared in Rod's room with her syrupy smile. "Doctor Larkin has signed your discharge form. So tomorrow you'll be leaving here. Have you decided where you want to go?"

With no hint of interest or eagerness in his voice, Rod asked, "Is your offer still open?"

"Indeed it is," Carol said, looking like the proverbial cat that ate the canary.

And so it was that Rod left the Millborough Rehabilitation Center and moved in with Carol Bennett, having no idea of the dangerous trap he was walking into or the diabolical person that she truly was.

But as much of a danger Carol Bennett posed to anyone who crossed her, Rod would prove to be the last man that Carol would ever collect.

40.

Indeed, Attorney Travante's letter about the death of her father had stirred up untold layers of emotions and memories that Martina had hastily buried in the deepest chasms of her mind, many of which she had not even dared speak of when baring her soul to Chloe Renfrew. Some were just too painful and best left undisturbed. But thoughts of Julie regularly filtered through her mind and always made her smile. Many times, she wished Julie could see Roddy. After all, Julie was instrumental in helping her escape from Millborough and saving her baby. Was Julie still married to Freebird, she wondered, and did they have children of their own? Martina felt a sudden urge to talk to Julie. Surely, now she could.

When Martina had first gotten settled into her Aunt's and Uncle's house she had several times attempted to write a letter to Julie, but she was embarrassed by all that was going on with her father's case and the stories of sexual abuse that were circulating around Millborough at the time. Then her Aunt Catherine told her she didn't think it was a good idea to let anyone back there know where she was staying. Her Aunt was afraid that some zealous reporter from the Millborough Gazette would somehow get her address and the Denault house would be under siege. Even Shotgun took Martina aside and suggested that she not communicate with anyone in Millborough until, as he said, "all of that salacious *fol de rol* died down." Martina had a vague idea of what the word "salacious" meant, so her letter to Julie was never written. Martina felt bad about breaking the pledge she had made to keep in touch with Julie, but she had no choice back then.

Now, with Martino dead, there was no longer a need for Martina to keep her whereabouts a secret. And, surely, the interests of the people of Millborough had long since moved on to more current gossip. Or so Martina thought. It didn't matter to her anyway; she had no intention of returning to Millborough. Attorney Travante did indicate that Martino's estate could be disposed of without her having to go back there. Maybe Julie could come to San Francisco for a visit? But, first, Martina would have to find Julie. She doubted that if Julie and Freebird were still together they would be living in the same apartment over the garage on the McDonough property. How, Martina wondered, could she track down Julie? An idea began to take shape in Martina's head. Attorney Travante might know where Julie was now living. If Travante's investigator could find Martina in San Francisco he could certainly find

Julie, who was probably still living in Millborough. Anyway, it was worth a try.

Martina should have known better. After only five minutes of conversing on the telephone with Vittorio Travante, he had smoothly talked her into returning home to dispose of the assets of Martino's estate. Her Aunt and Uncle tried to talk her out of going back to the scene of such harrowing events in her young life, but Martina could not be dissuaded. The Denaults were certain that Travante had something up his sleeve, and called upon Shotgun to talk to Martina, with the hopes their bombastic friend, whom Martina adored, could override Travante's obvious spell. Even Shotgun, with his glittering and substantial cache, was unable to talk Martina out of returning to Millborough.

"What can I do?" Shotgun told the Denaults. "She is of age to make her own decisions and she is adamant

41.

Martina scanned the giant overhead screen that listed the flight departures from San Francisco's Airport for perhaps the fiftieth time. Her flight to Newark, the only town closest to Millborough with a major carrier airport, was not scheduled to take off for another fifty minutes, but she was eager to get going. Her Uncle Jack and Aunt Catherine had insisted on driving her and Roddy to the airport, and she was glad for their company. Out of nervousness, Aunt Catherine fussed needlessly with straightening the collar of Martina's turquoise jacket. Uncle Jack was off somewhere showing his excited grandson the airplanes parked on the runway outside the concourse windows.

"Are you sure you're ready to go back to Millborough?" Her Aunt asked, trying not to show the true fear she felt about Martina returning to a place so full of unhappy memories.

"I'll be fine, Aunt Catherine…thanks to you and Uncle Jack," Martina assured. "Besides, I think it's time I went back and faced down the demons. With Martino dead now, I have nothing to fear."

"Are you sure you don't want me to come along with you? I could look after the baby while you take care of business."

Martina noted the worried frown on her Aunt's face and placed a reassuring hand on the older woman's arm. "I won't be gone but a few days, Aunt Catherine…and I'll be staying with Julie and her husband, so I won't be alone. And Julie has said she can watch Roddy while I meet with Vito."

Although her Aunt nodded in agreement with Martina's assurances, her expression gave away the uncertainty she really felt about her niece making such a trip. Catherine reached over and brushed aside a lock of Martina's hair, not because the lock was out of place but only because she wanted an excuse to lovingly touch her niece. Catherine loved the girl as if she were her own daughter, and was extremely proud of the poised young woman and wonderful mother Martina had become. It was tragic, Catherine often thought, that her sister Jacqui did not live to see Martina blossom into a beautiful woman. But many times, when Catherine looked at Martina, she was sure she was looking at Jacqui. Even now, as she watched Martina scanning the flight information screen, Catherine was amazed at how Martina more closely resembled Jacqui than she herself did, and she was Jacqui's twin. Catherine's biggest fear was that Martina would be detained longer than intended in Millborough, and the fretting Aunt began to imagine a multitude of reasons that could delay the young woman's return. Sometimes, estate matters could drag on indefinitely. What if Martina simply decided she wanted to move back to Millborough, to be closer to her old friends? The thought of Martina and Roddy living clear on the other side of the country panicked Catherine. In a last ditch effort to assure Martina's return, the older woman suddenly blurted, "I have a great idea, Martina…."

Hearing the cagey tone in her Aunt's voice, Martina wondered what new plot the resourceful woman had hatched to either keep her from leaving or make sure she returned. "What's that?" Martina asked, turning to look at her aunt.

"Why don't you leave Roddy with Uncle Jack and I, and that will give you more freedom to get everything accomplished quickly with Attorney Travante and allow you more time to visit with your friends?"

"Oh, that's very sweet of you Aunt Catherine." Martina smiled indulgently at the hopeful woman. "But Julie is really looking forward to seeing Roddy…and he is still kind of nursing."

Her Aunt grimaced at the mention of Roddy still nursing. "Really, Martina! I can't believe you have not weaned that child by now." Suddenly, the woman's face brightened. "If you left Roddy with us he would most certainly be weaned by the time you get back."

"Nice try, Aunt Catherine, but I couldn't stand to be away from my son, even for a few days. I'd miss him terribly."

Her Aunt looked crestfallen. "Well…I'm going to miss you both terribly, too."

Feeling guilty, Martina threw her arms around her disconsolate aunt. "I'm going to miss you, too, Aunt Catherine…but I'll be back in just a few days."

"If you are not back here in a few days you can be sure that I will be on the first plane out of here and go get you," her Aunt said with a no-nonsense tone.

Martina smiled at her Aunt's admonition, but knew the woman would be true to her word. It warmed Martina's heart to know how much Aunt Catherine loved her and how protective she was. It struck the young woman that her Aunt had been more motherly to her than Jacqui, who, it seemed to Martina, had functioned like an older, more sophisticated sister. On an impulse, Martina threw her arms around her Aunt and hugged the older woman so tightly she almost lost her balance and toppled over onto her niece.

"Good heavens, Martina!" Catherine sputtered with surprise, but clearly flattered by her niece's sudden display of affection. Tears of both joy and sadness pooled in her eyes. She had been blessed to have Martina and Roddy come into her life just when she was feeling the emptiness of not having had children of her own; it was hard for her to let them go away, even for a few days.

"Mama! Mama! Ay-pane!" Shouted Roddy, wide-eyed with excitement, as he ran toward them, with Uncle Jack close behind. The little boy ran to his mother and wrapped his chubby arms around her legs. Martina bent down and scooped up the excited child. "Big pane," the wide-eyed boy told her, extending his arms as wide as he could for emphasis.

Martina loved seeing the expression of amazement in her son's big blue-green eyes and couldn't help but playfully nibble at his flushed cheeks. "We're going to be getting on the big airplane pretty soon and go up...up...and away," she told the uncomprehending boy, who was nevertheless further excited by the animated tone of her voice. Wiggling down from his mother's arms, the little boy ran back to Uncle Jack and tugged at his pant leg. "Me up! Ampa!"

Obviously delighted with the notion of being Roddy's "Ampa," Uncle Jack picked up the boy and cuddled him, while Catherine affectionately rubbed the child's back.

Martina thought she saw tears in her Uncle's eyes, too. She felt guilty about upsetting her Aunt and Uncle, and for a moment, albeit a brief moment, she thought about not going.

But then she envisioned Julie and Freebird, who would be waiting for her at the airport with their year-old daughter, Jody, and the guilt quickly faded from her mind. While she was torn about leaving her Aunt and Uncle, Martina ached to see her friends. There was so much of the past to catch up on. And after Vittorio Travante was gracious enough to utilize his investigative resources to find Julie and Freebird, Martina then felt locked into returning to Millborough. Had Vittorio not been able to locate her friends she probably would not be going back.

Aunt Catherine had a few choice words to say about Vittorio Travante's motivations, none of them were very flattering.

When the voice on the public address system announced the boarding of passengers for Martina's flight, the three family members simultaneously looked at each other with frozen expressions. The dreaded moment of tearful embraces had come. After Martina boarded the airplane, Jack and Catherine Denault stood in front of the large concourse window and watched until the aircraft disappeared from their view. It was probably the worst moment of their lives.

Luckily, Martina was assigned a window seat and was able to entertain Roddy by pointing to things outside until the airplane was aloft, and then there was nothing but milky white clouds to look at. Roddy, who was confined to his mother's lap, soon tired of the clouds and his confinement. It was now after one o'clock in the afternoon, well past the toddler's naptime, and he was winding down from all of his earlier excitement. In Roddy's young world it was the perfect time for curling up against his mother's warm breast. But the child was befuddled by the blouse his mother was wearing; it had no buttons in front or any other kind of opening that would allow him access to the objects of his desire. In his frustration the little boy began to fuss and pluck at the front of his mother's silk turquoise shell. Martina tried to pacify him with a bottle of apple juice but Roddy was not interested in anything that came from a fake nipple. He began to whimper and thrash about, accidentally hitting the man seated next to them with his little balled up fist.

"I'm sorry," Martina apologized to the man, noticing that he was young, probably in his late twenties, and quite handsome.

When he had first taken the seat next to her, Martina had not paid much attention other than to note he wore an expensive looking suit and dark sunglasses. Now, she noticed he had on a black turtle neck jersey, was tanned and rather sexy. But knowing how her exotic looks seemed to entrance men for the wrong reasons, she quickly looked away from the man and busied herself fishing around in her tote bag for a storybook to read to Roddy. The book interested the little boy for all of two seconds, after which he pushed it aside and shouted, "No!"

Then he resumed trying to find some way to get to his mother's breast. Flustered and embarrassed by her son's pawing and crankiness, Martina was just about to take the boy to the rest room to nurse him when the man in the black turtleneck jersey handed her a Tootsie Pop. Since lollipops were few and far between in Roddy's diet, the child was completely placated and remained pacified for quite some time.

"Thank you so much," a grateful Martina said to the man.

The young man smiled and nodded his acknowledgement. "I reckon I know something about little boys," he told Martina, "I have a couple of them myself." But that wasn't true. The man was just trying to ingratiate himself with Martina. Extending his hand toward her, he said, "My name is Ty Lockwood."

Martina shook his hand quickly and let go of it. "Nice to meet you. I'm Martina Denault and this cranky little boy is my son, Roddy."

Ty looked at Roddy, who was now absorbed with the sweetness of the Tootsie Pop, and smiled. Getting right to business, Ty asked, "Are you going east for a vacation or do you live there?"

"Just visiting," Martina responded, saying nothing further.

Ty nodded, not surprised by her laconic response. Not only was this Martina beautiful, more so than he had imagined from the description of her that he was given, she was also very smart. He wasn't sure what intrigued him more: her tanned, exotic beauty, those amazing green eyes, or her secretive nature. He had to admit that she was the most provocative package he had seen in a long time. Reminding himself not to show too much interest in the gorgeous woman beside him, he settled back in his seat and closed his eyes. After all, he was being paid by Shotgun Mitchell to only make sure she arrived safely at her destination, connected with her friends, and had no other problems while in transit. He was also supposed to make certain she boarded her return flight to San Francisco in three days. He had been duly warned by Shotgun to keep his hands off the merchandise. And if there was one thing Ty Lockwood knew about Shotgun Mitchell it was never to cross that crazy son-of-a-bitch.

When Roddy finally drifted off to sleep Martina shifted his little body to a comfortable position on her lap and tried to relax. Sleep would be impossible for her, she knew, but now that the boy was asleep she could at least get lost in her thoughts. Her mind automatically drifted to the emotional telephone conversation she had had with Julie two days ago. Thankfully, Vittorio's office had been able to locate her friend's telephone number without much difficulty since she and Freebird still lived in Millborough. Excited and nervous, Martina's hand shook as she dialed the number. The phone rang only twice before it was answered and the voice that said "Hello" was unmistakably Julie's. Martina thought her heart would burst; it was so incredibly wonderful to hear Julie's voice again.

"Julie…it's Martina."

"Ohmygod! Ohmygod! Martina! I knew you'd keep the pledge." Julie exclaimed, just before she burst into tears of joy. "Where are you? What happened? Your baby?" So overcome by the surprise of hearing

224

from her old friend after such a long time, Julie was reduced to fractal sentences before becoming completely speechless with emotion.

Sniffing back her own tears of emotion, Martina was only slightly more articulate. "I'm sorry I couldn't call sooner…what with…we're fine. The baby… he's—" Then she burst into bittersweet tears as well, because hearing Julie's voice brought back a flood of happy memories of their days together at Scenic Drive and, naturally, of Rod.

When they had both exhausted their excitement and emotion enough to allow a half-way intelligible conversation, Martina told Julie, "Mr. Travante…Martino's lawyer…he helped me find you. I was happy to hear that you and a Freebird are still together."

"Oh! Martina! We are just the same as ever…except we have Jody now…our little girl…and you won't believe it, Martina, she looks just like Freebird."

Hearing that, Martina began crying again. They had missed so many important happenings in each other's lives, memorable occasions that could never be recaptured, and the thought of those missed events saddened her. When Julie heard Martina's recent round of sniffling she, too, began crying anew.

Finally, Martina forced back her tears, and said, "This is stupid…to be on the phone with each other after such a long time and do nothing but cry…we've got to stop crying and talk." Julie agreed, but Martina could still hear her sniffling. "Okay, Julie," Martina announced, "before we go crazy asking each other a bunch of questions over the phone, let me tell you that I'll be in Millborough in a couple of days and I'm hoping we can spend at least a day together while I'm there."

"What? Spend a day?" Julie exclaimed, her sniffling replaced by near outrage. "If you don't stay with us while you're here you can forget about seeing us at all."

So, Martina readily agreed to forego Travante's hotel reservation in favor of staying with her friends. And since there was no point in trying to catch up on each other's lives over the telephone, especially when they were each bursting into tears at every other sentence, they decided to wait until they saw each other in person to continue with their update. After making plans to meet at the airport in two days, they each hung up the phone feeling as though they were in a fog, yet exhilarated by the anticipation of soon seeing the other again.

42.

After landing at the Newark Airport, Martina and Roddy then boarded a puddle-jumper for another flight to the Greenwich Air Terminal, which was the closest airport to Millborough. The Greenwich Air Terminal was such a "mom and pop" operation it could have been easily set down inside the main terminal of the San Francisco International Airport with plenty of room to spare. The fact that it was smaller and less crowded made it easier for Martina to immediately spot Julie and Freebird as soon as she entered the waiting area adjacent to her flight's arrival gate. The minute the two long lost friends saw each other they each broke into an excited dash. Julie had the advantage because she was not balancing a child on her hip and lugging a huge tote bag, as was Martina, so she was able to sprint across the terminal like a gazelle.

Freebird sauntered quietly at a short distance behind, proudly holding his little girl in his lean, sinewy brown arms, patiently watching as the reunited friends hugged and carried on in the wild frenzy of joy he had expected.

Calmly standing off to the side, cuddling his precious little Jody, Freebird's body language may have appeared passive, but his well-trained eyes observed every detail. Certainly, Freebird was overjoyed to see Martina again; he had once loved her as a sister and offered many prayers for her during the days she was recovering from her father's beating. But when she disappeared he wondered about the strength of her heart and her love for Rod. With all of the confusion and rumors surrounding her disappearance he didn't know what to believe. The worst of it was seeing Rod all tore up because she had left him when he needed her the most. No explanation. Just gone. And the pain of watching Rod's once giant spirit dissipate into nothingness, and then to stand by helpless while Rod become a mindless druggie, was unbearable to Freebird. It was hard for Freebird to keep his mind open and not feel that somehow Martina was responsible.

But still, in those dark days of Rod's spirit-death, he reasoned that everyone's path was determined by the Creator for a specific purpose, and no one could be judgmental of another without being judgmental of the Creator. The only thing he was sure of was what Julie had told him the night Martina split town: that Martina had to get away because she was pregnant and her father was insisting that she get an abortion. Then came the ugly rumors about Martino Fiasconi being the father of his own daughter's baby, and how he was pressuring Martina to have an abortion to keep the truth from coming out about his molesting her. Back then, Freebird had to wonder about the possibility the rumors might be true. After all, he had witnessed, firsthand, the viciousness of her father's jealousy when he found out she was dating Rod. What other evil would prompt Martino Fiasconi to beat Martina senseless and shoot Rod?

But now, seeing the little boy Martina was holding in her arms, Freebird's throat tightened with emotion. Carefully studying the boy's face, there was no doubt in Freebird's mind that the little boy was Rod's son; the resemblance to his friend was amazing. He could now confirm that the rumors of Martina being impregnated by her father were based only on evil minded gossip. Underneath his patient, calm demeanor his heart suddenly took flight, like an eagle released from a cage. He knew immediately what he had to do.

Julie snatched Roddy from Martina's arms and began kissing the face of the astonished child. "Oh, Marty— He's much too pretty to be a boy," she proclaimed, admiring the boy's cherubic face and rosy cheeks. Julie was struck by how much the little boy looked like Rod, but she was afraid to bring up Rod's name just yet. Suddenly remembering Freebird and her own baby, Julie grabbed Martina by the arm and pulled her over to where Freebird was standing.

When Martina turned her attention to Freebird, whom she associated closely with Rod, she could not control the full extent of her emotions any longer. She threw her arms around the young man and his baby, and sobbed against his shoulder. A tear or two escaped from Freebird's eyes as well and ran down his stoic, tanned face. After a few tearful moments Martina realized her crying was upsetting the children, so she quickly pulled herself together. Martina looked up at Freebird's handsome face, and managed a tentative smile. "I really am happy to see you, Freebird," she said, trying to make light of her burst of heavy emotion.

The young man inclined his head toward her and kissed her cheek. "I am more than happy to see you, Martina," he responded. His tone was soft but held a cryptic note.

Martina caught the enigmatic note in his voice and tried to read his dark, intelligent eyes, but they yielded no clue. She could sense he had something more to say to her but the airport was not the place.

Suddenly, a deep, familiar voice, coming from behind Martina, said, "It was very nice traveling across country with you, Ms. Denault."

Martina turned, surprised to see the good looking young man from the plane, Ty Lockwood, standing there. "We may run into each other again one day," Lockwood added, and loped off before Martina could think to respond.

"Who's that?" Julie asked Martina, eying the suave looking stranger.

"He sat next to me on the flight from San Francisco," answered Martina, watching Lockwood as he walked across the terminal, wondering what he meant by "run into each other again." Then, shrugging off the comment, she immediately turned to Freebird and asked, "May I hold Jody?" Freebird smiled and relinquished his second prized possession to Martina, Julie being his first. But as soon as Freebird's arms were free he motioned to Julie to give him Roddy to hold.

Preoccupied with the baby his mother was now holding and fawning over, the little boy did not object to the change of arms.

"Mama!" Roddy's voice sounded like a plaintive wail. Realizing her son probably thought he was being exchanged for another child, Martina moved closer to show Jody to Roddy. "Look, Roddy…this is Jody…she's going to be your little girlfriend." Roddy looked at the baby and babbled something in his incomprehensible juvenile language. The three parents laughed at his response.

"Uh-oh, Julie!" Freebird remarked. "If he's anything like his Daddy we'd better keep our little girl under lock and key."

While they all laughed at Freebird's observation, Martina couldn't help but also feel a pang of sadness because her little boy did not have his Daddy. But, now, at least the subject of Rod McDonough had been brought up, as it eventually had to be.

During the forty minute ride from the airport to Julie's and Freebird's house in Millborough, the conversation between the three friends was non-stop and oftentimes simultaneous. With so much of their lives to catch up on, there was an excited rush to cover all of the important events that had happened to each other since the last time they were together. Martina learned that Julie's mother finally found the husband she had so diligently searched for and moved in with him, giving her house to Julie and Freebird. "It was such good timing," Julie commented, "We were expecting the baby and needed a bigger house with a yard. Freebird built Jody her own personal little playground in the back yard…so she and Roddy will have a great time playing together out there."

"Roddy will love that...he loves going to the park and being with other children," Martina said, really wanting to know the circumstances of them leaving their apartment on the McDonough estate, but not knowing if she should ask. Mulling it over for a few moments, she decided to broach the subject through a back door. "So...how long have you been living at your Mother's house?"

"About a year and a half," said Julie, turning to look at Martina in the back seat, who was struggling to keep Roddy on her lap. "You look tired, Marty...but we fixed up the guest room just for you. There's a big ole bed for you and Roddy and when we get to the house Freebird is going to grill us some steaks for dinner, we've got special food for the kids, and...if you want...you can lie down and rest for a bit."

"Mmmm. Stretching out flat sounds real good to me after sitting for nine hours, but I think I'll be too wired for a nap."

"No! No nap!" Roddy chimed in, shaking his head emphatically. The two young women looked at the serious-faced boy and laughed.

"Oh, Marty— Roddy is such a beautiful little boy. He looks so much like..." Julie hesitated, unsure if she should bring up Rod's name.

Just then, Roddy started whining and pawing at the front of Martina's silk blouse. Martina tried to distract the boy with one of the new toys she had brought along just for that purpose, but Roddy pushed the toy aside and began protesting in earnest.

Flustered by her son's behavior, Martina tried to calm him by promising the object of his desire when they got to "Aunt Julie's house." But Roddy would not be pacified with promises and bellowed his frustration.

Surprised by Roddy's sudden tantrum, Julie asked Martina, "What does he want?" She had not seen the little boy tugging on the front of his mother's blouse. Rather than confess to Julie that Roddy was still nursing and having to listen to any more preaching about it, Martina simply said, "I think he's just tired from the trip."

From his vantage point in the driver's seat, however, Freebird had been intermittently watching the little boy in the rear view mirror. He noticed Roddy pulling on Martina's blouse and heard him whining with escalating frustrations because he was unable to get his way. Freebird couldn't help but chuckle quietly to himself. Like father, like son, thought Freebird, remembering how much Rod was obsessed with women's breasts, especially Martina's.

Entering Julie's living room was like stepping back in time for Martina. The furniture and decorations were almost exactly as they were the last time she had been there. And the guest room, where she and Roddy would be sleeping, was Julie's old bedroom, where the two friends hung out many a night when they were in junior high and high school. The room was now devoid of the many posters and photographs Julie had taped on the walls during their high school days and was now painted a soft purple. A quilted bedspread, featuring clusters of purple lilacs and a sprinkling of mauve, blue, and yellow flowers on a white background, and matching window curtains, made the room cheerful and inviting. The room actually seemed larger now that all of Julie's mementoes were gone. Freebird lugged in Martina's two suitcases and set the largest one down on a wooden bench that was placed against one wall. The smaller one, he set on the floor, next to the bench.

Julie, who was holding her baby daughter, and Martina, with Roddy clinging to her pant leg, stood next to the double bed reminiscing about what used to be where in the room. Freebird quietly slipped out of the room to go fire up the grill, thankful for the excuse to get away from all the excited girl talk.

"Whatever happened to that ugly giant panda you had in here? The one you won at the state fair eons ago?" Martina asked, laughing as she remembered Julie carrying the huge panda around the fairgrounds; it was as tall as Julie and probably weighed nearly as much as she did at the time.

"Oh, that thing! When we cleaned this room out Freebird hung it from the tree out back and used it for target practice with his bow and arrows," Julie said, not telling Martina that Freebird had pretended the panda was Martino Fiasconi. Then Julie said, "You may want to freshen up and change into more comfy clothes before dinner. There are towels in the guest bath for you and Roddy…so make yourselves at home and do whatever you have to do. Come to the kitchen whenever you're ready…that's where you'll find me most of the time these days."

Martina laughed at her friend's remark. "I know what you mean by that. I'll get Roddy and myself washed up and changed and then I'll be right out to help you in the kitchen." Kissing Julie on the cheek, Martina said, "Thank you so much for inviting Roddy and me to stay with you and picking us up at the airport."

"Please, Martina…don't even mention it. Freebird and I were so happy to hear from you after all this time…we wouldn't think of you staying anywhere else. You've always been like my sister-" Julie's eyes suddenly filled with tears and her voice became stifled from the emotion that welled up inside of her. Martina stepped forward and hugged her friend, too emotional herself to speak. Words seemed inadequate at the moment, anyway.

After Julie left the room Martina closed the door. "C'mon, Roddy," she called to her son, who was now busy investigating the tote bag full of toys and books, let's get you changed and ready for dinner. After folding down the pretty bedspread, she removed her jacket, kicked off her shoes, and then stripped down to her bra and panties. It felt good to be free of her airplane clothes.

Picking up her son and sitting him on the bed, she removed his shoes and wrinkled clothes. Taking off his diaper, she coaxed, "Let's go potty and show Mama what a big, big boy you are." Martina led the boy into the adjoining bathroom, where she boosted him up on her knee in front of the commode, but the child didn't seem to know what was expected of him. And she was obviously ill equipped to demonstrate what she wanted him to do. She wondered how she was ever going to potty train him? The little boy soon tired of being suspended in front of the bowl, wiggled from his mother's grasp, and ran back to where he had scattered the toys from the tote bag onto the floor. Martina sighed and dampened a washcloth to wash off his bottom before putting on another diaper and dressing him for dinner. As she knelt next to the little boy, wiping him with the damp cloth, she heard Freebird's voice outside the bedroom windows, which overlooked the back yard.

Suddenly, Martina knew who she could ask to assist her with her son's potty training.

43.

It was a warm, clear mid-August night; perfect for sitting outside on the patio. Martina looked up at the canopy of stars and marveled; she had forgotten the beauty of the night sky in Millborough. Through an open window the magical strains of Carlos Santana's guitar, probably the *Abraxas* album, could be heard every now and then, the volume so low as to be barely audible. Martina recalled Freebird's love of Santana's music and smiled, thinking: the more things change the more they stay the same.

The three friends had just finished eating a delicious dinner, and the children had been fed, bathed, and bedded down for the night without a squabble. Martina and Julie had just collapsed in lounge chairs after a long, exciting, emotional first day's reunion. Freebird was draping a tarpaulin over the sandbox for the night, "in case it should rain." The air around them was heavy with anticipation, as all three looked forward to finally having some uninterrupted time to talk. Each of them wondered how they were going to tactfully open that hastily closed door to the past. Certainly, they had to go back and start from the day they were last together, no matter how painful it might be to revisit that place in time they were all quite happy to have left behind them. Each had questions that only the other could answer.

"That was an excellent dinner, Honey," Julie complemented Freebird. "I think you outdid yourself tonight."

Freebird, who had just sat down next to his wife, leaned over and kissed her on the lips. "My pleasure, Sweetie."

Martina smiled at the couple, happy to see that they had not changed one bit since they first got together. They still acted like newlyweds, which is what they were when she last saw them. Back then, she was a newlywed, too. It was impossible not to think about Rod and the fact that he was missing from this wonderful tableau, but Martina refused to spoil the moment by being morose. "You guys have done wonders with this yard.

All of the plants and flowers are beautiful. And this patio is so nice," Martina commented, admiring the decorative pattern of the various sized blocks.

"It's all Freebird's doing," Julie said. "He spends a lot of time out here in the yard. He put in the patio and all of the plants. Until we moved here I had no idea he was such a handyman. Most of the plants you see in the yard came from cuttings he got from where ever he saw something growing that he liked. And the stonework for the patio, he did it all himself. He's amazing, Marty. He can do just about anything."

Freebird beamed in the glow of Julie's testimonial, smiling contentedly.

It was then Martina thought to ask him for his specialized assistance with Roddy. "Well...uh...I could sure use Freebird's help with a little situation," she told them.

Hunching forward in his chair, concerned Martina's need had something to do with the reason she had come to Millborough, Freebird's expression became serious. "What can I help you with?"

Martina saw the concerned look on Freebird's face and realized the young man was anticipating something of a more serious nature than what she had in mind. Nevertheless, she did need his help and he was the only man around she could ask. "I need help with Roddy...I'm trying to potty train him but all I can do is point to the toilet bowl and he thinks I want him to look at the water in there. I need you to show him what he's supposed to do." Martina thought Freebird would crack up laughing when he heard why she needed his help, but his expression became even more serious.

Looking her straight in the eye, Freebird said, "I think his Daddy is the one who should be showing him how to do that."

Martina gasped. Why would Freebird say such a cruel thing to her, she wondered? Rod was dead. Her son had no Daddy. She felt as though she had just been slapped across the face and looked as stunned as she felt. The young couple saw the stricken expression wash across Martina's face like a dark wave running across the surface of the ocean. It didn't take Freebird but a second or two to figure out from her expression that Martina did not know that Rod had survived his injuries, although just barely. He remembered the misinformation about Rod's death that initially circulated after the shooting, and realized that Martina must have also received the same misinformation, but apparently she was never told of Rod's recovery. Realizing his words must have sounded harsh and insensitive, Freebird sprung out of his chair and went over to Martina, knelt down and took her hand in his. "I'm so sorry," he apologized to the visibly upset young woman. "I thought you knew Rod was alive."

Hearing that, Martina felt her body go numb, like she had been plunged into a vat of icy water and hit by a bolt of lightning at the same time. Her heart pounded out of control, her eyes were open but registered nothing, and there was a loud roaring in her ears.

Julie, who was now crouching beside her husband, put one hand on Freebird's shoulder and the other on Martina's knee. "We thought you knew, Martina," she echoed Freebird's words, but they fell upon deaf ears. Martina was in shock.

Rapidly assessing the situation, Freebird stood up and pressed an index finger against each of Martina'a temples, holding them tightly against her skin while he closed his eyes and appeared to be concentrating very hard on something. Julie had no idea what he was doing, but within seconds Martina began hyperventilating and then burst into tears. Freebird and Julie knelt by her side until she regained some degree of composure. After several moments of trying to catch her breath Martina tried to stand up, but fell back heavily into the lounge chair, the trembling of her body and the expression of disbelief and confusion on her face confirming to Freebird that she truly did not know about Rod. "I'm sorry, little sister...I didn't know you didn't—" Freebird's voice stopped abruptly when Martina asked, "Alive? Rod is alive?" Then, as her mind began to process the full implications of what Freebird said, her sea green eyes widened with sudden realization. "Where is he? Can we call him? I have to see him?" She had managed to pull herself to the edge of her chair. "They told me Rod had been killed when his motorcycle crashed ...after...he was sh...shot—" Her words seemed to stop as though they had hit a cement wall head on.

"Who told you that?" Asked Freebird, hoping to now finally learn the reason why Martina left Rod when he needed her the most—when it was her turn to take care of him the way he had taken care of her after her father had beaten her so severely.

"A detective from Millborough. He had flown out to California after the shooting to talk to me. He told my Aunt and Uncle that Rod had been killed. I overheard him telling them." Martina covered her face with her hands, as if feeling the despair of that moment all over again. "I just wanted to die, too. The only thing that kept me from losing it was knowing that Rod's baby was growing inside me. The baby and Chloe Renfrew kept me going."

"Who's Chloe Renfrew?" Freebird and Julie both asked, sounding like a Greek chorus.

"She's the psychologist my Aunt took me to see for counseling. She helped me work through a lot of stuff...depression mostly."

The couple nodded sympathetically. They certainly understood why Martina would have had to see a shrink after all she had been through with that crazy father of hers. Julie was especially aware, as she used to spend a lot of time at Martina's house until the strange dramas of Martino and Jacqui became too much for even her to deal with.

At first, Freebird had not been judgmental of Martina's actions when he learned she left town the same day Rod was nearly killed; he knew she was in a bad situation herself – she was pregnant and feared for the safety of her baby. And Julie had assured him that Martina had no way of knowing what had happened to Rod, since her friend had just escaped from the abortion clinic where her father had taken her, and was hiding out somewhere across town when the shooting probably occurred.. He and Julie didn't even find out about Rod's shooting and crash until the next day, when it made the local news on the television. Nonetheless, each time he went to see Rod in the hospital and heard his injured friend pitifully call Martina's name, his stomach would churn with anger and frustration. At those times he wanted to go out to California, find Martina, and drag her back to Millborough. Now, however, as he stood in front of the distraught young woman, he realized that she had been just as much a victim of her father as was Rod. He reached toward her and placed a comforting hand on her arm, not knowing how to tell her that Rod might not want to see her.

The agonizing implications of what Freebird had just told her were beginning to unfold and magnify in her mind. Bitter, stinging tears welled up in her eyes. "All this time I've been raising my son alone, thinking Rod was dead—" she said, fighting back another resurgence of tearful emotion. "Roddy could have been with his father." Grabbing Freebird's forearm, she asked, "Is he still living up on Scenic Drive? I would like to go see him…I've missed him so much."

Lowering his head so he would not have to look at her imploring eyes, Freebird said, "I will need to talk to him first, Martina…he's kind of messed up."

Martina shot him a worried, inquiring look. "What do you mean messed up? Like from the accident?"

Freebird shook his head. "No. Not exactly that. He thinks you ran out on him and…uh…he's living with another woman." He didn't want to come right out and tell her that Rod had told him he never wanted to see Martina again.

As though someone had pushed her, Martina fell against the back of her lounge chair. The thought of Rod living with another woman brought on another spate of tears. It was the worst news anyone could have told her.

Julie tried to comfort Martina by saying, "He thought you had left him."

"But you knew what had happened, Julie," Martina sobbed. "Didn't you tell him?"

"Yes, I did," Julie responded defensively, "but he wouldn't believe me, Marty. He was just coming out of a coma and he was in a bad way. He had a broken arm and leg, broken ribs…a ruptured spleen. He was really messed up…physically and mentally. He kept asking me where you were and I didn't know what to tell him. Someone…I think the police…told him you had left town. He got really depressed after that. He thought you left because you were ashamed of the baby."

"Why would I be ashamed of his baby?" Asked Martina, her voice choked with emotion.

Freebird raised his arm to Julie, indicating that he wanted to answer that question himself. Kneeling down in front of her again, he calmly told Martina, "Because Rod didn't know it was his baby. He didn't even know you were pregnant."

Although Freebird's tone was not accusatory, Martina felt a need to explain. "I never had a chance to tell him. I had only just found out I was pregnant that morning and I was going to tell Rod the news when he came to pick me up in the afternoon but…." She couldn't finish the sentence.

Picking up another thread of the story, Freebird said, "Let me tell you what was happening back then and maybe you will understand where Rod was coming from. Like Julie said, he was really messed up. The head injury he got in the accident did a number on his memory and he couldn't remember a lot of things. He didn't even recognize me and Julie at first, when we finally got to see him in the hospital…and that was about three weeks after the accident because he was in intensive care all that time, in a coma. It took a while for things to come back to him. But when the newspaper got onto the story of your father shooting Rod…that's when all kinds of stories started coming out. Every day there'd be a big front page story about Rod's shooting. One story said your father shot Rod because Rod talked you into getting married and you were too young to know what you were doing. Another story told about how your father had a court case against Rod to get you back, and the court took you away because both your father and Rod were unfit. It was all such a load of crap."

Freebird stopped talking and stood up to stretch his legs for a few moments. It was obvious that retelling the story had brought back some of the anger he must have been feeling at the time.

Then, pulling his chair closer to where Martina was sitting, he sat down and went on with his account. "After you left town…the word had gotten out about your father taking you to a medical clinic…supposedly for an abortion. The rumors flying around Millborough were that your father had gotten you pregnant and he was trying to get rid of the evidence. (Martina dropped her head into her hands.) Rod eventually heard those rumors."

It felt like a load of sand had fallen on her chest and her lungs were being crushed. She no longer even had the breath to cry. For several moments she merely sucked in air. Finally, when she was able to speak again, she asked, "Did Rod actually believe I was pregnant with my father's baby?" Her expression showed she was shocked and hurt that Rod, of all people, would think such a thing. How could he have forgotten all of those wonderful, languorous afternoons they had spent together, making love?

Freebird registered the hurt on Martina's face. "Like I said…his brains were kind of scrambled in the accident and he had forgotten a lot of his life. He's gotten better since then but he's still not a hundred percent himself."

"So, what you are saying is that he is mad at me and will probably not want to see me." Her comment was a statement, not a question.

"That's why I want to talk to him. One look at Roddy and he's going to know that little boy is his son. He'll be so blown away by Roddy that he'll forget all about everything else," Freebird said, smiling at the thought of telling Rod until he saw a frown harden on Martina's face. "What's wrong?" he asked her.

"What about his girlfriend?" It was hard for Martina to conceive of her beloved Rod living with another woman, but the searing pain of jealousy she felt was very real.

Freebird shrugged. "I don't know Carol very well. She's not real friendly to me."

Julie, who had been sitting quietly over the last many minutes that her husband was talking with Martina, suddenly chimed in, "Carol isn't friendly to any of Rod's friends. If she had her way she'd keep him locked away from the world…and I don't think they have a real thing going anyway."

Martina gave her young friend a quizzical look. "What do you mean about not having a real thing?"

"I feel like it's just a relationship of convenience for Rod," Julie said, scrunching up her face as she carefully chose her words. "Carol was one of Rod's nurses when he was in the hospital. I think Rod got attached to her because she took good care of him…. I remember her buzzing around him when we'd go to see him. My impression is that she forced herself on him at a time when he needed someone to lean on."

Freebird mumbled his agreement. He didn't pass judgment on many people but he never could find anything to like about Carol Bennett. There was something about her that was not right. But he would never get close enough to her to find out exactly what it was that made him uneasy. He preferred to keep his distance from the woman.

"It's almost like he just doesn't care anymore…there's none of his old spark," added Julie, who then immediately wished she had not made that comment when she saw Martina drop her head in her hands and begin sobbing again. Hoping to stop Martina's crying, Freebird said, "I'll go see Rod tomorrow morning. I'm pretty sure what I have to tell him will be a shot in the arm for him."

Martina looked up at Freebird and managed a half smile. She, too, was sure Rod would be interested in knowing he had a son. But would he want to see Roddy after all this time, and would he even want to have anything to do with her. Maybe he would think she was just after child support. Her thoughts prompted her to say, "Just let Rod know I don't expect or want anything from him…for Roddy, I mean. I would just like him to spend time with his son and be a father to him…if he wants."

Before going to bed that night, Freebird brewed a cup of hot herbal tea for Martina. "This will relax you and help you to sleep."

"I'm going to need it. This has been an excruciating day," she said, still reeling from the shock of learning Rod was alive.

"Tomorrow is always a clean slate," Freebird reminded her.

44.

The familiar white Corvette, now covered with a heavy coating of dirt and tree droppings, was parked in the driveway outside the small clapboard house Rod shared with Carol Bennett. Rod's current residence was a dingy, ramshackle dwelling that bore no comparison whatsoever to the house on Scenic Drive, but he had vehemently refused to return to live at his family's estate when he became well enough to leave the hospital. Rod's parents had stayed there for several months, while Rod was hospitalized, but now the mansion stood empty. Freebird understood that the memories of Martina's presence in that house were too strong for Rod to deal with, especially in his vulnerable frame of mind. For that reason, Freebird had no doubt, it was easy for Carol Bennett to talk Rod into moving in with her. The one thing Freebird could not comprehend was Rod's acquiescence to Carol; he was almost robotic in his submissiveness to her.

Turning into the driveway, Freebird was relieved to see that Carol's car was gone. He assumed the sergeant-major, as he privately called her, was at work, which meant he would not have to engage in a battle of wills with her in order to get Rod out of the house. But Rod, too, was another obstacle. It was extremely difficult to get him motivated to leave the house, even on one of his better days. Freebird knew enough to call his friend earlier that morning and do some cajoling and persuading, which took about twenty minutes before Rod would agree to go out to breakfast with him, and it was now getting closer to lunchtime.

Rod barely cracked a smile when he opened the door in response to Freebird's coded knock, a carryover from their Viking's days. Looking over Rod's shoulder at the inside of the house Freebird could see that the interior was dark as usual, and he caught a whiff of its funky, unclean odor. Stepping outside, Rod closed the door behind him and blandly said, "Good to see you, old buddy. Thanks for the invite." But Freebird knew that Rod's unenthusiastic reception was as good as it got these days, and he simply nodded in response. It was enough that Rod even consented to go out to breakfast with him. The two men climbed into Freebird's rusted, two-tone blue F150 pickup. They had not previously discussed where they would go for breakfast, but Freebird had a plan. He had already decided to take Rod to North Hampton. Rod had more or less dropped out of the bike club after his accident but his brothers still kept his stool reserved in front of the makeshift bar at the clubhouse, just in case he should turn up again. They even placed a red cloth over the seat of the stool, so that no one else would sit on it. If there was one thing Bikers truly loved it was a tribute to a maimed brother. The only thing better than a maiming was the death of a brother, preferably as the result of a flaming motorcycle crash. It became instant legend, and then they would all rush over to some tattoo parlor and have memorial tributes to their fallen brother prominently inscribed on their bodies, the size and placement of which depended on what skin space might be available at the time. This tattoo tribute was *de rigueur* even if they didn't particularly like the fallen brother. In Rod's case, however, he was the club's president and well liked, so they went all out for him.

This morning, though, Freebird was taking his friend to a restaurant that was just around the corner from the Clubhouse, where they used to spend a lot of time before they met Martina and Julie. There was a reason for taking Rod there. Freebird was hoping it would trigger the old, lively spark in his friend. And maybe after he told Rod about the existence of his little son the spark would become a huge bonfire of desire to see the little boy.

Recognizing the familiar route they had always taken when driving to North Hampton, Rod asked, "Why are we going to all the way to North Hampton for breakfast?" With the words of his response already in mind, Freebird coolly stated, "Because they'll be no reporters from the Millborough Gazette snooping around there." He knew Rod would not argue with that, because North Hampton was the kind of transient place where no one took the trouble to learn anyone else's real name.

Rod nodded, obviously pacified with Freebird's reasoning. Ever since his shooting he shied away from the streets and shops of Millborough. Despite the passage of more than two years he was still the object of stares and gossip around town. So whenever he absolutely needed to go out he preferred the anonymity of the neighboring towns.

There were only two other patrons eating breakfast at Foley's BLD (an acronym for "Breakfast, Lunch and Dinner") when Rod and Freebird entered. One was an old lady with frizzy maroon hair, who was sitting in a booth and having a grand conversation with herself, as she ate her fried potatoes and scrambled eggs. The other was a skinny man sitting at the counter, drinking his coffee and listening intently to Art Foley expound on the vices and virtues of mankind. Foley turned to look at Rod and Freebird, and said, "Where the hell've you two assholes been? Haven't seen your ugly mugs for a coon's age. Thought maybe the Feds finally caught up with yooz guys."

Freebird laughed and said, "The Feds are pussies compared to your rotten cooking. We're just now recovering from the food poisoning we got the last time we ate here."

Foley waved his hands at them in a "go to hell" gesture.

"Yooz guys wanting the 'Greasy Spoon Special' as usual?"

"Bring it on!" Rod yelled over his shoulder in a sudden burst of his old self, but then seemed to sink right back into the dullness of his lethargy. The brief ignition surprised Freebird, who was not expecting such immediate results from his strategy.

Leading the way to their usual booth near the back wall of the small diner, Freebird felt encouraged that what he had to tell Rod would be well received. Foley brought them two beat up mugs and a large carafe of strong coffee, muttered something about how he had missed their bullshit, and then disappeared back into the kitchen. The two young men made small talk until Foley reappeared with two plates heaped with fried potatoes, three over easy eggs, fried ham, and a side of flapjacks dripping with butter and syrup. Not much was said between them while they concentrated on eating their food, but as soon as Rod set his empty plate aside Freebird announced, "I've got something important to tell you, Rod."

Rod, who had been staring into to his coffee cup, looked up and noted the serious expression on Freebird's face. "What's wrong?" He asked, automatically assuming something bad was coming his way.

Freebird flashed a quick smile. "Nothing is wrong…but something has happened that I need to tell you about. It has to do with Martina…." A scowl immediately darkened Rod's face at the mention of Martina's name. Freebird's hands shot up in a "Hold it!" gesture to Rod, and then he resumed speaking. "I know you don't like talking about her, but this is something you have to hear. Okay?" When it came to the subject of Martina, Freebird knew he had to tread very lightly. He tried to read Rod's expression, to gauge his receptiveness, but received no signals either way. Freebird concluded he could proceed with caution.

"I'm sure you know that Fiasconi died. (Rod gave no indication of knowing or not knowing.) Martina called us out of the blue. We were really surprised to hear from her. She told us she was coming to Millborough to take care of the estate. Julie invited her to stay at our house. We picked her up at the airport last night and—"

"Good for her! I don't need to hear any more," said Rod, suddenly agitated and looking like he was about to jump up and leave.

"I think you do good buddy." pressed Freebird. "Because she has your son with her."

Rod blew out a puff of air that sounded like a hiss. "My son? I doubt it!" Rod grabbed the edge of the table and was about to slide out of the booth. Freebird grabbed his hand and jerked it hard.

"Rod! Listen to me! The boy is your son! The minute I saw him I knew he was your blood. Do you think I would be here now telling you this if I was not sure?"

Rod stared at his friend, incredulous, but made no further attempt to leave. He trusted Freebird with his life and knew Freebird would never knowingly do anything to hurt him. "What does she want from me? Money for the kid?"

Freebird gave Rod a dark look. "No, man! She just wants the boy to know who his father is."

Rod stared blankly at Freebird for a moment. He knew his friend would not lie to him. Could it be that Martina's rumored baby was his? He did have some recollections of those long afternoons of lovemaking on the days she was released from the Juvenile Intervention Facility to visit with him, and he knew that neither of them had ever taken any precautions to prevent her from becoming pregnant. Back then, he secretly hoped that she would get pregnant, thinking that maybe then the court would recognize their marriage as legitimate and they could have some kind of a normal life.

Realizing that what Freebird was telling him could possibly be true, a slight measure of hope and excitement crystallized inside of him. But such positive feelings had been dormant within him for so long Rod was unable to process them right away. In truth, he was afraid of hope and excitement; they could only lead to hurt and pain.

Relaxing his grip on Rod's hand, Freebird could surmise his friend's conflicted feelings. "It's entirely up to you, Buddy. But he's a beautiful little boy and if you saw him you'd know he's your blood."

"What's his name?" Rod asked, obviously considering Freebird's words.

"Roddy."

"She named him after me?" Rod said, surprised.

"She loves you, Rod."

"Then why did she leave me, Freebird?" Rod's question came straight from his broken heart and carried with it all of his bottled up bitterness and pain.

"She was young, afraid, confused…her father had just dumped her at some kind of a clinic…to get an abortion. Then some asshole Millborough detective told her you had been killed. She even had to go for psychiatric counseling to get over the whole thing. You really need to talk to her, Rod. If for nothing else, to just understand why she left. She was so shocked last night when I told her you were alive she almost passed out." Freebird could see that Rod was mulling over what he told him. For good measure, he added, "I don't think life has been easy for her either, Rod."

Rod sunk back in the booth, his mind completely log-jammed with thoughts and confusing emotions. "My God!" He whispered to himself. Slowly, it was starting to sink in that he might possibly have a child. He wanted to believe it but needed his own proof. "Are you positive about the boy being mine?" He asked Freebird again.

"Well…let me put it this way…not only is he the spitting image of you, he takes after you in a certain other way that really convinced me he is your kid."

Rod looked up at Freebird, curious. "What way is that?"

"He likes to suck on his Mama's tits and pitches one hell of a fit if she won't let him," Freebird said, flashing Rod a knowing grin.

Rod's expression suddenly grew concerned. "Why won't she let him?" He was now thinking about how much he had enjoyed fondling and sucking Martina's breasts.

"Jesus, Rod! He's eighteen months old. He's getting kind of big for doing that." Then Freebird added, "That's why he needs his Daddy…to teach him how to be a man. He needs a man to show him how to do other things, too."

Freebird's last statements seemed to hit home with Rod, who had a lot of good memories of spending time with his own father. "When can I see him?" asked Rod, suddenly feeling eager.

"When do you want to see him?"

"Today. Now."

Freebird nodded and got up from the table. "Let's go," he told Rod, smiling and feeling great happiness for his friend. More than anything, he hoped that once Rod saw little Roddy he would snap back to his old self. He sure missed his old friend.

45.

On the outskirts of Millborough, Freebird stopped at a gas station payphone to call Julie and tell her he was bringing Rod to the house to see Martina and Roddy. "Get yourself and Jody ready and we'll go to the park for a while, so they can be alone together. They really need to talk," he told his wife and hung up the phone. Freebird took his time driving home in order to give Julie and Martina enough time to get themselves and the babies organized. He couldn't help but be pleased with the way it turned out with Rod; Freebird never expected Rod would want to see Martina and Roddy this soon, if at all. He figured he must have done something right. Perhaps it was a good idea to take Rod to North Hampton after all.

"Just one favor." said Rod, "Stop by Carol's so I can pick up my car. That way, you won't have to take me home later."

"No problem," Freebird said with a broad smile, unable to conceal his happiness.

When Julie announced that Freebird was on his way home with Rod, Martina went into a panic. She plucked Roddy out of the sandbox and hauled him into the bathroom for a quick bath and change. "Daddy's coming," she excitedly told the crying boy, but since he never had the experience of a daddy he didn't understand why he was in the bathtub when he wanted to be back in the sandbox. Further adding to the child's frustration, once he was scrubbed, dried, and changed into one of his dressy outfits he was unable to escape from the bedroom. Martina had locked the bedroom door, so Roddy could not run back to the sandbox and get himself dirty again. He hung from the unyielding doorknob and screamed while Martina changed into a long, colorfully patterned Gypsy skirt that accented her lithe body and a coordinating purple Spandex top with a low cut neckline that accented her ample breasts. After applying her make-up, she then pulled her long, thick hair over one shoulder and quickly plaited it. Just as she finished tying the end of her braid, Julie knocked on the bedroom door and announced that Freebird's truck and Rod's Corvette had just pulled into the driveway.

The thought that she would be standing in the same room with Rod within seconds caused her to break out in a nervous sweat. She ran back into the bathroom to dab the back of her neck and forehead with a cool facecloth. When Roddy trailed behind her into the bathroom she tried dabbing his face, too. By then, the child had stopped crying but his cheeks were beet red and his long eyelashes were wet with tears. She picked him up and held him close, kissing his warm face. "Okay, Roddy. It's show time," she told the child. Opening the bedroom door, she could hear Freebird and Julie laughing in the living room, and then she heard the familiar sound of Rod's voice. Her entire body began to vibrate.

Julie had warned her beforehand that Rod had lost a lot of weight since the accident, but Martina was not prepared for the gaunt version of Rod McDonough who now stood in the living room. Her heart ached to see him so pale and thin. For a brief moment their eyes locked, and then Rod's gaze naturally fell upon the little boy in Martina's arms. Instantly, Rod knew the child was his son.

Not knowing what Rod's reaction to seeing her and Roddy would be, Martina stood stalk still, watching his expression. When she saw the tenseness of his expression soften, she knew he had recognized his own likeness in Roddy, and she relaxed her guard.

"Hello, Rod," she said, her sultry voice was soft and tentative, and her sea green eyes gentle and hopeful.

Inclining his head to acknowledge Martina's greeting, Rod was momentarily tongue-tied by the close proximity of the woman who haunted his days and nights, and he thought she looked more beautiful than ever. And he could easily see that the little boy she held in her arms was every bit a McDonough. Knowing the moment called for him to say something, he was surprised to hear the words, "It's nice to see you again, Martina" come spilling out of his mouth. Despite having nurtured a hard-held anger toward Martina for so long, the physical presence of her and the little boy – his son – now standing only inches away from him, quickly overpowered and then extinguished his animosity. And as his anger dissipated, he started to feel the lively beat of his heart again.

Freebird and Julie looked at each other and knew it was time for them to leave. Quietly, they slipped out the front door with Jody. The only one who noticed their departure was Roddy, who pointed at his new little friend and cried out, "Yoee!" Martina laughed at the cuteness of his expression and kissed his cheek. "Jody will be back soon," she assured him. Then, turning to face Rod, she told the boy, "This is your Daddy...can you say 'Hi' to your Daddy?" Roddy looked at the stranger for a moment, uncertain. "Say 'Hi Daddy!'" Martina gently coaxed. Deciding to be shy, Roddy buried his face in his mother's shoulder. Then, slowly, the boy turned his head to peak up at Rod and broke into a wide grin. For a moment, the little boy and his father smiled at each other, making their first acquaintance.

Clearly mesmerized, Rod's eyes glowed with amazement, as he visually familiarized himself with every feature and physical characteristic of his son, noting his baby-fine, curly brown hair; the big, intelligent blue-green eyes that were studying him, as well; the turned up McDonough nose that would surely look like his one day; the way his perfect little bow-like lips surrounding the tiny thumb he was sucking; his pudgy fist and the smoothness of his off-white skin; the rounded belly and chubby, solid legs. So absorbed by his immediate need to know every aspect of his little boy, Rod automatically reached out to touch the baby-soft skin of Roddy's pudgy arm. As if Roddy knew this was an important moment in his life, as well as the life of the man who was gently stroking his arm, the little boy stayed quietly molded against his mother's body and curiously eyed the stranger.

If the first glimpse of his son had awakened Rod's heart, the sensation of touching his little body had the effect of recharging his mind and, ultimately, his spirit. Rod was suddenly overcome by the realization that he and Martina had created this amazing, perfect little boy from the incredible love they had once shared. Unable to hold back the intensity of his emotions any longer, tears filled his eyes and ran down his face. He made no effort to wipe them away—they seemed an affirmation of this wondrous moment, and he was grateful to be feeling such joy again.

Tears were something Roddy could relate to, even though he didn't yet comprehend that people also cry when they are happy. Seeing the tears on Rod's face, the little boy released his thumb from his mouth and extended his chubby arm toward Rod, and with a look of concern, he said, "No cwi." Those were the first words his son spoke to him and they were words of comfort. The sound of his son's baby voice, so innocent and caring, filled Rod's heart with a rush of love he had never experienced before. It was not the same kind of love he had felt for Martina; this strange, new feeling was a different kind of love, more protective and unconditional. Paternal. And Rod would never forget the sound of his son's baby voice or those first two words the child said to him for as long as he lived.

Rod took hold of the little hand extended toward him and held it in his palm, studying the perfect little fingers. He ached to hold the boy in his arms and feel the weight of him against his own body. As if sensing Rod's desire, Martina whispered into the boy's ear, "Give Daddy a big,

big hug." The little boy sized up Rod for a moment and then leaned out toward him. Rod gingerly took the boy in his arms and held him close, simply feeling his nearness and smelling the scent of his skin. When Roddy tried to wiggle free of Rod's embrace and held out his arms to his mother for her to reclaim him, Martina told the little boy, "I'll bet your Daddy will play in the sandbox with you." Hearing the magic word sandbox, Roddy's eyes widened with excitement. The boy looked at Rod and pointed in the general direction of the backyard. The word "sandbox" was too much of a tongue twister for the child, so he jiggled his body and said, "Go-see."

Delighted by the interaction with his son but at a loss to understand his language, Rod looked to Martina for translation. "What did he say?" he asked, laughing at the boy's excitement.

"He said he wants to go outside and play in the sandbox with you," Martina answered, with tears brimming in her own eyes. She was so happy to see Rod alive and holding his son she could hardly believe the scene before her was really happening. She ached to touch him, put her arms around him, but her desires would have to wait. There was a gap between them that could not be quickly bridged, she knew. She also knew that this was not the time for her and Rod to talk about the past or their feelings. This moment belonged strictly to Roddy and his Daddy.

"Come," she told Rod, wiping her tears with her hands. "I'll take you to the sandbox."

46.

The sight of Rod sitting in the sandbox with Roddy and building sand forts was much too funny for Martina not to laugh. She ran back inside the house to get her camera, and on the way back out she stopped in the kitchen to pour two tall glasses of iced tea and fill Roddy's sippy cup with fresh apple juice. When she stepped out onto the patio, balancing the glasses, the little cup, and the camera on a metal serving tray, Rod joked, "Look, Roddy! Here comes the pretty waitress with our drinks."

Roddy looked up and laughed as though he understood his father's joke. The little boy pointed at Martina and said, "Mama!"

"Yes, Roddy. That's your Mama," Rod said, smiling warmly at the boy. Then pointing to his own chest, he told the child, "Daddy! I am your Daddy!" To Martina, Rod's tone sounded like an affirmation and her heart flooded with relief and happiness to hear him acknowledge Roddy as his son.

Roddy listened intently to his father's words and then pointed to Rod's chest with his stubby little index finger and said "Dah-dee."

Rod's face lit up like a 300-watt bulb. "Did you hear that, Martina? He said Daddy!" Rod reached over and picked up the child and thrust him upward over his head. Roddy giggled and kicked his chubby little legs with excitement.

Martina grabbed her camera and began snapping photos. She was ecstatic to finally see her little family together, even if it was just for Roddy's sake. After taking nearly an entire roll of sandbox shots, Martina set the camera down on the picnic table and realized that in her rush to take the photographs she had forgotten all about the drinks. Picking up a glass of iced tea and the little blue sippy cup, she walked over to the sandbox to give Rod his drink. She had intended to give the apple juice to Roddy herself, to make sure he drank it, but Rod took the sippy cup from her hand as well as his glass.

He examined the sippy cup and chuckled. "Haven't seen one of these in a long time." He looked over at Roddy and saw the boy was busy covering his plastic soldiers with sand. "Hey Little Buddy," Rod called to the happy and contented child. "How about some juice?" The child took the cup from Rod's extended hand, took a long sip, and handed it back. After babbling something that remotely sounded like a "thank you," Roddy went back to his play. Rod smiled at the boy's serious, little old man behavior. He could easily see that Martina was a very good mother and was doing a good job raising him. The child looked healthy and happy and seemed very well behaved for being just a little tyke. Rod couldn't help but feel a strong sense of loss for having missed Martina's pregnancy, the birth of his son, and the past eighteen months of the little boy's life. But now was not the time to bring it up; Freebird had cautioned him to tread lightly because Martina was just getting over the shock of finding out he was alive. And there would be time later to talk about the past; he would make sure of that.

So, for the rest of the morning, Martina and Rod kept their conversation light and restricted to the present. At noon, Martina stood up from her patio chair and announced to Roddy that it was time to get washed up for lunch. By then, the toddler had worked up quite an appetite from all of his excitement and rolling around on the grass with his "Dah-dee," so he followed Rod back to the patio without a fuss. Rod fell into one of the chairs, looking exhausted. He had sand stuck to his sweaty skin and grass stains on the knees of his jeans, but his big smile brightened his gaunt face. "I'm out of shape," he told Martina. Adding, "That little guy kicked my ass."

"Ash," repeated Roddy, who stood between them.

"Whoops!" Rod said, embarrassed. "I'm going to have to watch my vocabulary around him."

Martina nodded in agreement. "He's very smart...and he doesn't miss a trick. He reminds me a lot of his father." Pulling Roddy onto her lap, she began removing his sand-filled shoes and socks.

Rod smiled at her reference to him. Automatically, he leaned over and started helping Martina take off one of Roddy's shoes, examining the tiny little sneaker with an amused expression on his face.

After dusting the sand from between Roddy's toes, Martina stood him on the patio and removed his sandy clothes and soggy diaper. Rod marveled at the wonderfully rounded physique of his little son, certain that he was the most beautiful baby that had ever been born. With his brown curly hair, bright blue-green eyes, rosy cheeks, and chubby bottom, Rod thought he looked like a cherub straight out of a Rubens painting. The tears were suddenly back in Rod's eyes and along with them came a sizeable lump in his throat. His love for this little boy, who only just came into his life, seemed to be growing with every second he spent with him. And there was no doubt in his mind that Roddy was his son; the boy was the carbon copy of him at that age.

"Okay, Nature Boy! Time for a quick bath," Martina said, gathering up his clothes.

"I need to use the rest room," Rod told her. "Where is it?"

"Good!" She told him. "Please take your son with you and show him how the big boys pee. I'm at a bit of a disadvantage when it comes to potty training a little boy, and this diaper routine is getting really old."

"Are you sure that's a good idea?" Rod asked, visibly concerned. "I mean...I wouldn't want to do the wrong thing and then have him turn out...you know...." Rod swished his wrist for emphasis.

"For goodness sake, Rod. Where did you ever get an idea like that? Don't make a big deal about it. Just leave the door open and he'll watch what you're doing and that's it. After he sees you using the potty, he'll want to use it, too, since you are now his new best buddy."

Rod shrugged and followed Martina to the guest bathroom. "Just give it your best shot," Martina said, oblivious to the pun she just made.

"Very funny," Rod said, over his shoulder, as he lifted the toilet seat, and as Martina predicted Roddy followed his Daddy into the bathroom.

When Rod emerged laughing, with Roddy in tow, she asked, "How'd it go?"

"Well...he's a keen observer. He wanted to give it a shot, as you say. His heart is in the right place but unfortunately his equipment is a little low to the ground. He needs a little stool to stand on. But I stood him up on the rim and he did his business like a champ."

Martina looked down at the little boy, who was sucking his thumb and smiling sheepishly. "Did you go potty like a big boy?" She excitedly asked Roddy, who merely giggled a response. "What a good boy you are," she praised the toddler "Let's get in the tub, young man." Picking him up, she carried him over to the tub and turned the water on. Then, turning to Rod, she asked, "Would you like to help with his bath?" She saw his face brighten at the invitation. "You can soap him down," she suggested, thinking it would be a good bonding experience for both father and son.

Taking the soapy washcloth from Martina's hand, Rod knelt beside the tub and began washing the boy from head to toe, carefully avoiding the genital area. Thinking he was finished, he continued to kneel and watch Roddy play in the water with his plastic bath toys Rod was completely fascinated by the child's imaginative interaction with the various toy animals.

"You missed a spot," Martina commented to Rod.

"Where?" Rod looked over the boy. "I got his neck and ears...in between his toes."

"You missed the most important area on a baby...the diaper area," she advised.

"Maybe you should do the washing," Rod told her, somewhat embarrassed. "He's more used to you doing it."

Martina could see that Rod was uncomfortable with the idea of touching his son's private parts, and wanting to immediately dispel his phobia, she tackled the subject head-on. "Don't you think boy's can become overly attached to their mother's, too? It's really all in the way you deal with it, Rod. Babies are born innocent. It's the parents who have the hang-ups. You are not going to influence his masculinity one way or the other if you just wash his body." She took the washcloth from him and rolled her eyes in disbelief.

Rod considered her words for a moment and recognized she was right. "I guess it was the way I was raised," he explained. "My father was a man's man and expected my brother Travis and me to be the same way when we grew up. He didn't even hug or kiss us good night when we were kids. That was just his way, but we knew he loved us from the way he spent time with us, teaching us to fish and hunt."

Watching the way Martina tenderly talked to their son as she washed him, Rod marveled at how much she had grown and matured since having Roddy. He could see that she was an exceptional mother and noted the way the boy responded to her. It seemed to him that her entire day was involved with the care and feeding of one little boy, and he couldn't help but wonder what kind of a social life she could possibly have. The thought had crossed his mind that Martina might be in a relationship with another man and he felt a stab of jealousy. Yet, if she were, he could not fault her for it, since she had believed she was a widow. And she was, after all, a beautiful young woman, living in San Francisco, which was known far and wide as a happening city. Nevertheless, Rod could not stomach the thought of his wife being with another man, or someone else raising his son. Freebird had not been able to give him any information on her status in that regard, and Rod was aching to know if there was any hope of them getting back together. He needed to know.

"So...what do you do for excitement when you are not feeding, bathing, or changing little Master McDonough?"

Martina almost laughed at the transparency of Rod's question. "What you really want to know is whether or not I am involved with another man," she said, wringing out the washcloth and setting it on the ledge of the tub. "Let me explain something to you right now—just so we don't ever have to have this discussion again. Yes! My life centers on Roddy, because I'm his mother…and a single parent. I'm not seeing anyone in particular. In fact, I don't date at all. I tried going out on dates a couple of times but it wasn't for me. I've already found the love of my life…and you know the ending of that story better than I do. I know about the rumors that went around Millborough after I left. But I can assure you that Roddy is your son and no one else's." She paused and stared him straight in the eyes, then added for emphasis, "End of story!"

"End of story," said Rod, feeling chagrined for prying, but nonetheless ecstatic to know there was no man in her life.

"Now, let's get our little Master McDonough out of the tub. It's getting way past his lunch time and he'll soon be needing a nap." Grabbing Roddy's towel from the bar, she handed it to Rod, who then wrapped up the boy and brought him over to the bed to dry him off.

Digging around in the suitcase that contained most of Roddy's clothes, Martina pulled out a T-shirt and a pair of training briefs. "Since Roddy is using the potty now, he can wear big boy briefs," she announced with an excited tone that was meant as praise for the little boy's recent achievement.

When Rod finished dressing Roddy, he picked the boy up and started tossing him in the air. Roddy squealed with excitement, yelling "Mo! Mo!" Rod understood he was saying "more."

Martina watched, concerned that it was nearly an hour past Roddy's lunch time but hesitant to spoil their fun. She enjoyed seeing the natural way the father and son played together. It was like Roddy knew that Rod was more than just a stranger who came by to play with him.

It wasn't long before Rod was out of breath from the tossing and catching and had to quit. "I must really be out of shape," Rod remarked, surprised by his lack of stamina. He continued to hold Roddy in his arms, not wanting to let him go. Looking at the boy's rosy, happy face, Rod spontaneously gave the boy a kiss on the cheek and hugged him a little tighter. He felt his heart surge with such paternal love and pride he was amazed by the intensity of the feeling. Closing his eyes, Rod concentrated on the warm, wonderful soft feel of his son.

Unaware that his father had run out of steam, Roddy squirmed and tried to break free of his father's embrace. "Mo! Mo up!" the little boy cried, pointing to the ceiling. Martina smiled, seeing the obvious pleasure on Rod's face. "I'm going to fix us some lunch," she said, then remembered all the water Roddy had gulped when he was in the tub. "You might want to take him potty again...especially after getting him so excited."

Rod looked at Martina, puzzled. "What does his excitement have to do with his going potty?"

"I don't know, Rod. He gets excited and then he has to pee. That's just what he does."

Rod shrugged and looked at Roddy with amusement. "Is that what you do when you get excited, boy? You pee? I sure hope you grow out of that habit by the time you're old enough to chase women."

Martina headed for the kitchen and was half way down the hall when she heard Rod calling her back. He sounded panicked. She ran back to the bathroom to see what he wanted. "What's wrong?" She cried, as she entered the bathroom. Roddy was standing on the rim of the toilet and Rod was holding him steady.

Pointing to Roddy's briefs, Rod exclaimed, "These briefs don't work. They have no opening in the front. Are these little girl's panties, Martina?"

"That's the way they make training briefs for little boys Roddy's age. He doesn't have the coordination to use regular boy's briefs." Reaching over to Roddy, Martina pulled his briefs down to his knees. And while she and Rod were arguing the finer points of training briefs, they suddenly heard the sound of water splashing in the toilet. Turning to look at Roddy, they saw he was peeing.

"See! They work!" said Martina.

47.

Martina sat next to Roddy, who was enthroned in Jody's highchair, and patiently helped the boy spoon the noodle soup into his mouth. In between feeding Roddy, she snatched bites of her ham and cheese sandwich. Rod sat on the other side of Roddy, eating his sandwich and studying Martina's profile. In so many ways, she seemed different to him. She had always been mature for her age. Even when she was seventeen she was more adult in her manner and way of thinking than some of the women he had dated, who were in their twenties. Now, she seemed so confident and at complete peace with herself. Her sea green eyes radiated her inner joy and her skin glowed with a healthy sheen. And motherhood had changed the shape of her body. The skinny girl with the ample breasts and narrow hips had matured into a lissome woman with fuller breasts and slightly broader, but still very proportionate, hips. Rod imagined Martina would be one of those women, who would always be sexy and glamorous, even when she was well past what was considered a woman's prime. Her beauty would be ageless.

From where Rod was seated he had an unobstructed view of Martina's cleavage and the way her breasts strained against the front of her Spandex top. He wondered if motherhood had changed the appearance of her nipples, which he had always found so erotic. He hoped not. The sudden desire to lie naked with her and see every inch of her new mother's body came upon him like a ravenous ghost from the shadows of his memory. But even if such an opportunity arose, things were different now. It was not just him and her, with uninterrupted hours to do as they pleased. Now, he realized, there were the needs of a child to consider.

Martina had noticed Rod's frank stare and asked, "Will you be able to stay a little longer? Roddy will be going down for his nap and I'm hoping we can talk then."

"I'll stay as long as you want me to, Martina," he responded, his tone soft and sincere. Then seeing that her sandwich was still half eaten, he suggested, "How about if I try my hand at feeding him…so you can finish your sandwich before it gets stale?"

His offer reminded her of how thoughtful he had always been, before all of the trouble. It was his sensitivity she had found so surprising and attractive when they first met; she did not expect it from a biker she had met in an alley in North Hampton. Her thoughts of the day they met brought a dreamy, romantic smile to her sensual lips, which Rod mistook as gratitude for his offer to feed Roddy.

"Oh— Thank you, Rod. But there's no playing around when he's eating. We don't want him to get the idea that eating is just more playtime."

Rod stood up and saluted. "Yes, Ma'am!" he acknowledged, in the manner of a Marine recruit.

"I'm serious, Rod. We want Roddy to be a good eater and not play with his food."

Rod looked at his son and saw the boy was intently shoveling a spoon full of noodles into his mouth with the help of his fingers. "Point taken," he said, more seriously. Although, he was actually dumbfounded by all of the rules and regulations for the governance of one little boy.

Martina rose from her chair and absentmindedly patted his arm. Her touch, albeit innocent and light, surprised and encouraged him. Rod stood in front of her, hemming her into the narrow space between the chairs and table. Looking up at him, she saw reflected in his eyes all of the same emotions that she, too, had been struggling with—the pain of their separation; the joy of seeing each other again; the desire to be close to each other again; and the fear that it might now be too late to recapture any of the closeness they once shared. Had too much happened to each of them since being apart that would now prevent them from being together? They stared at each other for a few moments, each wondering about the possibilities. Then, Rod reached out and brushed her cheek lightly with his fingers, as though testing the realness of her. The contact with her smooth, caramel skin sent a shockwave of desire through his body. Suddenly, his arms were around her and his mouth was pressing down hungrily on her lips.

For the briefest of moments, Martina was willingly carried away by the familiar ecstasy of Rod's touch and the warmth of his body against hers. But as his kissing and caressing became more heated and urgent she knew she would have to stop him for the sake of their son. She suddenly worried that the child might get frightened by what they were doing. Just then, as if Martina had psychically tuned in to the little boy's thoughts, he started fussing and calling for her Pushing against Rod's chest, she tried to break free from his embrace. But Rod, who was not used to sharing Martina's affections, held onto her more tightly. "Rod! Please stop!" She tried to sound forceful enough to get Rod's attention without upsetting the baby even more than he was. "We can't do this now. We've got the baby to take care of." At first, Martina thought he was not going to let her go but, then, slowly, he loosened his hold and backed off. He seemed somewhat confused by his own behavior. Martina had never known Rod to be so possessive, but she attributed his unwillingness to let her go to their separation and all that he had been through. And since she had assumed a heavy load of guilt for what her father had done to him, her heart went out to him.

"I— I'm sorry!" He said, after regaining his composure, giving Martina a quick, uneasy smile as he handed her the plate with her half-eaten sandwich. Then, slipping into Martina's vacated chair, he eyed the little boy with the mixed emotions of any new father: knowing he loved this child, who was a part of him and the love he had for his mother, yet resenting the fact that he now had to share Martina with him. He was faced with the realization that any relationship he would have with Martina from now on would be forever changed, and he would have to adjust to it accordingly. Would they ever again be able to spend long, sensual afternoons in the bathtub without interruption, he wondered. Was he even ready to accept the reality of being a parent?

48.

Certainly, it was not the lack of physical desire for Rod that caused Martina to resist his advances. If only he knew the seconds that turned into endless days and nights when she nearly went crazy with the desire to just simply feel the touch of his hand—just once. Martina's desire for Rod had never ebbed; if anything, it grew stronger every time she looked at their son. And that was the reason she was resisting him now; she was alarmed about where kissing him would lead. They both had Roddy to think of. She knew that Rod didn't understand that just yet but, in time, she hoped he would. She saw his injured look when she pushed away from him. Martina remembered what a difficult transformation it was for her to rebuild her own life around a new baby, but she had had the benefit of a day-to-day adjustment. Rod, on the other hand, had to do a crash course.

When Martina finished her lunch, she wiped off the table and put the dirty dishes in the dishwasher. Then, she wiped Roddy's face and hands with paper towels and cleaned the mess in the tray of the high chair. Rod watched as she efficiently put the room back in order. Her constant movement made him almost dizzy. When she had finished, he thought perhaps they could then sit in the living room and talk. He should have known better. There was a whole new set of procedures for getting the boy settled down for his nap. First, Rod had to take him potty one more time. Then Martina tried to put a diaper back on him for his nap, but Roddy didn't want to wear a diaper and pulled it off, protesting loudly. Rather than make an issue of it, Martina sat down on the bed, adjusted the pillows behind her, and slipped off her Spandex top. The sight of her bare breasts was like the answer to a prayer for both of the McDonough men. Completely caught off guard, Rod sucked in a deep breath of air and blew it back out. Not only had motherhood increased the size of her breasts they were more erotic than ever. And while Rod merely gaped, his bare-bottomed son wasted no time in scrambling up onto his mother's lap and immediately latching on to the handiest nipple with his mouth and fondling the other with a chubby hand. Settling right in, the little boy closed his eyes and seemed to float off to Nirvana. His diaper outrage now forgotten.

Rod sat at the bottom of the bed and watched with envy as his son peacefully snuggled at his mother's breast and Martina gently stroked the little boy's face. Rod thought about pitching a fit himself. Not only did the little tyke command all of Martina's attentions and usurp the afternoon bath scene, he was now the sole proprietor of those beautiful breasts. Feeling his stare, Martina looked at Rod and saw the bereft expression on his face. She motioned for him to come and lie down beside her. Taking a cue from his son's playbook, Rod wasted no time stretching out alongside of her. Martina took hold his hand and gently squeezed. It was her subtle way of making him feel included and letting him know that she would always have time for him, too. Turning to face him, she smiled, contented beyond words that he was there with her. With her beautiful, full lips so close, Rod could not restrain himself from touching them with his own. She did not stop him this time. Instead, she parted her lips to receive his tongue and caressed it with her own. After several minutes of exchanging their tender kisses, she whispered, "Let's put Roddy in the crib in Jody's room."

Rod hoisted the sleeping boy into his arms and watched as Martina put the Spandex top back on and tug it into place. Gathering up her long skirt, she then scooted off of the bed. He observed that she was no longer shy with him about her nakedness, as though her breasts were now only utilitarian containers for the delivery of nourishment to their son and no longer available for erotic purposes.

When she stood up, he drank in her flawlessly smooth skin, her luminous green eyes, and the way her long skirt swayed around her ankles. He could easily envision her on the South Seas island of her ancestors, standing on the white sands of a tropical cove with a sea-green ocean that matched her eyes. Her exotic beauty never failed to captivate him. Some day, he told himself, he would love to take her to that island. But, for now, he followed her across the hall to Jody's nursery, where he gently placed Roddy in the crib, covering his bare bottom with a blanket Martina had brought with her. Silently, they stood beside the crib for a few moments, watching their sleeping child, and taking in the immensity of their creation. Then, taking hold of Rod's hand, she led him back to the bedroom, where they stood facing each other, now suddenly unsure of how they should begin the journey forward. The intensity of their episode in the kitchen reminded Rod of the lie he had been living. Ever since the moment he learned that Martina had left him he steeped himself in an anger toward her that he fabricated as a diversion from the truth. It was easier for him to deal with the pain of her absence by telling himself she was "nothing but a no good whore." But in that deep inner self, where a person's true beliefs are held, Rod knew Martina was no such thing. The simple fact was that his ego, which had been wounded far worse than his body, was humiliated by the ugly rumors circulating Millborough about Martina and her father. Instead of going after his wife and standing by her as he should have, he had succumbed to self-pity. He had been stupid and weak. And for his stupidity he had paid dearly: The loss of two years of being with the woman he truly loved and missing the birth of his son.

Just thinking about his little boy and the fact that he was now a father brightened his thoughts immeasurably and brought him quickly back to the present. By some miracle, he was now standing in the same room with Martina and he had no intention of letting his ego get in the way again. Rod couldn't help but draw the conclusion that he and Martina were put together again for a reason; with her coming all the way from California it was simply too extraordinary to be a mere coincidence. Their being together now was beyond coincidence – it was meant to be. He was convinced.

They stood quietly, searching the depths of each other's eyes for a long time before any words were spoken.

"He's a beautiful little boy...our son," Rod said, finally breaking the silence. His voice was soft, conveying much emotion and pride. Lowering his head, he started to say, "I only wish—"

Martina cut him off. "Don't say it!" Her tone was soft and comforting, but she did not want their first meaningful conversation to go astray with recriminations and what-ifs. She reached toward him and placed her slender index finger against his lips, and then said, "There is no time for wishing that things had been different...the point is that we are here now and where do we go from this time forward?"

For a moment, Rod studied the fine aspects of her face and then locked his gaze upon her phosphorescent green eyes. Releasing a deep sigh of emotion, he took her in his arms and held her gently against his body. "I want us to be together again," he whispered with deep, tremendous feeling as he caressed her hair with his lips. "I've been so lost without you...I can't let you go again...I can't let my son go...."

Becoming too emotional to continue, Rod's words dissolved into a heavy sigh. Martina felt the heaving of Rod's chest and automatically began stroking his shoulders and back. Then her own tears erupted and for the next several minutes they could only cling to each other for support.

Finally, Martina said, "When you talk about being lost without the person you love, I know exactly what you mean. When I landed in San Francisco I was so miserable without you. Then I was told you were dead. You cannot imagine the awful emptiness I felt, thinking you were gone forever from my life. I wanted to die, too. If it weren't for our baby I don't think I would have made it, Rod. And my Aunt Catherine and Uncle Jack…they took me right into their home and treated me like I was their daughter. They had this quiet, steady life and here comes this pregnant teenager, whose father had just been arrested for shooting her boyfriend, and the Millborough Police are telling them that my baby might be my father's child. My life was a mess. My aunt and uncle didn't even know I was married or pregnant when I got there. They learned about it all from the police. But through it all they stuck by me and helped me through the worst time of my life. And when Roddy was born they were so thrilled. They consider Roddy their grandchild and they spoil him rotten with love. They didn't want me to make this trip back here. And I almost didn't come." She paused, her mind suddenly commandeered by the thought of how close she came to not being in this moment and not knowing Rod was alive.

Rod tightened his arms around her. "I guess it all comes down to the hand of fate," he said. "I could have easily died. I was close enough to it. But here I am and here you are. We're suddenly brought back together again. How does something like that get orchestrated?"

Martina shook her head. "I don't know, Rod. It's one of life's mysteries. It must be fate."

"Is the hand of fate really the hand of God, I wonder?" He paused briefly to collect his thoughts, and then he went on. "I've never bought into any religious belief system, but when something like this happens it makes you wonder about a higher power."

She sighed heavily. "I would have to believe there is a higher power at work in a situation like this. There just has to be."

He studied her face for a moment, his expression serious and contemplative. Then, lowering his lips to hers, he began kissing her. Gently. Reverently.

49.

While Rod was in the bathroom Martina sat on the edge of the bed thinking about all that had transpired since Freebird brought Rod to the house that morning. It was like three days' worth of activity compressed into only several hours. Suddenly feeling exhausted, she flopped over onto the pillows and stretched out on her back. Instantly, her body felt like it was melting into the mattress. Still suffering the effects of jet lag from yesterday's long flight, all of this heavy emotional stuff with Rod had really taken its toll. Her energy level was already zapped and the day was not nearly over. Roddy would be up from his nap and rearing to go in another hour or so, and she and Rod had yet to have their "talk." And talk they must, especially if they intended to get back together. But right this second, she needed to close her eyes for just a minute. Martina heard the bathroom door open and the sound of Rod's stocking-muffled footsteps coming toward the bed.

"May I join you?" he asked, sounding a bit tired himself.

"Absolutely!" She motioned to the empty space next to her and felt the mattress move under his weight as he snuggled up against her. His face was damp and she could smell the fresh scent of soap. She shifted onto her side to face him and they immediately locked in an embrace.

There was none of the frenzied removal of clothing that almost always preceded their couplings, such as when they lived together on Scenic Drive. Probably because they were too physically and emotionally exhausted to summon that kind of frenetic energy. They simply took it slow and easy, each fully aware that they were no longer the same two people they were before their separation, and this moment simply did not call for the kind of raw passion they ignited together in the early days of their marriage. The very fact that they were together at all was almost too overwhelming for them to comprehend. When Martina first slipped her hand under Rod's shirt she was shocked to feel how thin and spare his body had become. It was as though she was touching the body of a stranger. He didn't feel at all like the way her hands remembered him. Used to the feel of brawny muscles, her fingertips now encountered an unfamiliar terrain of boney protuberances and a cascading rib cage. An aching sadness came over her, and as she burrowed against him protectively her cheek brushed against an unusual fleshy bump on his chest. Instinctively, she brought her hand to the spot, which was a few inches below his left shoulder, and traced the crinkled surface of the area with her fingers.

Immediately, she knew what it was and despite all of her months of counseling with Dr. Renfrew the reality of touching the scar on Rod's body filled her with a terrible guilt and shame.

Rod felt Martina's fingers exploring the scar where the bullet exited his chest after her father shot him in the back. Hearing her gasp of realization, he quickly removed her hand from the scar and held it in his. From the moment she had unbuttoned his shirt Rod prepared himself for her reaction, not only to the dissipation of his body but especially to the bullet wounds. So it was not unexpected that she would become emotional by those things. He was glad the moment was behind them but, now, he needed to put the matter of the shooting permanently to rest.

"Martina!" He said, squeezing her hand to get her attention. Feeling her nod her head in response, he continued, "Don't be upset. It doesn't hurt me any…and actually I'm pretty lucky."

"Lucky? How?" She asked, still choked up with emotion.

"I was lucky that your father was a lousy shot," he said, trying to make light of the moment. He hoped a bit of levity would change her mood. When there was no reaction from her right away he then worried that his attempt at humor had missed the mark. When after a few seconds the sad expression on her face dissolved, almost giving way to a smile, he released a sigh of relief. Taking heart, he added, "And I'm even luckier to have you right here in my arms…and to have a beautiful son…who is taking a long nap so we can have this time alone together." He paused to scatter kisses across her forehead, and then reminded her, "Aren't you the one who said we shouldn't get hung up on recriminations?" Then, before Martina could respond, Rod playfully rolled her onto her back and pressed his lips to hers, telegraphing his intentions with the sensual in and out movement of his tongue. Simply tasting the sweetness of her mouth was almost more than Rod could bear. But there was also the familiar essence of her body. The spicy patchouli fragrance of her hair. The remembered whole deliciousness of her. These subtle energies of taste and smell all combined to tantalize and awaken his senses. Even the warmth that emanated from her body enveloped and excited him. Hungry to see and taste her entire body, Rod slowly peeled away her clothes.

50.

"Please don't be upset," Martina encouraged Rod with a soft, comforting tone. Her crestfallen husband stared up at the white flocked ceiling, while she attempted to resuscitate his wounded ego. After several intrepid attempts to rise to the occasion he was vanquished by the one formidable enemy he should have anticipated – a traitorous penis. And he was taking it hard. Continuing with her assuagement, she brushed her lips against Rod's ear and murmured, "You've been through a lot Rod...."

Rod did not answer her. He continued his dejected stare, feeling embarrassed and useless. He knew Martina meant well but her words of comfort only made him feel worse. The fact was that he knew exactly why he could not get it on with her; his impotence had nothing to do with what he had gone through after he was shot. At least not in the sense of lingering health issues relating to the chain of physical injuries he suffered as a result of that incident. He did not need an epiphany from on high to understand that it was the opiates he allowed himself to become hooked on after the shooting, when he had found out Martina had left him.

Rod's lack of response only fueled Martina's efforts to comfort him. When that didn't work she then attempted to slake him with a more practical observation. "Perhaps it's for the best, Rod. We're not using anything to keep me from getting pregnant again...." Her words broke off, leaving him to factor in his own conclusion.

Enough was enough, she finally decided. He needed to snap out of it. Martina then rested her weary head on his chest and closed her eyes. Within seconds, his arms went around her. She sighed, contented. Satisfaction comes in many forms.

"An interesting take on it," he said, his voice a bit gravelly and somewhat sulky.

Martina patted his flaccid organ and assured, "You've got to admit that you are capable of making babies."

Her remark seemed to restore some of his eminence as Master of the Domain. Suddenly, she found herself playfully pinned to the mattress as Rod grabbed hold of her wrists and hovered over her. "Yes," he said, affecting his best leer. "We certainly have evidence of that...and luckily...my sweet...I have a reliable back-up appendage I can use for pleasuring you." That said, he lowered his head to her taunting breasts and began to demonstrate the versatility of his tongue.

Martina giggled and squirmed with the delight of his antics, but within a short time his tongue play became quite serious as he slowly and sensually made his way to the even more erogenous regions of her body, where her earlier efforts to rouse his spirits and self-esteem were satisfactorily rewarded. Of course, Martina rewarded Rod in kind and he did achieve a happy ending of sorts. And while their bittersweet afternoon delight may not have risen to the elevation of past such interludes, it was enough for them at the moment. Enfolded in each others' arms, they had just started drifting toward a peaceful nap when they heard a little voice calling from the direction of Jody's bedroom.

"Mama! Up! Up!" It was Master of the Domain, Jr.

Martina started at the sound of Roddy's voice. "Stolen moments," she said with a wistful tone. "I suppose this is all of the time we get to ourselves for the rest of the afternoon...I'd better go get him before he pees in Jody's crib."

"I'll go get him," Rod said with a sheepish grin. "Since I'm his pee instructor." He rolled to the side of the bed and stood up.

Martina laughed, happy to see his sense of humor resurfacing. "But you're naked, Rod," she kidded. "Aren't you worried about him seeing you undressed?" Looking down at his nakedness, he remarked, "But we have the same basic equipment. Mine's just a little bigger and hairier." Considering himself for a moment, he then said, "Maybe I should put something on...I might scare him."

"Don't be silly...he needs to get used to seeing us naked together."

Hearing that, Rod took heart. He knelt at the side of the bed and placed his hand on one of her breasts, gently rolling her nipple between his thumb and index finger. "Does that mean you want me in your life, Martina?"

"Was there ever any question about that, Rod?"

Just then, Roddy started crying. "Mama! Mama" He wailed.

"Hold that thought," he told her. Standing up, he left the room.

As Rod walked away, Martina noted the thinness of his body, which actually made him look like an undeveloped teenager, and vowed to fatten him back up. Decidedly, she liked his muscular physique much better.

Rod carried his son back into the room and took him into the adjoining bathroom. "Daddy's going to you make you your own little stool to stand on when you go potty," he told the boy, as he held him up on the rim of the toilet. The boy looked up at him and said "Dah-dee." Rod smiled down at the boy, pressing his cheek to the top of Roddy's head, feeling as though his heart would burst with the love that surged inside of him for his newfound son. Martina heard Roddy say, "No-cwi-Dah-dee," his little voice halting between each juvenile word. Then she heard Rod say, "Daddy's not crying …he's happy because he loves you and Mommy."

51.

Later that afternoon when Freebird, Julie, and little Jody returned home, the McDonoughs had just barely gotten out of bed and dressed. After retrieving Roddy from the crib, the three lolled on the bed and Roddy entertained his parents with his antics. At five o'clock, they decided they had better get up and dressed before Mr. and Mrs. Clayton J. Terry, III, and daughter returned home.

"So, what did you guys do today?" Julie asked, as she plunked down on one of the patio chairs. She could see that Martina was glowing.

Roddy and Jody were busy playing in the sandbox, chattering in their nonsense juvenile language. Rod and Freebird had gone to the store on the pretense of getting more beer but, more specifically, to talk in private about Rod's first day with Martina and Roddy.

"Well...thanks so much to you and Freebird for giving us your home for the day...we had a very nice day, Julie."

"So I see, Marty...your face is glowing like a hundred watt bulb or something. You look so happy. What'd'ya all do?"

Martina blushed. "Well...we talked...Rod played with Roddy in the sandbox. You should've seen the two of them sitting in there together. I took lots of pictures. It was hysterical. We gave Roddy a bath afterward and then had lunch. After that, we put Roddy down for a nap...then Rod and I went down on each other."

Not expecting such a candid report, Julie jumped forward to the edge of her chair. "What? Are you serious?"

Martina snickered. "You're the one who said I was glowing."

"But I didn't expect that to happen so soon. I mean...."

"Julie— It was like we had not missed a beat. We've never stopped loving each other. We've never even been with anyone else."

"Really?" Julie scrunched up her face. "What about that Carol-person he lives with?"

"I don't know about her and I don't care. I know he loves me...and that's all that matters."

Julie nodded. "I know Rod loves you. He's been pining away for you all this time. I could see it."

"We haven't talked about our future, though," Martina said. "Other than to agree we want to get back together. But...honestly, Julie...I can't come back here to live. It's a small town and the gossip has been nasty. And it wouldn't be good for Roddy."

"I know, Sweetie," Julie agreed. "But where would you live? You can't go back to California. Freebird and I would die missing you. And Jody…she just loves little Roddy. You can't separate them!"

Martina thought of her Aunt Catherine and Uncle Jack, who had given so much to her, and felt torn. "I don't know, Julie. Rod and I are going to have to talk about that. I just know I cannot live here…not now and not ever."

Hearing Freebird's truck pull into the driveway at the side of the house, the two young friends looked at each other. Julie said, "If you and Rod want to go out after dinner to talk in private, we'll watch Roddy."

"Thank you, Julie. But you and Freebird are like our brother and sister…any talk about where we live should include you guys. You are family to us."

Julie jumped from her chair and ran over to hug Martina. "Oh! Marty! You have no idea how much I have missed you. When I was having Jody, I wanted so much for you to be there with me—"

"Really!" Martina cut in, excited. "I wished you were there, too, when I was having Roddy."

The two young women were hugging each other when Rod and Freebird came around the corner of the house and into the backyard. Rod elbowed Freebird. "I wonder what they're talking about?" he asked.

"Probably the same thing we were talking about," Freebird responded, smiling widely.

Rod walked over to Martina, put his arm around her shoulder and kissed her on the lips. "Missed you," he said.

She smiled up at him. "I missed you, too."

Rod looked over at the two toddlers in the sandbox, "I guess we're chopped liver, now that Roddy has Jody to play with," he commented.

"Don't complain," Martina told him, "He's learning to socialize and we all get some time to visit."

Freebird passed out cold beers to everyone and then went to fire up the barbeque grill.

Rod sat down and pulled Martina out of her chair and onto his lap. They gazed into each other's eyes the way new lovers tend to do and smiled as though they both knew a secret that no one else was privy to. His hand automatically slipped under her skirt and went straight to the triangle of pleasure. Martina immediately slapped his arm away.

"Rod! There are children here and we are visiting with Julie and Freebird," she chastised the stricken man.

"Since when has fondling your wife been socially unacceptable?" Rod countered.

Martina gave him a look of disapproval. "There are different degrees of fondling, Rod…and grabbing your wife's private area in public is not acceptable. You're not in high school any more."

Rod looked at Freebird and shrugged. "I guess she put me in my place," said Rod. He looked at Martina with an exaggerated pout. He knew she was right and that he had been out of line.

Turning to Julie, Martina proudly announced, "I think Rod has potty trained our son. Every time Rod has taken him to the potty, he's peed and he hasn't wet himself all afternoon."

Rod said, "He's a smart little guy. All you have to do is show him once and he picks up on it right away." Rod looked up at Martina and asked, "Maybe I should take him again now…it's been awhile." She nodded her assent.

"Roddy!" Martina called to the boy, who was having too much of a good time to pay attention. She slid off of Rod's lap and walked over to the sandbox. "Roddy, let's go potty."

"No!" The little boy told her, emphatically.

"Yes!" Martina insisted. "Now!"

The boy got up and climbed out of the sandbox. Then, running straight to Rod, he cried, "Dah-dee! Pot-tee!."

Rod gave Martina a wry expression. "Oh, that's just great! Now he associates me with the potty." As Rod marched his son into the house, Martina, Julie, and Freebird laughed uproariously. Secretly, although, Rod was delighted that the boy came to running to him, even if it was just for the menial task of taking him to the potty.

52.

Martina was betwixt and between. She wanted Rod to move out to San Francisco with her and he insisted that he couldn't because of his business ties to the Millborough area – he still worked at his family's construction company. Freebird was non-committal, as usual, but Julie was adamant that Martina live close by. They had just finished eating dinner and were sitting at the picnic table on Freebird's and Julie's patio, discussing Martina's options.

"I can understand if you don't want to live in Millborough," said Julie, who was sitting directly across the table from Martina, "but please don't move back to California...I want our babies to grow up together, Marty."

It was a persuasive appeal. Martina looked at Roddy and Jody, laughing and playing together so compatibly with a giant beach ball, and couldn't help but agree with Julie. But, then, there were the feelings of her Aunt and Uncle to consider; they had been so kind and wonderful to her and were her only remaining family. It would devastate them if she took Roddy so far away from them. And Rod's position also had strong merit; he had an established business reputation not just in the tri-county area surrounding Millborough, but throughout the state, with numerous multi-million dollar commercial construction projects in progress. He could not just pack up and run out on his brother Travis. And in San Francisco, he would be just a little fish starting over in a big pond.

"I don't know, guys," exclaimed Martina. "There are too many bad memories for me in Millborough."

"But there are so many neat little towns nearby where you could live," Julie bargained. "You won't ever have to come to Millborough, Marty. Just stay close enough to where we can visit often."

Martina took hold of Julie's hand and sighed. "It's a big decision to make. There's my Aunt and Uncle to think about...and I also have my job to consider, too."

Rod looked over at her, surprised. It was the first time he had heard anything about Martina having a job. "I thought you stayed home with Roddy?"

"I do stay home with Roddy...but I also have to earn an income to support us. Anyway, I only work part-time and he usually comes along with me."

"What kind of work do you do that will let you bring a baby with you?" Rod asked, his interest peaked.

"I do modeling…but now, it's mostly just catalogs and newspaper ads for Macy's. Since having Roddy, I won't do the out of town assignments anymore. Macy's is local and steady…and, sometimes, Roddy models the kid's clothes. Then he gets to keep the clothes and also gets paid for it. He even has his own bank account, where all his paychecks are deposited and he is saving for college."

"That's so fantastic!" Julie said.

Rod frowned, feeling excluded again. "You didn't tell me you do modeling."

Martina placed her hand on his arm and reminded him, "The subject hasn't come up yet, Rod. Give it time. Between the sandbox, giving Roddy a bath, lunch, potty, and…other things…when have we had the time to discuss anything about our jobs? I thought we could do that tonight after we put Roddy to bed." And, then, to let Rod know she was aware that he also had not told her about certain aspects of his own life, she added, "Or do you have to get home to your girlfriend."

Rod lowered his head. "It's not what you think…Carol is not my girlfriend. She's more of a roommate." His tone was slightly defensive. Martina reached over to where his hand rested on the table and covered it with hers.

Nudging Julie, Freebird said, "Why don't we take the kids inside and get them ready for bed." Martina started to get up, but Freebird told her, "Stay there and finish your drink. Julie and I can handle the kids." Rod took hold of her arm and gently pulled her back down onto the bench they shared.

When Freebird and Julie disappeared into the house with the kids, Rod said, "I guess I need to back up to the beginning…the day of the…uh…accident—"

Martina cut in, her voice sounded thin and sad. "You can say the day of the shooting, Rod. I know Martino shot you and that's what caused you to crash your bike. Don't worry about sparing my feelings…I can't feel any worse about what he did to you."

Rod heard the guilt and sadness in her soft voice and said, "I hope you're not blaming yourself for what Martino did, because you had nothing to do with that."

Martina lowered her head, tears filling her eyes. "I think I did, Rod…that was the morning I found out I was pregnant. I was so excited about having your baby and couldn't wait to tell you. Without even

271

thinking about how he would react to the news, I told him…that's when he went nuts and dragged me to that clinic that did the abortions…." Looking up at Rod, her tear-stained face reflecting the anguish she felt inside, she said, "It was my stupidity that set him off. So I did have something to do with it."

Rod placed his hands on her shoulders, and with a firm voice said, "No! You did not! It was Martino's decision to shoot me − not yours. Don't you assume any blame for his actions." Pulling her against his chest, he felt her body shaking as her sobs broke loose. Knowing she had to release this emotional torment, Rod could only comfort her with his gentle embrace.

When she regained control of her voice, she said, "I'm so sorry, Rod. I didn't know he was so crazy. I should have listened to your warnings and stayed away from him."

Rod squeezed her more tightly and pressed his cheek against the top of her head. His voice, too, was choked up when he told her, "You have no reason to apologize to me…and I don't want to hear any more about it. Maybe we shouldn't talk about it anymore…just bury it in the past."

"We can't bury it, Rod. It's too big to bury. We can move on and be happy together in spite of it, but there's this whole block of your life that I know nothing about. And I'll always be wondering about it. I need to know what happened, just so I can fill in the missing pieces in my mind. I think that if we deal with the emotions of it now, they won't come back to haunt us later on." Martina looked up into his eyes to see if he was considering what she had said.

Cupping her face in his palms, Rod bent close and kissed the tip of her nose. "I suppose you are right about dealing with it now and then growing from it. But…to be honest, Martina, there's a whole block of my life that I don't know anything about, either. After I was shot and crashed my bike I was out of it for a long time. All I remember about that afternoon is getting the phone call from you, and you telling me that you were over at your father's house. I was pretty upset with you for going there after what he had done to you, but I knew that idiot counselor the judge appointed was pressuring you to reestablish contact with him…and Martino was so good at running guilt trips on you and manipulating you to do what he wanted. So, when you called me and said you were at your father's house I just wanted to go get you out of there and bring you home.

"I don't know how Martino knew which route I was taking over there...I guess he just got lucky. He pulled up behind me...almost beside me, to my right. I saw him stick the gun out the window and then...pow! (Rod gestured the shooting of a gun with his hand) Good thing it was a small caliber pistol...but it did knock me for a loop, and that's when I went off the road and hit a tree. Some poor old couple driving along behind me saw the whole thing. The wife stayed with me while her husband drove to the closest gas station and called for an ambulance. They were the ones who gave the police Martino's license plate number and a description of his car.

"I was taken to the hospital and had emergency surgery. I also had a broken arm and leg. That's how I met Carol...the woman you think is my girlfriend. She was one of my nurses. I was in a bad, bad way, Martina. When I finally became conscious the first thing I asked about was you. Freebird and Julie were there in the room at the time. Julie told me what had happened to you. I was depressed and became angry with you for leaving me. I felt like my life was over. Then my doctor told me I might be stuck in a wheelchair for the rest of my life and that hit me real hard. That's when Carol jumped in and suggested I see an orthopedist she knew...a Doctor Larkin. Larkin had me doing all kinds of therapy. It was painful but I actually liked the physical pain, because it dulled the pain in my heart from missing you so much.

"But those stories about your father and you were all over town. I began to think that you ran away because the rumors were true. I even believed that your father took you to the abortion clinic because he wanted to destroy the evidence of his getting you pregnant. All I could think about was the way he had beat you, and it made me wonder if he did it because you had given him up for me and he was in a jealous rage about it. Julie argued with me until she finally got fed up and basically stopped coming to see me.

"Back then, I was so messed up mentally and physically that I wasn't thinking rationally. It seemed like all of my love for you had turned into solid hate. One minute I wanted to fly out to California and find you; the next minute I wanted nothing to do with you. It was about that time I began hitting up Carol for mind numbing drugs, which she was more than happy to supply. She had her own motives for keeping me high. The drugs she supplied to me were like a carrot hanging from a stick, and she used them to get me to follow her home. But Carol's motivation was not inspired by love. Carol likes to possess and control.

She gets off on it. It's her form of sex. And between my depression and her drugs, I was easily possessed and controlled.

"I've been trying to kick the drugs on my own, but it's been tough. I'm thinking I may have to get professional help. I still have pain in my leg and hip and I need pain pills for that, but I don't need the stuff Carol's been feeding me." He turned to face her squarely. "I won't lie to you, Martina...I'm a drug addict. Up until today...when I saw you and Roddy...I didn't have much incentive to kick. The stuff is too easy for me to get. I know I need to get away from Carol and take back my soul...but it's easier said than done. So...that's the block of my life you wanted to know about. I hope you won't think less of me for it."

Rod's account left Martina quiet and thoughtful, but not emotionless. She took his hand between her palms and held it tight, while a plethora of thoughts, feelings, and impressions whipped around in her mind. How could she possibly judge him for his weakness after all he had been through? Especially when it was her own father's evilness that altered the course of Rod's life—and hers as well.

"I could never think less of you for your pain, Rod. It's not like you brought this on yourself." She hugged him fiercely, tears streaming down her face. A sudden sadness took hold of her as she thought about the wreckage of their lives, and just as suddenly she shook it off. "We can get you help for the drugs." Her voice was filled with hope.

Rod noted that she had said "we", and was encouraged. "I will get help, Martina," he assured her. "Our son will not have a hopeless drug addict for a father. I want you and Roddy to be proud of me." Rod told her about the rehab clinic in North Hampton and of his plans to get help there. Martina reminded him that his drug problem was something they could solve together, and they both took comfort from that knowledge.

Martina looked up at him and smiled. Her happy expression belied the anxiety she was feeling inside about what she had to tell him. She wondered how proud would Rod be of her when she finally told him the truth he needed to know about her. The truth she should have told him long ago, before they were married. If they were to start over with a clean slate and build a strong relationship she needed to be as candid with him as he was with her. The time, it seemed, had finally come to tell Rod the whole truth. Come what may. Would he think less of her? She had to take that chance.

Martina's typical style of handling difficult matters was to face them head-on. She sat up and squared her shoulders, then started off by saying, "There's a whole block of my life that you don't know anything about either, Rod. Things that I should have told you a long time ago. It's the real truth about Martino and I (she faltered for a moment) that you need to know if we are to go forward and be free of the past." With an opening like that there was no going back, but Martina did not intend to renege this time. She took a deep breath and gathered her resolve, determined that Rod should know everything. She saw that she had his full attention.

"I guess I too should start at the very beginning…back to the time I became an embryo and the actual reason I was conceived in the first place.

"I always knew that I was Martino's grand experimental child. I had been told that from birth. Martino wanted to mold me into some kind of intellectually superior person, who was a tribute to his free thinking philosophy. He felt that the rules of society were Neanderthal and restricted the development of the mind. So Martino and Jacqui never imposed any rules on me…other than to make sure I did not harm myself. I was taught that the three of us were a unit, with equal rights and powers between us. I even slept in their bed until I was practically a teenager, when I started to feel uncomfortable about it. As soon as I was old enough, Martino began schooling me on his philosophies. I spent several hours a day with him while he lectured me about everything from Plato to Alfred North Whitehead and existentialism to nihilism. I could speak fluent French by the time I was five…Jacqui was my language tutor. I was even taught Latin…since Martino considered Latin to be the 'language of all the masters of great thought'. While most kids were out playing hopscotch or jumping rope I was learning the theories of Kirkegaard and Nietzsche." A wry smile formed on her lips, and she said, "Did you know that morality does not exist? Morality is an abstract concept designed to control the masses and our existence is pointless." Another deep sigh punctuated her narrative.

"After Jacqui died it was a foregone conclusion that I would simply assume her role. We were now a unit of two. Martino just naturally felt I was to be his companion. After all, I was his creation and too good for the common world. Martino took Jacqui's death very hard. He was out of his mind with grief most of the time…crying and depressed. He couldn't even work, so he took an indefinite leave of absence from the University. I thought he was going to lose his mind. I don't know what I was thinking…I just wanted to help him feel better. I felt so bad for him. And I was afraid too…of becoming an orphan if he did not get over it.

"Martino and Jacqui had a different kind of love—if you want to call it that—from most married people, but they were really two of a kind. They had strange tastes that would probably seem weird to other people but…for them…their strangeness was very compatible. They were really good together in their way…so I knew he was really lost without her. I became afraid that I would lose him too. I was only fifteen and taught to be suspicious of the outside world." Martina stopped for a moment, summoning the words to go on. Rod merely studied her face and gently held her hand.

"Everyone always commented about how much I looked like Jacqui…so, one night, after listening to Martino crying in his room for what seemed like hours, I went to her dressing room and found a nightgown that Martino had always liked seeing her in. I put it on and went to him, thinking that if I could remind him of Jacqui, then, I could make him feel better.

I don't know if he knew it was me or just wanted to believe it was her…but I went to his room and got into bed with him…I wanted only to comfort him. I didn't stop to consider if I was crossing any lines. I was never taught about crossing any lines imposed by society…and I just wanted him back to the way he was when Jacquie was alive. I did not realize back then that there might be unintended consequences to what I was doing.

And I won't lie and say that I didn't enjoy some of what we did. Martino could be very tender…at least back then…in the early days of it.

"After that first night, he wanted me to… to be with him every night. In the beginning it was just touching and holding him…but then…he got to where he wanted more. He wanted me to be his full-fledged mistress. I had seen Jacqui and Martino having sex many times…from as far back as I can remember. They never closed their bedroom door and a lot of times they'd just do it wherever they happened to be in the house and whenever they felt like it. It didn't matter to them if I was there. As I got older, I learned to read their body language and stayed in my room to avoid seeing them. I realize now that their behavior wasn't right…or even what society considers normal…but that was the environment I was born into. I also know now that Martino's idea of sex wasn't quite…normal. I never saw him really make love to Jacqui. He didn't do the things to pleasure her…not

276

the way you did to me. But I didn't know that until I married you. Not once, that I can recall, did he ever look her in the eyes and kiss her when they had sex. He always did it from behind…it was like he didn't want to see her face or make the act personal. That's why I was so freaked out about going to bed with you the night we got married. I didn't know any better than what I grew up seeing in my house.

"The first time he tried to…do that to me…I freaked out and he pulled back. I ran to my room. I wasn't going to let him treat me like a dog, the way he did Jacqui. He came to my room and apologized and said he would never do that again if I would just go back to bed with him, because he couldn't stand to be alone. So, I did sleep with him at night, but I couldn't really sleep because I never trusted him to keep his word…especially since he always slept naked. Then I met you and that changed everything. I didn't want to play the Jacqui game anymore or be the child of superior intellect. I wanted to live in the world like everyone else. Martino didn't like it when I started dating you. But, later, he came to me and said that he understood that I needed to be with people my own age and all. When he started dating a woman from the college I thought he was getting his life back on track. But he wasn't. He still wanted me...body and soul. He was just a ticking time bomb…."

It was very difficult for Rod to listen to her revelations without showing any emotion, but he knew he had to remain impassive and allow Martina to continue with her story. Nothing she was telling him now was surprising in any way. Rod had always suspected Martino had an unnatural craving for his daughter. There were too many signs of it to be ignored. And even if it were she who had initiated the first contact by getting into bed with him, Rod considered that her motives were pure. Martino was nothing more than a sick fuck, taking advantage of and manipulating a distraught young girl.

Martina had been watching Rod's facial expressions while she confided her deepest secrets to him. Other than Chloe Renfrew, she had never told anyone else these things, mostly because she feared a reaction of disgust. If Rod was disgusted by her revelations he certainly hid his feelings well. She noted only that his jaw seemed clamped tight and his gaze had shifted upward, into the darkening sky above her head when she recounted the bit about her father's attempt to have sex with her.

Rod merely nodded his head slowly, pensively, when she finished her narrative, his hand still gently holding hers. After several moments of silence Rod encircled her with his arms, gently and protectively. His voice was barely above a whisper when he said, "That explains a lot about why things blew up the way they did." He heaved a deep sigh. "Thank you for telling me. I know it was hard for you."

"I'm sorry, Rod. I didn't know how to tell you before. I was so stupid to think—"

"Stop, Martina!" He said, cutting her off. "I'm the one who's sorry...sorry you had to carry that burden alone." Shifting his position, he held her at arms length so that he could see her face. He looked into her eyes with unnerving intensity, and continued, "Surely you know that what your father did to you would be considered criminal...and he had to know what he was doing was not just a crime against nature but a betrayal of your trust," Rod explained with a gentle voice. "Even if you want to think of yourself as the aggressor, he was still the adult. He was supposed to be your protector." Resting his forehead on her shoulder, he let out a heavy sigh. "I got off easy with just a bullet in the back compared to you...but he'll never hurt anyone again."

There were many things Rod could have said about those dark days leading up to their separation and the details she had just recounted, but he saw no point to rehashing long passed events, and Martino, who had been the only problem in their relationship, when they were together, was now dead. The only important issue to be considered between them at this moment, at least as far as Rod could see, was how were they to go forward? Could they reclaim their love? Their marriage?

And, most importantly of all the issues now facing them, what would be best for their son. He could not imagine living separately, on the other side of the country, from them.

They sat quietly, embracing, for several moments, processing each other's words, thoughts tumbling wildly in their heads.

Finally, Rod spoke. "What's to become of us , Martina? Do we have a chance again? I still love you as much as ever...and I am crazy in love with our son. I want to be in your lives forever." His words became a plea.

Martina drew closer to Rod and hugged him as tight as she could. "We want you in our lives too...forever, Rod. You have no idea how much I have wished for you and cried for you since that night. I still feel like this is a dream...being here with you. Like it's not even real. It's like my prayers have been answered but it's just too unbelievable for me to absorb."

Looking up at him, she said, "If this is real, Rod, and I am not imagining all of this…you can be sure that I am not letting you out of my sight or out of my hands again." She squeezed him harder for emphasis. Martina's words were heartfelt. It was true that she was having trouble believing what was now happening to her was real. These kinds of second chances just did not happen to people every day. Martina was sure she was either experiencing a miracle or a very convincing hallucination.

"I can assure you this is as real as it gets," Rod said, his tone a cross between marvel and conviction.

53.

"Where the fuck have you been all this time?" Carol screamed when Rod finally returned to her house from his reunion with Martina. She eyed him suspiciously. "I called here from work about fifty times and got no answer. Then I get home and you're not here. Here it is after four in the morning and you're just getting home. I suppose you were out running around with that asshole Indian?"

"Sorry. I should have left you a note," was all he said to the irate woman, and then went to his room and closed the door behind him. Flopping down on the bed, sandy clothes and all, he wanted only to be left alone to think about everything that had happened to him in the last sixteen fantastic hours. But Carol didn't want to leave him alone. She barged into his room and continued her rant. She knew her yelling would bring on one of his headaches and he would need the drugs she kept hidden from him. The drugs that numbed his pain and kept him dependent upon her. Carol looked upon Rod's addiction to the drugs she gave him as an insurance policy—her insurance that he would never leave her. But she didn't count on him being introduced to an even more powerful addiction: the instantaneous love he felt for his son…and the love he had bottled up inside for Martina.

"You miserable sonofabitch!" Carol yelled, standing over him in the near dark. "I'm here worrying about whether you are dead or alive and all you've got to say is 'sorry.' Well that's just plumb fuckin' ducky."

Her rant continued off and on for another hour, but Rod willed himself to not get a headache. Instead, he pictured Roddy's innocent little face and heard his son say, "No cwi," and his remembrance of that tender moment between him and his amazing little boy strengthened him. He lie still, with his eyes closed, while the irate woman wandered in and out of his room, calling him "a good for nothing junkie" at one time and an "ungrateful bastard" at another, as well as numerous other unflattering names, and peppered Rod with every expletive she could think of. While she raged, Rod crept inside of himself and visualized Martina the way she looked when he left her only an hour ago, when she was lying naked on her bed.

Carol stomped back into Rod's room, about to scream at him for ignoring her when she suddenly had an uncharacteristic change of heart. Looking down at Rod's supine body she felt an urge to touch him, to see if she could make him notice her sexually. Perhaps, she reasoned to herself, if their relationship was more intimate Rod would have no need to leave her house at all. Reaching down, she attempted to grab hold of him. Like a flash, Rod's arm shot out and pulled her hand away. "Don't you ever touch me!" He yelled angrily, as he jumped up from his bed. Thinking Rod was going to hit her, Carol automatically recoiled and brought her free arm up to cover her face. Pushing her aside, Rod quickly walked from the bedroom and headed toward the back door. Behind him, he heard Carol screaming, "Get out of my house! Get out! Don't ever come back here again or I'll call the police."

Jumping into his Corvette, he dug around under the driver's seat for the keys and started up the car. He couldn't go back to Martina in the middle of the night and disturb everyone there, so he threaded through the streets of Millborough and made his way to Scenic Drive.

54.

On the morning Rod walked out of Carol's house he didn't bother taking anything with him other than his wallet, his dirty Corvette, and the clothes he wore. He had no intention of ever going back there again. What few possessions he left behind belonged to a version of himself that no longer existed, so he would have no use for them anymore. He hoped the clothing he had left long ago at the Scenic Drive house was still there or he'd be in a hell of a fix. It was sometime close to six o'clock when he reached the big stone house on Scenic Drive, and the sun was spreading its first tendrils of dawning light across the sky.

Pulling into the driveway for the first time since his accident, he never thought he would ever again be happy to see the house he once shared with Martina, but now that she was back in his life he could withstand the memories of her brief residence there. In fact, he now hungered for those memories.   Stepping out of the Corvette, he immediately looked up at the balcony over the sunroom, the place where Martina used to sit, reading and waiting for him to come home from work. He felt a stab of loneliness because she and Roddy were not there with him now, but perhaps he would bring them over later, after he picked her up from Vito Travante's office. Rubbing the soreness in his low back, he limped along the brick path to the back porch. Between playing in the sandbox with Roddy and playing in bed with Martina his muscles, which had lain fallow for far too long, were now reacting to their sudden, extended usage. He vowed to start pumping iron again and build himself back up to the way he was before the accident.

More worrisome than his back and leg pain was his inability to perform sexually. Although Martina tried to soothe his humiliation by assuring him that they were both tired from the long, emotional day, Rod knew better. Before yesterday, he had no reason to be concerned with that particular side effect of his drug addiction and never even gave it a thought. The relationship he had with Carol was never a sexual one, and he was relieved when she gave up on trying to entice him into her bed. So, his lack of a sex drive had never been an issue. Now, it was a problem he needed to take care of immediately. Today, while Martina was busy meeting with Travante and taking care of her father's estate matters, Rod planned to contact a drug counseling center over in North Hampton, one that Freebird had told him about. If he had to, he would check into one of those new resort-like rehab places, where they weaned you off of your drug of choice and put you on a nutritional diet. Whatever it took to get back into his former shape he was ready to go for it. Much too wired to even think about catching a few hours of sleep, Rod entered the familiar, old house and headed straight upstairs to the shower. Stripping off his shirt and jeans, he stood naked while he waited for the hot water to start flowing from the shower nozzle, grateful for the gas heated water because the electric power had been turned off. Even though he hated to wash away the wonderful, musky aroma of lovemaking that still clung to his body, he knew the hot water would feel real good on his stiff and aching muscles. He would replace the scent of Martina's essence as soon as possible, he thought, smiling to himself.

The chills and tremors started shortly after Rod showered and dressed. He knew immediately what was happening to him and he knew there was going to be some rough going ahead.

With the telephone at the house now disconnected, he literally ran to his car, drove to the nearest pay phone, and called his brother Travis for help. Then he sat in the Corvette and waited, not daring to drive himself to the drug counseling center in North Hampton. By the time Travis arrived, less than twenty minutes later, Rod was shivering uncontrollably, his nose had already started to drip, and he was practically incoherent.

Travis pulled, shoved, and pushed Rod onto the floor of his cargo van and immediately drove his brother to the Emergency Room at Millborough General.

Travis instantly recognized the tall, stocky Wesley Couch, the former quarterback of his high school football team. It was a good ten years ago since he had last seen him, but he had heard Couch was now a doctor at the local hospital. Couch, who now wore his frizzy blond hair closely cropped and the white lab coat of a doctor, was on duty in the Emergency Room when Travis brought in his very agitated and raving brother, to have him admitted for treatment. After shaking hands and briefly exchanging the usual long time-no see pleasantries, Doctor Wesley Couch's smile quickly transformed to serious concern when he looked at Rod. Setting down the clipboard with Rod's intake chart attached to it, the young doctor removed his cigar-sized flashlight from a pocket in his lab coat and began examining the pupils of Rod's eyes. Apparently deciding he did not want anyone staring at his dilated pupils, Rod took a limp, uncompleted swing at Doctor Wes Couch.

Even if Rod's fist had made contact with the Doctor, it is doubtful it would have had any impact on the solidly built man.

"Sorry, Wes," Travis apologized as he grabbed Rod's flailing wrists and immobilized his arms.

"Do you have any idea what he's on?" Asked the young Doctor, greatly concerned that Rod's eyes were rolling uncontrollably and his body was jerking spasmodically. "I'd like to give him something to counter it, but I'd sure like to know what I'm up against."

Travis nodded and bit his lip. He didn't like the idea of ratting out anyone but he never did like the way Carol Bennett treated his brother, and Travis knew she was the source of Rod's drugs. Numerous times, he tried to get Rod to leave her and move in with him, but Rod always stubbornly refused.

Travis could now see why Rod was so adamant about staying with Carol; she had him hooked. Worried about Rod's worsening condition, Travis had no choice but to tell Wes about Carol. "I don't know exactly what he's on but he's been staying with one of the nurses who works at this hospital...a Carol Bennett...since his motorcycle accident and she's been giving him something for pain. Perhaps we can call her and find out what it is?"

Wes nodded, thoughtful. Then rushing to the doorway of the examining room, the erstwhile high school quarterback called to someone in the hall. A young woman with short, dark hair, and wearing the standard issue white nurse's uniform appeared. Travis heard Wes say, "Find out if Nurse Carol Bennett is on duty. If she's not, call her at home. I need to talk to her S-A-P." The young nurse nodded and rushed away. Turning to Travis, Wes said, "I can give him something mild to calm him down in the meantime...but I'm hoping we can find out in short order what he's using. He's obviously detoxing and it's not going to be pretty. We may have to use restraints on him, to keep him from hurting himself...or someone else." The two men stood watching Rod, who was rolling his head from side to side and sweating profusely, while his body jerked uncontrollably. Wes asked, "Do you want to stay with him for a while?"

"Yes. I can't leave him alone like this," Travis responded, unable to take his eyes off of his brother.

"Okay. We're going to be moving him to a room on the third floor and I'm going to authorize your staying with him...as long as you can handle it. But don't feel bad if you can't...he's probably going to be vomiting, losing control of his bladder, screaming and crying for his mother and the Virgin Mary herself before it's all over. And there will be two male nurses keeping an eye on him for the duration…and I will monitor him throughout his withdrawal…so anytime you feel you want to leave, just go ahead and leave…don't worry about him."

As if on cue, Rod vomited all over himself, the bed, and the floor. Two male nurses entered the room, covered Rod's shaking body with a blanket, and wheeled him out of the examining room.

"Give them about twenty minutes or so to get him up to his room and cleaned up," Wes told Travis, patting him on the shoulder and easing him out of the examining room. "We'll check with the nurse's station down the hall here (Wes pointed to their right) and find out which room he's going to be assigned to." Wes grew thoughtful for a moment and then commented, "Darn shame. Darn shame. Your brother was always a straight arrow. People just don't realize how habit forming these pain medications can be."

As Travis and Wes Couch approached the bustling nurse's station, the young nurse with the short, dark hair called to Wes, "Doctor Couch! I've not been able to get in touch with Nurse Bennett. She's not on duty and she's not answering her home phone, either."

Acknowledging the young nurse's information, Wes told her, "This is the patient's brother, Travis McDonough. We go back a long way. Will you please make sure he finds out which room his brother is assigned to…and he has my permission to stay with his brother as long as he wants to." To Travis, Wes said, "I've got to order some blood tests for Rod…so we can determine what's in his system. In the meantime, we'll give him something to keep him comfortable. I'll catch up with you after I take care of all that."

"Thanks, Wes," Travis said, truly thankful the doctor was someone he knew, who would really look after Rod. Watching Wes Couch prance away, Travis remembered how everyone on the football team used to call him "Twinkle Toes" behind his back because he had a rather mincing gait when running across the field with the football tucked primly under his arm. No one ever teased Wes about it to his face, especially since he was chosen All Star High School Quarterback statewide for three seasons in a row, and also because Wes was bigger and more powerfully built than most of the other guys on the team. If Wes knew anything about his "Twinkle Toes" designation, Travis was sure glad his old team mate didn't bring it up today.

"Mr. McDonough!" The young nurse's voice broke into Travis's thoughts.

"Uh— Yes, ma'am," Travis responded, noticing for the first time how the young woman's pixie hair style nicely framed her fine-boned face, which was lightly sprinkled across her nose and cheeks with freckles. He thought of her as having that healthy all-American girl look. When she smiled at him, Travis suddenly found himself tongue-tied. Quickly, he scanned her name tag and committed the name "Nancy Farnsworth, R.N." to memory, although Travis wasn't sure just then what he would do with that information.

"Doctor Couch has instructed me to give you the number of your brother's room," she advised Travis, "but with all of the construction going on up in that new wing I think it would be best if I actually took you there…so you won't get lost."

Travis smiled back at Nurse Farnsworth and felt like his body was floating and bouncing along on electrostatic air currents as he trailed along behind her to the elevators, watching her perky little butt animate the back of the crisp, white skirt of her uniform. He calculated that she was probably only two or three inches over five feet in height, and admired her petite, compact build. He liked the way her white hosiery outlined the muscles of her slender legs. She looked so spotlessly clean and fresh. Unable to think of anything clever to say to her on the elevator ride up to the third floor of the hospital's new wing, Travis stood red-faced, with his hands folded together in front of the notoriously unpredictable McDonough appendage, and sneaking sideways glances at the pixie-faced young woman.

Nancy Farnsworth could feel the heat emanating from Travis McDonough's body. She also saw his not so surreptitious glances. She had never before felt the desire to escort anyone to a patient's room, but this young man seemed to grab her interest. He was so neatly dressed, wearing a camel colored leather jacket, a light blue shirt, dark blue pants, and camel leather loafers. Nancy always had an eye for a sharply dressed man. There was just something about his round face, with its rosy cheeks and big brown eyes that she found so attractive. Travis was endowed with the same boyish good looks as his brother Rod, the kind that nurturing women always found so irresistible.

The elevator stopped at the third floor and the young nurse smiled at Travis and said, "Follow me this way." She turned to the left and started down a sterile looking hallway that still smelled of new carpet and fresh paint. There was none of the people traffic and medical accoutrements in the hall usually associated with hospitals, and just as Travis was thinking how the new wing looked abandoned, a tortured

286

scream pierced the stillness of the empty hallway and he stopped short. He knew it was his brother who had screamed. The fine hairs on the back of Travis's neck stood on end. Nancy Farnsworth turned to see why the young man had stopped walking and saw the expression of alarm on his face. She didn't have time to analyze her feelings just at the moment but she knew she felt a tenderness for this handsome stranger that she had never felt before. Walking the few steps back toward him, she placed her hand on his arm in a comforting manner and looked into his dark, troubled eyes.

"Maybe you would like to reconsider going in there…drug withdrawals are not easy to watch, even for those who are trained in detox," said Nancy, her voice soft and solicitous.

Travis was torn. He wanted to be there with his brother and help him through the hell he knew Rod was going to face, but Travis didn't know if he had the stomach to watch his brother suffering. The scream he just heard had already unhinged him. Finally, Travis concluded, "I've got to be with him," affirming the decision more to himself than the pretty young nurse.

Nancy looked up and down the hall, hoping to spot a chair. There were none in sight. "Perhaps if we put a chair out here in the hall, where you could sit, you'd be close by and could go in and out when you wanted," she suggested. Travis mustered an uneasy smile and a quick nod of assent.

Nancy walked over to the closest door and looked inside the room. "Here we go," she said and pushed the door all the way open, kicking down the brass door stop with the tip her spotlessly white shoe. She disappeared into the darkness of the room for a moment and soon came back out carrying a lightweight chair. Travis ran over to assist her, taking the chair from her hands. "We can set it outside Room 321," she advised, "which is just—"

She was about to point to a room only a few doors away when a young man wearing a white lab coat and carrying a tray containing small vials of blood suddenly emerged from the room she was pointing toward and closed the door behind him.

The young man with the tray nodded a greeting to Nurse Farnsworth and Travis as he hurriedly brushed past them. Travis carried the chair up the hall and set it down next to the closed door of room 321. He stood there, looking unsure of what to do next.

Suddenly, Nancy's professional training as a nurse was vying for control over stronger, more primitive desires—she wanted to touch the boyish face of Travis McDonough and feel his lips on hers. Embarrassed at her thoughts, she quickly stifled them and asked, "Would you like me to go see if it's okay for you to go in there?"

Travis nodded, relieved. "I'd appreciate it, Ma'am," he said.

Nancy liked the way he called her "Ma'am." It told her that he had manners and was respectful. Such qualities were important to her. She walked over to the door, opened it, and slipped inside. It seemed to Travis that she was in there a long time but it was actually only less than a minute. When she emerged her smile was reassuring.

"Doctor Couch has just given him a shot and he seems to be calming down. The nurses are cleaning him up a bit and getting him changed. When they come out, you can go in and see him," she reported in a nurse-like fashion, wondering if Travis was as well-endowed as his brother, whom she had just chanced to see naked.

"Is he going to be okay?" Travis asked, needing reassurance that Rod would get through his ordeal alive.

Nancy beamed him her most engaging, dimpled smile and flashed her white, even teeth, "He's in excellent hands, Mr. McDonough. They don't come any better than Doctor Couch."

One look at Nurse Farnsworth's all-American smile and Travis felt reassured, even though she did not actually answer his question.

Looking at her watch, Nancy saw that it was almost time for her lunch break. She had been trying to think of a way to let Travis McDonough know she found him attractive but did not quite know how to go about it without being too obvious. She would feel like an absolute fool if she came on to him and he rejected her because he was married or had a girlfriend. But her watch had just given her a great idea. "I'll be heading down to the cafeteria for lunch now…and maybe it would be a good idea if you grabbed a bite to eat…while your brother is resting. By the time you're done eating he might be awake."

Travis took heart. He didn't have Rod's gift for smooth talking women into giving him their telephone numbers, but he had been wracking his brain trying to come up with some reason to ask the pretty nurse for hers without being too forward. Now, she had solved his dilemma. "That's a great idea," he said, trying to control his enthusiasm. "I didn't even have time to eat breakfast this morning…what with my brother getting sick." Then, looking around at the seemingly deserted hall, Travis had second thoughts about leaving Rod alone. "Maybe I'd better not go…what if he wakes up and no one is around? He's kind of isolated up here." He saw her quizzical expression and wondered why she was looking at him that way.

"He's not alone up here. There's a nurse's station right outside his door in the main hallway on the front side of this wing. We're in a back access hallway...these rooms have two doors." Then Nancy realized that Travis was unaware of the new building's design and thought his brother was in an empty wing. Taking him by the arm, she said, "Let me show you how this new wing is designed for maximum access." Nancy opened the door to Room 321, which was a standard double room with an accordion type divider that could be pulled out to create a privacy wall between the two beds. Since Rod was the only patient in the room the divider was pushed back to the wall and Travis could see that his brother was sleeping quite peacefully. There was another door at the opposite end of the room, which was wide open, beyond which there was a well-staffed nurse's station visible through the open doorway, just as she said.

Breathing a sigh of relief, Travis smiled at Nancy. "I had no idea there was a regular beehive of people on the other side of the room. I feel better now about leaving my brother for a little while."

"Good!" She said, beaming a friendly smile. "Let's go get some of that marvelous hospital cafeteria food."

55.

Carol was sure Rod would come back for his regular morning fix, but when he didn't, she went looking for him. The first place she checked was the stone house on Scenic Drive, but his car was not in the driveway. She even peaked in some of the windows just to be sure he wasn't in there. There were no signs of life inside. When she drove back down the hill to the foot of Scenic Drive, had Carol turned to the right at that intersection she would have eventually seen Rod's Corvette in the parking lot of the Super Drug Store, just a few blocks up the road. Instead, Carol turned left and headed for the McDonough Construction offices. When she arrived at McDonough Construction she saw neither Rod's car nor Travis's van parked in the lot there.

Frustrated, Carol slammed the heel of her hand against the steering wheel and yelled, "That fucker! Where the hell is he?" There was only one other place she could think of. "He's probably over at that spooky asshole Indian's house," she announced aloud to herself. But Carol would not drive to Freebird's house to see if Rod was there. She wouldn't go anywhere near that whacked-out Sioux or Mohican or whatever the hell he was. "Scares the hell outta me," Carol muttered to herself, as she drove homeward, recalling how Freebird always gave her flinty stares that seemed to peer through the layers of her skin and muscle and disapprove of what he saw underneath.

It was obvious to Carol that the Indian didn't like her. What did she care about him, anyway? Except that he had a lot of influence over Rod. Every time that damn Freebird came around there was always trouble between her and Rod she agreed with herself. And she was sure Rod had been with Freebird all day yesterday and up until early this morning. And now, sure enough, there was trouble. Turning the corner onto her street, she hoped to see Rod's Corvette back in her driveway, but it was not there.

Fuming, Carol stomped around her dark, musty-smelling house and tried to organize her thoughts. Her mind would not cooperate. Only one unscrambled thought came through – I have to get Rod back, she told herself. Finally, out of desperation, she picked up the phone and dialed Freebird's telephone number. She was relieved when she heard Julie's voice.

"Oh…good morning, Julie…this is Carol Bennett." Carol's words flowed out of her mouth like warm syrup out of a bottle. For a moment, Julie was too surprised to speak. She always thought Carol hated her and Freebird, so why would she be calling their house? But Julie, being the kind-hearted soul that she could only be, courteously responded. "Hi, Carol...how have you been?"

Carol ignored Julie's pleasantry and pounced. "Is Rod there?"

"Rod? Oh— No. He left early this morning. I thought he went back to your house," Julie said, unaware of Rod's current situation.

"No. He didn't come home all night," Carol lied, playing the part of the concerned friend. "I'm starting to get worried about him...you know how he gets so depressed sometimes. I'm always afraid he'll...well...let's not even think such things."

"Well, he sure wasn't depressed last night," Julie said, in an effort to assuage the woman's concern. "Actually...Rod was more like his old self last night than he's been since his accident...now that his wife and little boy, Roddy, are in town...he spent all day yesterday with them. It was great to see him so happy and excited."

Carol froze on the other end of the line. Her thoughts darted wildly: Rod's wife is here? He has a kid? Where does that leave me? It was hard to keep her syrupy voice warm when she regained enough composure to say, "How wonderful for Rod? He never mentioned to me he had a child." Carol could feel herself being swallowed up in the darkest of dark moods she had ever experienced. She could feel a thick mass of venomous anger and hate forming in the back of her throat and it was now threatening to choke off her voice, if not her very breath. Struggling to keep her voice light and friendly, she lied again, "Oh, here comes Rod now. Thank you so much for your time. I'd better get off the phone." Dropping the receiver into the cradle, Carol stood in the middle of her living room and screamed her anguish until her throat became raw and her voice grew hoarse. Then, when she could scream no more, she ran into the kitchen, grabbed a finely sharpened boning knife from its wooden holder, and rampaged through her house, stabbing the walls and slicing the upholstered furniture until she eventually collapsed in a sweaty, crazed heap of madness. But she would soon rise and have in mind a well thought out plan to ensure her continued presence in Rod McDonough's life. *How dare he think he could simply toss me out onto the junk heap of his life, she thought.*

Other than one brief meeting with Carol Bennett at the hospital, when she was Rod's nurse, Julie really didn't know the woman. Julie was aware that Freebird did not like her, but he had never told her why he felt that way. On the phone just now, Julie thought that Carol sounded very friendly and nice. And Carol did seem very concerned

291

about Rod. When Carol quickly hung up, Julie shrugged it off and went on with her extra busy morning. With Martina gone for her meeting with Attorney Travante she had both Jody and Roddy to take care of, so there was no time for any telephone chatting anyway.

Besides, Julie was enjoying how wonderfully Jody and Roddy played together. She was even thinking about how great it would be if she and Freebird had another baby, a playmate for Jody. It seemed so much easier with two babies, because they entertained each other, and it gave her some time to catch her breath.

So, when Julie's telephone rang two hours later and it was Carol Bennett calling back, she had no reason to be the least bit suspicious. "Hi, Carol," Julie chirped.

Back in command of her syrupy voice, Carol fed Julie the story she had concocted to set her plan in motion. "Rod asked me to call and leave a message for his wife (Carol couldn't even remember Martina's name). He was kind enough to take my car over to the service station...I've been having problems getting it started...so...he was wondering if she and Roddy (Carol had picked up the boy's name from her earlier conversation with Julie) could meet him at his house on Scenic Drive...something happened with a water pipe over there and he said he would have to drive straight over there from the service station, to let the plumber into the house."

Later, Julie would have to admit that Carol's story did sound a bit odd, but at that moment she obediently took the message. Several hours later, when Martina called Julie, wondering why Rod had not shown up at Travante's office to pick her up as they had earlier planned, Julie unwittingly put Carol's demented plan into motion.

"Just hang tight for a moment," Julie assured, after relating the plumbing problem story to Martina, "and I'll come get you and drive you over to Scenic. There's no phone over there, so I've not talked to Rod. But I'm sure he is over there by now and waiting for you and Roddy."

"I'll keep an eye out for you," said Martina, thinking it was strange that Rod would want to meet her over there while he was dealing with a plumber, but she shrugged it off.

56.

After his lunch with Nancy Farnsworth, Travis was flying high. He went back upstairs to the third floor as though he was actually ascending to Cloud Nine. He couldn't wait for Rod to come around so he could tell him about how he had just met the woman he was certain was going to be the love of his life. And safely tucked in Travis's pocket of his Italian leather jacket was Nancy Farnsworth's telephone number. But Rod was still sleeping when Travis returned to his room, so he went to a pay phone to call his secretary, Naomi, and tell her he would be out of the office for the rest of the day and fill her in on Rod's situation.

"What's going on with Rod?" Naomi barked into the phone, her voice raspy from years of chain smoking and hard liquor. Travis had inherited the crusty older woman from his father and she was a formidable war horse. Naomi knew everybody in the building trades who was anybody and she pulled no punches. And while she may have had a fondness for Travis, Naomi had a deep, grandmotherly love for Rod.

"He's going to be okay…but he's still out of it," Travis told her. Naomi was considered a trusted family member, so Travis felt as though he could tell her anything.

"I'm going over there to see him and I'm going to kick his ass," she proclaimed to Travis. "He ought to know better than to be up to those kind of shenanigans."

"Yes, Ma'am," said Travis. "I'm going to kick his ass too, so you'll have to stand in line. But in the meantime, I'll be at Millborough General and you can call me here at the third floor Nurses' Station if you need me."

After his conversation with Naomi, Travis went back to Rod's room to continue his vigil. When Rod had still not awakened by three-thirty in the afternoon, Travis became antsy and decided to walk around. While he was pacing up and down in the hall, he suddenly thought of Freebird and decided he should call Rod's best friend and let him know Rod was in the hospital.

When Freebird answered the phone with "It's your dime and my time!"

Travis laughed at the Indian's utter coolness.

"Hey, man! It's Travis!"

293

Freebird was surprised to be hearing from Rod's brother. Travis seldom called him. "What's up, Travis," said Freebird, his suspicions aroused.

"Just wanted to let you know that Rod is in Millborough General—"

"What happened?" Freebird cut in, suddenly afraid for his friend. All he could think of was that Carol Bennett tried to kill Rod after he told her he was getting back with Martina. "Did Carol do something to him?"

"In a way, yah, she did do something to him. He's having bad withdrawals from whatever drugs she's been feeding him. He called me this morning...all strung out. I picked him up and drove him straight to the hospital. He's going to be okay...but he is real sick now...it's like he's possessed by demons from Hell."

Freebird blew out a heavy breath. "Like he hasn't been through enough crap...and now...just when things are looking up for him this happens."

"What do you mean by 'things are looking up?'"

Freebird realized that Travis probably didn't know about Martina and Roddy. "I guess Rod was too far gone to tell you...but Martina is here...visiting from California and Rod was with her all day yesterday and half the night. Looks like they might be getting back together."

"What! Martina?" Travis exclaimed, his tone conveying his shock and surprise. He wasn't quite sure if that was good or bad news, all things considered. "I had no idea he had seen her...he was hardly coherent when I picked him up. My God! Where is she staying?"

"She's staying here at our house...but there's something else, Travis...Rod has a son." Freebird could practically hear the cogs in Travis's mind clicking and whirring as the twice shocked man tried to assimilate the news Freebird just gave him.

Travis tried to respond but the connection between his brain and his voice box was temporarily compromised, so all he could do was sputter bits and pieces of words. "I don't— My God! What? A son?"

Freebird couldn't help but laugh at Travis's reaction. "Yes, a beautiful son...who looks just like Rod." Freebird threw in the last bit of information about the boy looking like Rod because he knew Travis had to be wondering if the child was really Rod's. Everyone in Millborough had been tainted by the rumors of incest, which especially troubled the McDonough family when the stories began circulating after Rod's shooting, provoking them to hire an attorney to protect Rod's interests. The perceptive Freebird suspected that Travis would have mixed emotions about Martina resurfacing and Rod seeing her again.

Finally, Travis asked, "How did Rod react to seeing her and…his son?"

Freebird chuckled. "Huh! It was Martina who had the biggest reaction…all this time she thought Rod had been killed by her father. It was a complete shock when she found out he was alive."

"My God! How did she get that idea?"

"From some dumb-ass Millborough detective back when Rod was shot. Then no one bothered to tell her he actually survived."

"How awful," Travis commented, remembering how Rod was so depressed about Martina's disappearance when he came out of his coma. "So they saw each other yesterday?"

"I'm sure there were a few major adjustments to be made but…really Trav… it was like they hadn't missed a beat. I mean…don't get me wrong … they still have a lot to work out between themselves, but they are both older and wiser…and the bottom line is they still love each other…and now they have a kid to think about also."

"This just blows me away," Travis commented, still trying to grasp the full import of it all. "I'd like to see her and the boy…are they there now?"

"Uh…no. I'm not sure where they are. I just came in from work and Julie and the kids are gone. Martina had a meeting this afternoon with that attorney who's taking care of her father's estate and Rod was supposed to pick her up from the dude's office. I'm thinking that since Rod was not able to show up or call, Martina must have called Julie to go there to pick her up."

Still reeling, Travis said, "Oh my God! This is unbelievable. And poor Rod…going into detox at a time like this…I just don't know what to say."

"Well…actually…anytime is a good time for Rod to detox. I've been after him for months to get away from that chick and her drugs."

"Do you have any idea what drug she was giving him…the doctor here at the hospital asked if I knew but I didn't even know Rod was taking any drugs at all."

"I think Methadone…but I'm not sure. That shit is worse than Heroin. I think Carol was stealing it from the Hospital," Freebird remarked with obvious disgust.

"I'll let Rod's doctor know—they said something about having to do a blood test on Rod to find out what he was using…." Distracted by another thought, Travis's voice trailed off and he was silent for a moment. Then he asked Freebird, "Would it be possible for me to come by tonight…after I leave the Hospital? I'd like to see Martina and Rod's boy. How old is he?"

"Roddy's about…well, I know he's not quite two years yet. But sure…you are welcome to come over any time. How does it feel to be an instant uncle?"

"You're right! I am an uncle." Travis started laughing, obviously pleased with the idea.

"Hang on, Trav," Freebird cut in. "Here comes Julie now. Let me find out what's going on." He set the telephone receiver down on the kitchen counter. Looking through the window next to the back door, Freebird saw only Julie, carrying Jody, walking from the car toward the house. He pulled open the door and went to meet her. "Where's Martina and Roddy?" Freebird asked Julie with a worried tone.

"I took them over to the house on Scenic Drive," said Julie.

"Why did you take them there?" Freebird asked, feeling the first inklings of foreboding.

"Because Rod had Carol call here earlier to tell me he had to go over to Scenic for some kind of plumbing problem. Carol said Rod wanted Martina to meet him over at the house—" Julie saw Freebird's expression change from worried concern to horror. "What's wrong?" She yelled as he turned and ran back into the house.

Picking up the phone from the counter, Freebird told Travis, "We've got big trouble. Carol's up to something and she's got Martina and Roddy over at your house on Scenic Drive. I'm going over there right now. Meet me there as soon as you can." Handing the phone to a dumbstruck Julie, Freebird instructed, "Call the police and tell them there's a possible…uh…confrontation going on at the McDonough House on Scenic Drive and they need to get there immediately." Seeing the look of horror on Julie's face, he didn't want to totally freak her out by saying the word "murder," but he was sure that was what Carol had in mind. Freebird then ran to his bedroom closet to retrieve the loaded gun he kept hidden in there on the shelf.

Unaware that she had been duped by Carol Bennett, Julie called to Freebird as he bounded out of the kitchen, "Why would there be a confrontation between Rod and Martina?"

"Not Rod!" Freebird yelled over his shoulder. "It's Carol. Just call the police like I asked. I have no time to explain now."

As Freebird ran out the back door, Julie was on the phone with the Millborough Police Dispatch, trying to tell the duty officer what fragments she knew of the situation, but the officer didn't seem to be convinced her friend Martina was in any imminent danger. "Well...all I can tell you," screamed Julie, "is that my husband is on his way over there now with a gun and he will use it if he has to." Julie's reference to a gun seemed to catch the dispatch officer's attention.

57.

Holding Roddy's hand, Martina helped the little boy climb the few steps up to the back porch of the old stone house. She had mixed emotions about being there, and wondered why Rod hadn't come out to greet them when Julie blew her car's horn. Nor was there a plumber's truck in the driveway. Stepping into the screened porch, Martina got a chill. The house was eerily quiet and she didn't feel Rod's presence nearby. She wished Julie had not left right away, but her friend was worried about getting home in time to cook Freebird's dinner. Where was Rod? Something was not right about this whole scenario.

The older model gray Chevy Impala in the driveway was Carol's car, but, according to Julie, Rod must have driven it there. Martina did not relish the idea of Rod driving her around in Carol's car. And she could not imagine that Rod would even want her to ride in another's woman's car. Peering into the familiar kitchen through the open back door, she called Rod's name. There was no answer. Perhaps he's out of earshot, she thought. But another voice coming from deep inside cautioned her to turn around and get out of there. Martina brushed the warning voice aside, telling herself she was merely being silly about the whole situation. Besides, it felt good to be back in the house that was the scene of so many of her happiest memories, when she and Rod were together and so much in love.

When Martina attempted to lead Roddy into the house, the little boy balked and pulled back. "No," exclaimed the child, his eyes wide with fright. "It's okay, Sweetie," she told him. "We're going to see Daddy." Tentatively, the little boy followed his mother into the shadowy kitchen, the sound of their shoes on the floor announcing their entry.

It was in the living room that Carol was waiting for Martina's arrival. She was sitting, almost leisurely, in a large upholstered chair that faced the kitchen doorway, so she would see Martina the instant the young woman approached. It was unlikely that Martina would see Carol in the darkness. The chair in which Carol had ensconced herself happened to be in a very murky area of the room. And with the shades all drawn so tight to the window sills, the room was even darker than the kitchen. Carol heard the footsteps of the unwitting young mother and the child coming her way. An evil smile spread across her diabolical face as she thought of the apropos phrase: *Step into my parlor said the spider to the little flies.*

The dark room beyond the kitchen terrified Roddy and he pulled back when his mother tried to lead him through the doorway. Martina stopped and groped the wall beside her for the light switch. It seemed strange to her that Rod would not have already turned on the lights, knowing that she was coming there to meet him. After flipping on the light switch and no lights coming on, it was apparent the electrical power had been turned off. Now Martina was convinced that something was amiss and started to turn to leave. Suddenly, a flashlight came on in the living room and its powerful beam hit her in the eyes, temporarily blinding her.

"Well, will you look who's here," a harsh, booming voice called out from behind the light. "If it isn't the little slut of Millborough and her bastard son."

Martina made the connection immediately and assumed it was Carol who was speaking, and knew she had to get Roddy out of there and to safety. But she had hesitated just a moment too long, giving Carol the edge for a surprise attack. Before Martina could escape, Carol jumped from the darkness behind the blinding flashlight beam and grabbed hold of Martina's long hair. Then, yanking Martina off balance, Carol punched her surprised victim in the stomach with such brutal force that Martina fell to the floor, gasping for breath. While Martina writhed on the floor in pain, Carol took advantage of the moment and began tying Martina's hands and ankles together with a length of rope she had brought with her just for that purpose. "I'm not interested in you anyway," Carol hissed malevolently as she roughly knotted the rope. "A worthless piece of ass like you can be replaced. But the kid...that'll hurt Rod more than anything." Then she muttered, more to herself than Martina, "I'll show that ungrateful sonofabitch he can't dump me like I'm some kind of trash."

Martina could hear Roddy whimpering nearby but she was unable to see him from her position on the floor. Furious with herself for being so stupid, she was heartsick that she had put her precious little son in such terrible danger, and now she was helpless to protect him from whatever the crazed woman had in mind. She tried to beg Carol not to hurt Roddy, but she was gasping so hard for air that it was impossible for her to form an intelligible word. Attempting to tear her hands free from the rope that bound them, Martina only succeeded in pulling the bindings even tighter. A terrible panic seized her mind as she continued to gasp for air and struggle to free herself. Suddenly, everything went black.

With Martina disposed of, Carol turned her attention to the crying child. "No need to cry, little boy," she said with a strange, detached voice. "We're going for a nice ride in the car...and Carol's going to take you swimming." The child, even in his innocence, sensed the woman was not to be trusted. He ran over to where his mother lie on the floor and huddled next to her inert body.

Laughing maniacally, Carol picked up the crying boy and carried him out of the house.

58.

Freebird arrived at the McDonough Estate just minutes before Travis and the police. He stood in the driveway and scanned the house and grounds with his keen eyes, and listened intently for the slightest sounds. The door to the back porch and the door to the kitchen, he saw, were wide open, but he heard no conversation coming from within. Cocking his 9mm revolver, the young man started walking toward the house. Midway along the brick walkway to the back porch Freebird saw one of Roddy's small toy automobiles lying in the grass. A bad feeling came over him while, simultaneously, a vision of a crying Roddy flashed in his mind. He knew immediately that Roddy had been taken from the house.

As he entered the house he heard a car speeding up the driveway, but Freebird did not allow it to break his concentration on the feel or his finely tuned senses. He was sure he heard someone breathing in the living room, and crouched behind the island counter in the kitchen until he could discern the situation. When the blurred image of Martina came into his head, Freebird knew immediately it was Martina's breath he heard and she was in trouble. He also sensed there was no one else in the house. When Freebird found Martina hogtied on the living room floor she was barely conscious. The sudden musty smell of Carol Bennett assailed his nostrils and he knew for sure it was she who had been there earlier and tied up Martina. Setting his gun down on the floor, he unsheathed his long skinning knife and sliced the rope that bound Martina's wrists and ankles. He was in the act of feeling her pulse when a man's voice behind him shouted, "Don't move! Put your hands up where I can see them."

Freebird had no doubt there was a cop behind him with the barrel of a gun trained on his back, so he slowly raised his hands. "I'm a friend," Freebird said calmly. "This woman needs an ambulance…and the person who injured her has kidnapped her little boy and is getting further away as we talk."

"Are you Clay Terry?" The authoritative voice asked.

"Yes. I had my wife call the police while I drove here," Freebird explained, adding, "The person you want is Carol Bennett and she is going to harm this woman's little boy if we don't find her quick."

"Stand up and turn around slowly…I'll need to see your ID," the voice commanded.

Just then, Freebird heard more voices coming from the kitchen and turned around to see another policeman come into the room, with Travis McDonough behind him. Seeing Martina lying so still on the floor, Travis became alarmed. "Oh my God!" He exclaimed. "She's not—" The policeman who was holding his gun on Freebird said, "She's unconscious." To his partner he hurriedly said, "Grady! Go call for an ambulance." Officer Grady ran back out through the kitchen, to the use the radio in the patrol car.

Travis knelt down beside Martina and took one of her hands in his. He saw the remnant of rope tied around her wrist and he shook his head sadly. Looking up at Freebird, he asked, "Carol did this?"

Freebird nodded a response as he handed the policeman his driver's license.

"Where's the little boy?" Travis asked, looking around the room.

"Carol's got him," said Freebird, giving the policeman with the gun an angry look. "And we've got to find her before she does anything to him."

"Who is this Carol Bennett and why would she take this woman's child?" asked the policeman, who was examining Freebird's ID.

Travis succinctly explained Carol's connection to Rod, Martina, and the kidnapped child. "We've got to find her and get my nephew back," Travis implored, his face pale and stricken.

"And where's your brother...the father of the child...now?"

The officer interrogated Travis.

"My brother is in the hospital...he's very sick," Travis responded tersely, offering no further information.

"Can you give me a description of Carol Bennett and the vehicle she's driving?" asked the officer as he handed Freebird's license back to him and holstered his gun. "We can issue an APB for her."

Travis and Freebird responded affirmatively at the same time, and the officer took down Carol's information from both of them. As they each told the cop all they could remember about Carol's physical appearance and her gray Impala, a wailing siren could be heard approaching the house.

Travis told Freebird, "I'll follow the ambulance back to the Hospital...so Martina will not be without any family there, when she wakes up. But I'm worried sick about the baby...."

Freebird could see that Travis looked like he was ready to freak out, and placed a hand on the man's shoulder. "Don't worry about the boy, Travis." Turning to the cop, Freebird asked, "May I leave now?"

The cop nodded and asked, "Where will you be if I need to get in touch with you later?"

"I don't know yet," said Freebird, looking distracted. "I'm going to find my friend's little boy." Saying that, Freebird strode quickly from the room, passing the incoming medical attendants wheeling a gurney into the kitchen. He knew that Martina would recover from what appeared to be a blow of some kind, but little Roddy was in a more lethal situation. And Freebird knew he had to get away from all of the activity at the McDonough house, so he could focus on Roddy and where to look for him.

59.

The footpath in the woods behind the McDonough Estate was well known to Freebird. He had traveled along that path many times to climb to the summit of the steep hill above Scenic Drive. The summit, he was certain, had once been the sacred ceremonial site of his ancestors, the Pequots. There was a small cave up there, hidden from the casual eye that had pictographs drawn on its walls by ancient hands. Freebird had studied and pondered the drawings many times. He thought perhaps the summit was once a place referred to as the hill of enlightenment, as the actual shape of the summit was depicted in a cave drawing with rays of light encircling it. Whether or not it was a sacred place in the past didn't matter; Freebird considered it his sacred place, where he could go and ponder mysteries and find answers. So, after leaving the chaotic scene in the stone house, he quickly sprinted up the path to the summit.

It seemed to take a long time for Freebird to quiet his mind and focus on the strange energy he could identify with Carol Bennett, but once he picked up the thread of dark emanations she released into the Universe he was able to see clearly where she had gone, and that Rod's little boy was perilously close to drowning. Shaking off his trance, Freebird rose and raced back down the path, and by the time he burst through the tree line behind the McDonough property he was running at his utmost speed toward his truck. The two policemen who were the first to arrive on the scene earlier, Grady and the one with the gun, whose name Freebird did not know, were standing in the driveway talking with two other officers, who apparently arrived while Freebird was up on the summit. The ambulance was gone.

When the four policemen saw young Indian come running out of the trees, his long black hair flying wildly out behind him, the two officers who had not seen him previously, simultaneously went for their guns.

"Follow me," Freebird yelled, as he ran to his truck. "I know where she's taken the boy."

Grady's partner shouted back, "How do you know? Come over here!"

"There's no time!" Freebird yelled back, "She's going to drown him." Jumping into his truck, there was just enough clearance for Freebird to back up and make a U-turn on the lawn and drive through the trees until he was around the two patrol cars that were blocking his exit from the driveway.

The four cops looked at each other and then paired off towards their respective patrol cars, to follow the strange young man. As Grady tried to keep up with truck, he said to his partner, whose name was Joe Duggan, "What the hell is going on here? How would that Indian know where Carol Bennett took the kid?"

Duggan shrugged and said, quite seriously, "Maybe he went up on the hill back there and consulted with the Great Spirit or something. How the heck would I know? Just don't lose sight of him."

60.

The needle of his gas gauge was on empty but there was no time to stop for gas. It would be getting dark in less than an hour and Freebird knew he would have to find Roddy before the sun went down, and he hoped his truck didn't run out of fuel before he made it out to Old Quarry Lake.

If it were not for the fact he liked to ride the deserted back roads on his bike, he would never have recognized the place that was shown to him in his vision up on the summit – the place where Carol took Roddy. As it was, he didn't recognize the water filled quarry pit at first. But there was that pyramid shaped pile of rocks next to the lake, and that was what triggered Freebird's memory. He had driven in there once on his motorcycle, just to look around, and actually took a swim in the lake. He remembered how it had a steep drop off several feet from its rocky shore, and he dove down as far as he could and never saw a bottom. Freebird shivered to think of Roddy being anywhere near that cold, bottomless pit of water. Automatically, he pressed his foot down on the accelerator and sped up on the open highway. Within seconds a red warning light flickered on in his dashboard, signaling he was running out of gas. He estimated the quarry was three miles up the road, and he prayed he would have enough fuel to make it to the lake once he turned onto Old Quarry Lake Road. For once, it felt good to have the cops chasing him.

Within fifty feet of the lake the fuel starved engine of Freedbird's truck began to sputter. He did not see Carol's car parked anywhere and suddenly grew worried that he might have wasted precious time and fuel in driving to the wrong place. Pushing his niggling doubts aside, he jammed on his brakes and the old truck skidded to a halt in the middle of the road. Grabbing his revolver, Freebird jumped out of the cab.

When his boots hit the gravel road he took off running in the direction of the lake, which he knew would be on his right as soon as he broke free of the high granite wall that formed one side of the semi-circular quarry lake. Finally, he saw the pyramid of stones ahead, off to his right, and beyond that was the lake. Still, he did not see Carol's car. Nor did he see any sign of the woman or Roddy. The sun was making its descent toward the western horizon, its yellow-orange orb still visible and fully illuminating the lake. Freebird reminded himself of the words he heard so clearly during his vision on the summit: As long as the sun is visible the boy will be alive. His heart pounded wildly in his chest. Did he misinterpret the signs he saw in his vision, he wondered. There was no time for any second guessing.

Squinting into the sun-drenched lake, Freebird noticed the bubbling and rippling of the water, right where he knew the drop off began. To his horror, Freebird immediately realized what Carol had done with her car. She had driven it into the lake, and he had gotten there too late to save Rod's son.

"No! No!" Freebird screamed as a shockwave of terror dropped him to his knees. "She wasn't supposed to do it now!" Currents of anguish, sorrow, and rage coursed through his body as he pounded the gravel road with his fists and terrible, mournful cries tore from his throat. He had failed to protect his best friend's son. He would never be able to face Rod again. How could he have let such a horrible thing happen?

Suddenly, from somewhere nearby, a child's halting voice urged, "No - cwi -bwird."

Not believing what he heard, Freebird looked up and saw little Roddy crawling over the rocks toward him, about ten feet away. He could see that the child's hair and clothing were soaking wet. Pulling himself up, Freebird ran to the boy and scooped him up into his arms, holding him tightly against his chest. Suddenly feeling the muscles in his legs weaken and tremble, the young man sat down on a nearby boulder, alternately hugging the child and inspecting his little body for possible injuries. But it appeared the child did not have even a scratch on him. Freebird studied the wet but otherwise calm little boy for a few moments, at a complete loss to understand what had just happened; he was certain Roddy was not anywhere near that lake when he arrived there. Freebird turned to glance at the placid quarry lake and saw a curious feathery mist hovering over the spot where he had seen the bubbles from Carol Bennett's sinking car. Suddenly, the mist swirled into a rotating vortex and plunged into the lake.

When the two police cars that had been following Freebird pulled up the scene the officers found Freebird sitting on a boulder, chanting and rocking the little boy, who appeared to be unharmed.

"Where's Carol Bennett?" Duggan asked the young Indian.

Freebird casually pointed over his shoulder, toward the lake. "In there," he said, clearly unconcerned about the watery demise of such an evil woman.

"Her car too?" Asked Grady, looking out at the glass-like surface of the lake, which was now serenely reflecting the blood red color of the setting sun.

Freebird nodded and continued rocking. Then, remembering his truck had run out of gas, he asked Duggan and Grady, "Can you guys give me and my little buddy a ride back to town? I'm flat out of gas."

61.

Other than feeling drained and weak, Rod sat up in bed, glad to be over the worst of his withdrawals. A pretty young nurse with short dark hair had just been in his room to fluff his pillows and told him she would let his brother know that he was awake and able to receive visitors. She acted like she knew Travis pretty well. Rod wondered why Travis had never mentioned anything about her to him. But, then, Rod had to admit that he had been inaccessible to family and friends for the last couple of years, so it was no wonder he was out of the loop with what had been going on in everyone's lives. But that, he knew, was about to change. As he looked out of the window across the room at the sunny day beyond, he was anxious to get back his strength and get on with his life. He thought of Martina and Roddy and felt a warming in his heart.

Of course, he was completely unaware that Martina was at that very moment in a room on the floor just below him, recuperating from a blow to the head, and Roddy was now back with Freebird and Julie, having been examined in the Hospital's Emergency Room last evening after being rescued at Old Quarry Lake. It was just as well Rod had no knowledge of what had transpired with his wife and son while he was in the throes of a detox. If he had been told, he would have crawled out of that hospital bed and demanded to be taken to them.

About three o'clock that afternoon Travis appeared at Rod's bedside with a basket of fruit. Rod had drifted into a light sleep but woke up as soon as he sensed another person in the room. "Hey, bro!" Travis said, plunking the fruit basket on Rod's lap.

"Oh! Hey, Travis." Rod reached up to hug his brother. "Thanks for coming to get me and bringing me here. I'm sure I was a total mess."

"You know I was glad to do that for you, Rod. It's good to see you looking clear-eyed again." Although, Travis thought his brother looked a bit worse for the wear he would never say so.

"I really would have preferred you not see me like that."

"We're brothers, Rod. You would have done the same for me."

Travis wasn't sure how to break the news to Rod about what Carol had done to Martina and Roddy, but he had volunteered to be the one, so he took a deep breath and stuck to the script he and Freebird worked out. "Uh…Rod…I've got something to tell you. Don't panic because everyone is okay…but your friend Carol is apparently gone…."

Rod gave his brother a quizzical look. "What do you mean? Gone as in gone away?"

Travis cleared his throat. "Uh— No. Gone as in dead."

"What! What happened?" Rod sat bolt upright, a shocked expression on his face. Although Rod did not ever love Carol, he did feel some connection to her; she had, after all, taken a medical interest in him and helped him to walk again. He felt he owed her something for that. But the rest of their relationship, as he well knew, was very destructive.

Taking a deep breath, Travis again assured Rod that everything was okay. "She apparently drove her car into Old Quarry Lake and drowned," he said, trying not to elaborate.

"She committed suicide?" Rod said, incredulous. "We had a fight before I walked out but I never thought she'd do anything like that."

"Don't feel bad for her, Rod. Just before she did it she tricked Julie into driving Martina and Roddy over to our house" Travis stopped short of telling Rod what Carol had actually done, adding only, "Her intentions were not good."

Rod attempted to get out of bed but he was so weak that Travis easily pushed him back against the pillows. "Martina and Roddy are fine. Don't worry. They'll be here to see you in a little while."

Rod heaved a deep sigh. "Jesus, Travis...." was all he could say.

"I'll be right back," Travis said, and left the room.

Down the corridor from Rod's hospital room was a small waiting area, where Martina, Roddy, Julie and Freebird were waiting for Travis to come and give them the okay to go in to see Rod.

"I only told him that Carol drowned herself in the pond at the quarry and assured him that everyone was okay." And then Travis remembered one other statement he made to Rod. "I also told him that Carol had tricked Julie into bringing Martina and Roddy over to our house...but I thought it would be best if Martina told him what she did...so he could see that she and Roddy are alright. That way, he won't get all upset. He's kind of weak right now."

Martina, who had a sizeable knot on the side of her head that was still throbbing, said, "I'll tell him what she did, but not until after he gets out of the hospital and is a little stronger."

"Good idea," said Travis, grabbing his little nephew and picking him up.

Freebird and Julie nodded in agreement. Then they all headed up the hall to Rod's room.

62.

"You know you can stay with me at the lake house and, frankly, I think it would be good for your health," Travis told Rod on the day before he was to be discharged from the hospital.

"But it's too far away from Martina and Roddy," Rod said, and then added, "Otherwise I would love to stay out there."

"Well, then, where else can you stay? It wouldn't be worth turning on the electricity at our old house if you're not going to stay there for a while. What's Martina going to do? Is she going back to California or is she going to move back here?" Travis queried his brother.

"Martina has already said she does not want to move back to Millborough…because of all the ugly gossip. She feels it will be bad for Roddy," said Rod.

Travis nodded. "Understandable."

From a corner of the room where he had been quietly sitting, listening to the two brothers talk, Freebird said, "He can stay at my house till he makes up his mind what he wants to do…and he will be close to Martina and his baby."

"Martina and the baby are welcome to stay at the lake house too," Travis said. "I wasn't excluding them from the invitation."

"Thanks. Both of you," said Rod. "Let me talk to Martina and see what her plans are. I don't even know how much longer she is staying, but I think she has one more meeting with Travante to sign some papers authorizing the sale of that mausoleum where her father used to live." He grimaced at the thought of Martino Fiasconi's torture chamber of a house; it was just another reminder of Fiasconi's evil and the place where Martina was abused and beaten.

"She'll be doing that tomorrow," Freebird said. "I heard her tell Julie this morning. Her flight back is the following day." Freebird didn't want to bring it up now, but he had also heard Martina say that after the terrible fright she had with Carol kidnapping Roddy, that she was doubly certain she would never move back here.

Rod winced. "Not much time left. I'm hoping she will move back here and we can live at our old house."

Travis and Freebird merely exchanged doubtful glances.

*****

311

It was his first day out of the hospital and Rod knew he should have been resting in bed, but he didn't want to miss out on spending as much time as possible with Roddy. Instead, he positioned a lounge chair on the sunny patio so he could watch his son and Jody play in the yard. Julie was there, too, to make sure Rod did not overdo it. She brought out a pitcher of iced water and cautioned Rod to keep himself hydrated.

"I hope Martina is not going to be tied up all day with Travante," Rod commented to Julie.

"I hope not, too. She'll be leaving tomorrow and we've hardly spent any time with her," said Julie, adding, "I'm glad you decided to stay here until she leaves so you'll have more time together."

"Maybe she can change her flight and stay a few more days. We have so much to talk about."

"That would be really nice," Julie agreed. "But she promised her aunt and uncle she would not stay any longer than she had to in order to take care of that creepy house her father lived in. I hope she can sell it right away and be done with it."

"I wouldn't care if that house of horrors burned to the ground. The sooner she is rid of that house, the better it will be. She told me that she can't even bring herself to go there to see what kind of condition it's in. She's having Travante handle it all."

"I wonder what her aunt and uncle will say when they find out about me?" Rod said.

"I'm sure they'll be shocked, but happy for Martina and Roddy...and happy for you," assured Julie. "They seem like really good people."

"I don't know, Julie. They won't be too happy if she and Roddy move back here to live."

Julie said nothing in response. She knew that Martina would not even think about moving back east now. Not after the incident with Carol. Martina was now too spooked about Roddy's safety. Even though Julie reminded Martina that Carol was no longer a threat, Martina told her that Carol wasn't the only nut running around Millborough. "What about all those sickos who said Roddy was Martino's kid? Any one of them might be crazy enough to hurt Roddy and me or even Rod, for that matter," Martina had countered. Julie could hardly argue with her about that. And once Martina told Rod the story of what Carol had done before she drove herself into the quarry pond, Julie was sure that Rod would move anywhere Martina wanted to go, including Timbuktu.

"No sense getting ahead of ourselves, Rod." Then, hearing the telephone ringing, Julie went into the house to answer it. "Keep an eye on the babies," she called over her shoulder as she ran inside.

*****

"I'm glad it worked out that Freebird could pick me up from Travante's office on his way home from work this afternoon," Martina commented, as she helped Julie set the kitchen table for dinner. It was now nearly eight o'clock. They decided to eat dinner later than usual so they could feed the kids, get them bathed and into bed. Rod and Freebird were out on the patio, where they could keep an eye on the grill.

Sidling up to Martina, Julie whispered, "When are you going to tell Rod about Carol?"

"How about tonight after dinner? But I want you and Freebird to be there when I tell him. Okay?"

"Are you sure?"

"Positive," Martina said. "You and Freebird are part of the story and can fill in a lot of the blanks."

"I just hope Rod won't be mad at me," Julie fretted.

"Mad? Why would he be mad at you?"

"Oh, c'mon. I let Carol trick me into bringing you and Roddy right to her."

"You forget that noise right now, Julie. You had no way of knowing what that woman was up to. You're a good-hearted person and would never suspect she would be capable of such evil."

"Thank you, Martina. But I should have been suspicious of her. Freebird's always said he didn't trust her."

"That's just it, Julie. You didn't know Carol, so how would you know to be suspicious? I probably would have believed her myself if I had taken her call." Martina placed her hands on Julie's shoulders, and looked her squarely in the eyes. "Do you remember the day after we got married when you got mad at me for saying that I did not deserve someone as good as Rod?" Julie nodded. "Well, I don't ever want to hear you say you were in any way responsible for what Carol did. Do you understand?"

Julie nodded to her friend, somewhat mollified.

"Good." Martina said. "Now let that be the end of it."

Martina then pulled Julie into a heartfelt hug.

313

"What's going on in there?" Freebird yelled into the kitchen through the patio door screen.

Martina looked over at him and smiled. "Just hugging the best little sister that anyone ever had."

63.

If Julie felt bad about Carol's evil deed, Rod felt even worse. Of course, he took all the blame upon himself. To his mind, he was the one who had brought the evil woman into their lives. After hearing all of the details about Carol's attack on Martina and then her kidnapping of Roddy, Rod was beside himself with anger and regret. It took a while to calm him down. Martina was the first to remind him what he had said to her about Martino, he's dead and can't hurt us anymore. The same reminder applied to Carol Bennett. While Rod was able to acknowledge the fact Carol was dead, he could not put aside the fact that if he had not been strung out on drugs he would have been able to protect his wife and son.

"You will just have to put it out of your mind, Rod," Martina told him later, when they had gone to bed. "Who would have ever thought she would do such a thing. Don't think about the evil she did, think about the miracle that none of us were harmed. She could have easily done something to you too, when you went back to her house after leaving here the other night."

Rod sighed and pulled Martina closer. "You're right, Baby. We can't live here. This place is not for us. We need to go someplace where no one knows us and we can make a new start."

Hearing him say that, Martina could hardly control her excitement. "Then you'll come back to California with me?"

"Yes. But you'll have to give me time to find a replacement at my job...I can't leave Travis with all of the projects I am working on."

"Do you know anyone who can take over for you?" She asked, trying to get an idea as to how long she would have to wait for him to join her in San Francisco.

"Actually, I do," he said, a note of relief filling his voice.
"And I'll call him tomorrow."
"Who is it?" Martina asked, feeling relieved herself.
"The man who started the business...my father."
"Do you think he will want to come out of retirement?"
"He will when I tell him what's going on." After a moment, he said, "And you better call your Aunt and Uncle tomorrow and let them know you are staying another week."

"I can't wait to tell them why. They are going to be blown away when I tell them about you."

"I hope so. Good thing we're not flying back there tomorrow. I wouldn't want them to see me looking like this."

"Never mind the way you look. We can never tell them about what happened to Roddy and me or they'd be here on the next flight and drag us right back. My Aunt was so afraid something bad might happen to us here."

She felt a shudder move through Rod's body. "I'm so sorry, Martina. When I think about how close you and Roddy came…it scares me that life is so fragile."

"Life is fragile for everybody, Rod"

"Yes, but we've had more than our share of fragility."

"Then that should be the end of it for us. The rest of our lives will be fragile free."

On that note, they drifted off to sleep with Roddy nestled between them.

64.

As promised, Rod contacted his father in the Bahamas the day after his discussion with Martina. It was a long conversation, as it had to be. There was a two year gap to fill in for his father. His father was ecstatic to hear he had a grandson and pleased to hear Rod sounding like his old self again, but was concerned about his involvement with Martina.

"But Dad, we still love each other and we have a beautiful son," Rod assured. "The only problems we ever had were caused by her father and thankfully he's dead. So now we have a chance to be a real family."

"Well, son, you're over twenty-one and you know what's best for you," Jim McDonough told his son. "You have a good head on your shoulders and I trust you to make good decisions."

"So you'll come back home and take over my job?"

"I'll be happy to help you out any way I can, Rod. Plus, your mother and I want to meet our daughter-in-law and grandson. We'll be home as soon as I can get the boat stowed. It'll be a few days."

"Thanks, Dad. I really appreciate your doing this."

"Truth be known, son...I kindda miss the business."

Rod hung up the phone and let out a loud whoop. He found Martina and Julie out in the back yard with the kids. Freebird had built a small swing using fencing logs and hung two baby seats from the top beam, and they were watching Jody and Roddy, who were both in awe of their new mobility, swing back and forth like pendulums.

"How'd it go?" said Martina, noting the big smile of satisfaction on his face.

"They're flying back in a few days and looking forward to finally meeting you and seeing their grandson."

"That's so great," Julie said. "But it's kind of sad, too. That means you'll both be leaving us."

"We'll visit each other," Martina said. "Who knows, when you and Freebird see California you might want to move there too."

"I've got to call Travis," Rod said, his mind obviously running at full speed. "And I've got to get the utilities turned on at the house on Scenic."

"Why don't you sit down in the sun for a little bit," Martina suggested. "You've been a bit too keyed up this morning and should take a rest. If you keep an eye on Roddy I'll make you a protein shake with lots of fruit in it."

"Okay, said Rod. Let me go get a chair. He was feeling a little peaked and didn't want to overdue it. He dragged his patio chair closer to Roddy. Watching his excited son as the swing went back and forth was just as exciting to Rod. Every time Rod jiggled the swing the little boy screamed with glee. Rod looked over at Julie and said, "This is really the best of life. Being with these little kids is kind of like going back in time and being a kid again yourself. They take you out of the messed up world of adults and make you see what's really more important…and that's just being with them, loving them and enjoying them."

Julie looked at Rod, surprised at how quickly he absorbed the role of being a parent. Just a few days ago he didn't even know he had a child. "Gosh, Rod. Isn't this amazing when you think about it. Here we are together again…you and Martina and Freebird and me…and now we have our babies. How these tiny little persons have changed our lives."

Rod nodded at the truth of her observation. "Our lives have been enriched because of them. They make us people of substance. They renew our lives. We get to enjoy childhood all over again just by watching them. Everything is a new experience to them. I guess what I'm trying to say is that they give us back wonder. If that makes any sense."

"Yeh, Rod. It makes a lot of sense to me"

"What makes sense?" Martina asked, balancing a tray with sippy cups, glasses of lemonade and Rod's frothy protein shake. She had him on a regimen of three protein shakes a day for nutrition and weight gain.

"We were talking about how having kids changes your life for the better," Rod said, as he fondled Roddy's curly head.

"But only someone who really understands what it is to be a parent would know that," Martina said. "I know that having Roddy sure changed my life. I can't even imagine life without him now."

"Speaking of that," said Rod, "I owe my life and the lives of my wife and son to Freebird. I don't know how I can ever repay him for all that he's done. And you, too, Julie."

Julie blushed. "Don't be silly, Rod. You have done great things for us as well. That's what families do. They watch each others' backs. We are a family and being scattered and apart for two years doesn't change that."

Rod stood up and pulled Martina and Julie into his arms for a three-way hug just as Freebird entered the yard through the back gate.

"What's going on here?" Freebird shouted, pretending to be outraged. "I invite Rod to stay at my house and I find him making himself at home with my wife." They all turned and laughed.

"We were just talking about you," said Rod.

"No wonder my ears were burning," Freebird joked, as he gave both Julie and Martina a kiss. "May I join in with this love fest?"

"Sure. Where's my kiss?" Rod asked, sitting down in his chair with mock indignation. Freebird bent down and gave Rod the usual biker brothers' hug.

"How you feeling, Bro?" Freebird sized up Rod's face. "Your color is better."

"Can't do much else but sit in the sun and drink these protein shakes," said Rod.

"What do you expect? You've got two years of sinnin' to make up for," Freebird teased.

"Your home early today," Rod noted. "What's up?"

"We always leave early on Friday's. It's tradition in the construction trade. The guys get their paychecks and head to the nearest bars to spend it. But not me. I have to come home early to keep an eye on you." Freebird knuckled Rod in the arm. "I suppose you can't drink a beer while you're drinking your formula?"

"No. Beer and milk don't mix to well. I'll have one with you later."

"We're taking the babies in for their lunch," Julie called over to Freebird and Rod. The two men watched their wives untangle the babies' legs and feet from the kiddy seats.

Freebird looked over at Rod. His expression was now serious. "Did you talk to Martina about where you're going to live?"

Rod emitted a deep sigh and nodded. He wasn't looking forward to telling Freebird what he and Martina had decided. "Much as I will hate leaving you and Julie and my other family behind, I've decided that it would be best if we made a fresh start in California. That whole thing with Carol really capped it."

Freebird nodded and looked away. "I can understand your decision. But I don't like it."

"Nor do I, Brother. Nor do I." Grabbing Freebird's arm, Rod said, "I don't know how to thank you...or even repay you...for saving Martina and Roddy. Every time I think about Roddy in that car with

319

Carol I get sick to my stomach. You saved my son, Brother. How can I ever thank you enough for that."

"Your 'thank you' is enough for me. You know that. Of course, I would do anything in my power to help you and your family. You would do the same for me and my family. Our families are one." Freebird paused for a moment to consider his next words. "To tell you the truth Rod...I don't know how Roddy was saved. When I got to the quarry pond I did not see anyone. Then I saw the ripples in the water and knew it was the car sinking down to the bottom of the pond. I thought I had gotten there too late. I completely lost it. How could I come back and tell you I was not able to save your little son. Then, like out of thin air, I heard Roddy calling me. I turned and there he was. I am still very mystified by it. I think your son is a shape shifter. I believe he somehow escaped from that car. Perhaps he became a fish and swam up out of the water. He was soaking wet when he appeared. But he was not even upset or scared. In fact, he tried to comfort me."

Rod sat quietly for a while, not knowing what to say. Freebird's account of finding Roddy at the quarry was too much for him to absorb at the moment. Finally, he thought to ask, "Did you see him in the water? Maybe he was in the water and just blended in."

"No, Rod. It happened just as I described. I did not see anything in the water except ripples from the sinking car. If I had seen Roddy in there I would have jumped right in to get him. Unless he came up out of the water when I had my face pressed to the ground. I was very upset. I didn't even know if I was in the right place. I was starting to doubt the vision Spirit had shown me. And then, like I said, Roddy was suddenly there. I can only thank Spirit. But I think the boy has special powers too." Seeing how white Rod's face had become Freebird didn't dare mention anything about the swirling mist that had appeared over the lake, he knew that would be too much for Rod to make sense of.

Rod quietly thought about what Freebird said for a few moments. "I still think you saved him. Even if you claim you didn't physically pull him out of the water. You knew where he was. Maybe Spirit intervened, but you were there for him with your special powers. You brought him home. And you found Martina too. You can't deny you saved them both."

"Your brother Travis helped also. If he had not called me from the hospital to tell me you were there, I would not have known Carol had lied to Julie. Carol told Julie you had gone to the house on Scenic Drive to meet a plumber. We would have been none the wiser if Travis hadn't called and told us you were in the hospital. I don't know how Carol knew that you were supposed to meet up with Martina later in the afternoon, but she seemed to have the timing just right." Freebird paused to ponder the miraculous intersession of Travis's telephone call. What had prompted Travis to call at just that moment? If he had called a minute or two later, what then might have happened? What if Travis had not called at all? Freebird sighed and looked at Rod for a few seconds before he spoke. "You, Martina and Roddy walk in Spirit's protection. That is the only explanation."

"I guess we're lucky," Rod offered.

"Where do you think that luck comes from?" Freebird said.

*****

The elder McDonoughs were back from the Bahamas and were hosting a "reunion" dinner Monday night for their family. The Terrys were of course invited, as they were considered family as well. On Monday afternoon Martina and Julie were busy in the kitchen preparing a broccoli casserole and a cake to bring to the dinner. Rod and the babies were napping, so they worked quickly to get everything done before, as Julie laughingly remarked, "all three kids" woke up.

"I'm kind of nervous about meeting Rod's parents," Martina confided.

"You shouldn't be, Marty. They're great people and I know they'll just love you." Looking up with her wide-eyed expression, she added, "And wait till they see little Roddy. They'll be just as goofy over him as you say your Aunt and Uncle are. Besides, your meeting them is long overdue."

Martina nodded, looking down at the eggs she was beating for the casserole's cream sauce. "I don't know, Julie.

Remember how they hired an attorney to protect Rod from any claims that the baby was his. It sure didn't seem as though they had any love for me then, even though I was Rod's wife."

"But they had never met you. They didn't know anything about you...other than your father shot their son," Julie pointed out, then assured Martina, "Once they meet you they will love you just the way we all do. And I told them that back when I met them in the hospital, when we went to see Rod."

Martina looked up at Julie, a quizzical expression on her face. "You met them before? What did you say to them about me?"

"Oh— We ran into them at the hospital quite a few times. They practically lived there when Rod was laid up. Maggie...Mrs. McDonough...she asked me about you. I told them how you and Rod and Freebird and I got married together and how much you and Rod loved each other. They wanted to know why you ran away and I told them about taking you to the airport and how you were scared to death of your father. Of course, they heard the ugly rumors around town. Maggie asked me if what they heard was true. I told her that it was just gossip and not to pay attention. I knew your baby was Rod's and told her so." Julie put down the mixing bowl she was holding and met her friend's querying gaze. "I told her you were a sweet and loving person."

Seeing tears flowing down Martina's face, Julie ran to embrace her. "Everything will be fine tonight," Julie comforted, "Maggie and Jim will just love you. We've all moved on from the past." Julie could not know that Martina's tears came from the haunting guilt she felt about the fact the ugly rumors were partially true. She knew she owed it to Julie to some day, soon, tell her the truth. But not today. Today, she had enough to deal with.

Everyone was dressed in their finest and ready to leave by six-thirty, and they piled into Julie's sedan. Rod sat in the back seat with Roddy on his lap; Martina sat next to him, holding the warm casserole dish on hers. She wore a ruby red silk blouse and matching challis skirt, and she had pulled her hair back and tied it at the nape of her neck. Rod eyed her and knew she was nervous. "You look very nice," he said. "That color red is definitely yours."

She smiled, tentative and nervous. "Thank you." Martina studied Rod's face for a moment. "You look good," she commented. "You are getting back your healthy color and I think you've even put on a few pounds."

"Exactly four pounds," Rod reported. "And I am starting to feel like my old self. In a week or so I am going to start working out again." He saw her worried expression. "I'll take it slow and easy. Don't worry."

Martina was not prepared for the jitters that assailed her when Freebird nosed the car between the familiar stone pylons that marked the McDonough driveway. It was a combination of nervousness at the prospect of meeting Rod's parents for the first time and the remembrance of the last time she was there. She quickly looked at Roddy and worried that he might react to being back at the house where he saw his mother attacked and where he was kidnapped by the maniacal Carol Bennett. But he seemed to be contentedly sucking his thumb and looking out the window.

Alerting Rod, Martina said, "We need to keep an eye on Roddy. He may have a problem with going into this house again...you know...since—"

Rod nodded his understanding. "Just be cool and he will see that we are okay with it."

When Rod and Martina got out of the car they could see that Roddy was staring wide-eyed at the house, looking like he was about to cry. Freebird was suddenly beside them. "Give me the boy," said Freebird, gesturing to Rod, who was holding Roddy tight against his chest in a protective manner. Rod had learned long ago to never question Freebird's actions, so he handed Roddy to his Shaman friend without hesitation. Taking the child into his sinewy arms, Freebird talked softly to the little boy in his native language. Rod and Martina could barely hear what Freebird had said, much less understand it even if they could. Then, it seemed that Freebird inclined his head to Roddy's ear and gently blew into it. Suddenly, the boy laughed and hugged the Shaman. Gently, Freebird handed the boy back to his father, saying only, "He will have no memories of it now," in his usual cryptic style. Rod and Martina merely looked at each other in wonder. They could see that Roddy was no longer frightened by the house. In fact, the boy was pointing at the lighted porch excitedly and jabbering in his own native language.

Freebird then took Jody from her car seat and stood waiting for Julie to join him, his stoic expression revealing nothing of what just happened. Julie appeared with the cake and a tote bag full of baby accoutrements. "Okay," she said brightly, "We're all organized. Let's go have a wonderful dinner."

As soon as they neared the door to the back porch, the aromas of cooking food struck them head on. "Something smells good," said Rod.

"I think a roast...maybe lamb," Martina chimed in.

Maggie and Jim McDonough came rushing out onto the porch to greet their family. There were plenty of hugs, kisses and moist eyes to go around, but Roddy and Jody were the stars of the reunion. Jim and Maggie fawned over both babies as though both were equally their grandchildren.

"Oh— They're so beautiful!" Maggie exclaimed with delight. "My goodness! Roddy looks just like Rod when he was that age. It's remarkable! And look at those great big brown eyes Jody has. She looks like her daddy, too."

Martina let out a long-held sigh of relief. Rod took her arm, "Mom! Dad! This is my lovely wife, Martina. He was happy to see that his parents did not hesitate to give her hugs and kisses too.

"We've heard so many wonderful things about you, my dear," Maggie exclaimed to Martina. "We must spend lots of time together and get to know each other better," she said, with sincerity and warmth, while holding onto Martina's arm.

"I would love that, Mrs. McDonough," Martina responded, feeling accepted already.

Maggie McDonough lovingly pinched Martina's cheek. "I want you to call me 'Mom'," she insisted. "I am your Mother by marriage and you are a part of our family."

Martina felt the tears well up in her eyes, but could not stop them.

Rod's father, who was now holding Roddy, immediately spoke up, "And I want you to call me 'Dad', Martina." Saying that, he gave her a kiss on the other cheek. "Welcome to our family."

"Well isn't this is a homey scene," said a voice at the back door. They all turned to see Travis and a cute young woman with short black hair standing in the door way.

"Travis!" shouted his Mother, excited to have her family around her again. "And this must be Nancy," she said, addressing the young woman holding Travis's hand.

Raising his voice over the din, Travis called out, "Let me introduce everyone to my sweetheart, Nancy Farnsworth." Practically in unison, the others all said, "Hi Nancy." Maggie and Jim swarmed toward their newly arrived son and his adorable girlfriend. The room was soon filled with exhilarated chatter.

As soon as Rod could get a word in, he introduced himself to Nancy. "I'm Travis's brother, Rod." He studied her face for a moment. "I feel as though I've met you before."

Nancy laughed. "You did. At the hospital. I am a nurse in the Emergency Room."

Rod felt his face flush hot. "Ohmygod! I hope I didn't leave you with a bad impression."

Shaking her head, Nancy replied, "Not at all, Rod. I'm glad to see you looking so well."

"I have my wife to thank for that." Rod called to Martina to get her attention. "Come here and meet Nancy."

Martina hugged Nancy like she was an old friend. "So nice to see you again."

"You two know each other?" said Rod, perplexed.

"We met at the hospital," Martina said.

"In a way, I have you to thank for meeting Travis," Nancy told Rod. "So I have lots of good thoughts about you. Don't worry."

Rod smiled. Relieved. "Have you met my brother Freebird and his wife Julie?" Rod gestured to the nearby couple, who were talking with Maggie and Jim.

"Yes. I met them at the hospital, as well…when they came to see you," Nancy said. "But this is the first time I have met your parents. They are wonderful." Nancy looked around, smiling at the convivial group and squeezing Travis's hand approvingly. This was just the kind of family she hoped to marry into.

The dinner was fabulous. Maggie McDonough heaped praises on Martina's broccoli and cream sauce casserole and Julie's deliciously light coffee cake. There were numerous toasts to the new members of the family, to the good health and bright futures of Roddy and Jody, and to the good fortune of Rod and Martina in their new beginnings in California. Of course, there were as many tears as there were joyful smiles.

"We've always wanted to travel to California," said Jim McDonough. "Now we'll have a reason to go and a place to stay." Turning to Rod and Martina, he asked, "Do you have a place for us to stay there?"

"We sure do," piped up Martina. "We have a large apartment in Pacific Heights in San Francisco and you are welcome to come and stay anytime."

Rod added, "Eventually, we'll get a house. They're way ahead of us on new housing design out there…I've been reading up on it. They're already into solar power and wind energy."

"Really." Jim McDonough said, perking up his ears. "I'd be interested in hearing more about that, Rod."

"I've got a few magazine articles on the subjects I'll give to you. I'm already checking into who the major construction players are out there," Rod told his father. "I want to hit the ground running when I get out there. I'd like to get with one of those ecologically-oriented builders I've been reading about."

Jim McDonough looked at Rod with pride and felt more reassured about his son's big move across country. And even though Rod felt pretty confident he would land on his feet in California, it felt good to have his father's confidence too.

Automatically, Rod put his arm around Martina and kissed her on the cheek. Roddy tugged on his father's shirt sleeve. "Dah-dee. Pot-tee," said the little boy. Rod stood up to take the boy to the bathroom. "Excuse me," he said to his own father, "I'm the newly appointed potty instructor."

"Well..." Maggie McDonough commented, "Isn't he doing good at his age to be potty trained."

Martina smiled at her mother-in-law and said, "Now if only I can get him weaned...."

Maggie McDonough cracked up laughing. "Sounds like he takes right after his daddy with that. I didn't think I'd ever get Rod weaned." Turning to her husband, Maggie slapped Jim on the arm. "Remember the trouble we had with Rod, Jim? Getting him to take a bottle."

"Oh, yeh." said Jim. "He'd pitch a terrible fit if she tried to give him a bottle."

Martina felt vindicated. "I'll have to tell my Aunt Catherine about that. She blames me for not being firm enough with Roddy. I'll admit I'm a softy...but ever since he's been spending time with Rod he seems less interested. It's Rod who got him potty trained. He wants to be a big boy like his Daddy."

Rod's Mother smiled, amazed by the turn of events. She was just happy that Rod was reunited with his wife and child, and all seemed to be going very well between them. And, after all, Martina did seem like a sweet and responsible young woman. She had certainly done a good job raising their grandson. The boy was healthy and well-behaved. And she had done wonders for Rod in just the few days they had gotten back together. After Rod and Travis had filled them in on all the details, Jim and Maggie McDonough decided they knew all they needed to know about the matter of the shooting, Martina's disappearance, Rod's addiction, and everything else. It was time to put it all behind them, and look to a more pleasant and family-oriented future with their sons, the lives they have chosen, and the women they chose to love. And, now, they were blessed with a beautiful grandson they did not know they had, so their focus was to spend as much time as possible with all of them.

"This has been a wonderful night," Jim McDonough announced. "How about another Scotch, Travis?"

"Just a short one, Dad. I'm not much of an imbiber."

"Well…if ever there was an occasion, this is it," said the elder McDonough.

"I'll drink to that," said Travis.

Maggie turned to Martina and said, "Let's get together for lunch, either tomorrow or Wednesday. I want to spend as much time as possible with you, Rod & the baby before you all leave. When is your flight scheduled?"

"It's next Sunday afternoon. At two o'clock," said Martina.

"Julie!" Maggie McDonough called across the table to the young woman. "I want you and Jody to come for lunch also."

"Thank you, Maggie. That will be fun," Julie said.

Maggie smiled at Julie. "At least I'll have you, Clayton and Jody close by."

"Don't run a guilt trip on us, Mom," said Rod, who had just returned to the dining room with Roddy.

Travis chimed in, "I'm not leaving you, Mom."

"C'mon you guys," Martina appealed, "You're making us feel like traitors."

Jim McDonough cleared his throat and they all turned in his direction. "Let's not make Rod and Martina feel bad. After what they have both been through in this town, it's no wonder they want to make a fresh start someplace else. None of us want them to leave…because we love them dearly. And who knows that they won't come back."

"Here-Here!" said Freebird, raising his cup of herbal tea.

65.

The remainder of the week flew by, but it was amazing how many family gatherings they managed to pack into those five days before Rod, Martina and Roddy were to leave. Martina made time every day for them to visit with Rod's mother and father.

They left Roddy with his "Amma2" twice while they went shopping to find some clothes for Rod to pack. He insisted on not buying too many slacks and shirts because he knew he would be gaining more weight. He bought some new black jeans and polo shirts, which he favored for casual dress. He also found some of his old T-shirts, dress shirts and suits at his parents' house, so he felt he had enough clothes for the present.

Martina had merely informed her Aunt and Uncle that she was coming home with a huge surprise and left them to speculate about what it could be. They were encouraged by the new ebullience they detected in her tone, as they had worried endlessly that the trip to Millborough would bring her nothing but painful memories.

"Perhaps she was able to sell the house," Aunt Catherine ruminated.

Uncle Jack proclaimed, "I think she met up with an old boyfriend."

"Don't be silly, Jack," Catherine chided, "Martina has always said she lost the only love of her life when she lost Rod. She's never even been interested in dating again."

"Things change, my dear," Jack said.

"Well, I don't know about that," said Catherine, "but I surely cannot wait for her and Roddy to come home. I don't care if she brings a pet elephant."

Jack merely nodded his assent.

* * * * *

All of the family showed up at the airport to give Rod, Martina and Roddy a proper send-off. Rod's parents promised to come out for a visit around Thanksgiving. Travis and Nancy said they would love to see San Francisco and take a side trip to Tahoe to go skiing. Freebird and Julie talked about going out to visit them for Christmas.

Maggie McDonough gave Martina a special going-away gift, a beautiful fire opal ring in an antique gold filigree setting. It had belonged to her mother. Martina was stunned by the beauty of the ring and what it signified − that Maggie had truly accepted her as a daughter. "I will treasure it always, Mom," she told Maggie, "and if I have a daughter I will pass it on to her when she is old enough."

Maggie hugged Martina, and said, "Are you and Rod planning on having more children?"

"Absolutely, Mom. Roddy shall have brothers and sisters."

Epilogue

About four months after Freebird's amazing vision and rescue of Roddy at Old Quarry Lake, the police were still perplexed about how he knew where to look for the child. Officers Duggan and Grady were sure Freebird had supernatural abilities that might be useful to the Department with their cold case investigations. Of course, they were careful not to allude to the precise reason they were recommending to the Chief of the Millborough Police Department why they should hire Freebird as a "Technical Advisor", citing only the young Indian's uncanny tracking skills.

Rod and Martina both recovered nicely from their respective ordeals at the hands of Carol Bennett, and Roddy seemed to suffer no ill effects either, thanks to Freebird's Shamanic ministrations.

When Aunt Catherine and Uncle Jack went to the airport to pick up Martina and Roddy, they were amazed to see that Martina had found a boyfriend whom so closely resembled Roddy. They were, of course, shocked when he was introduced by Martina as "Rod McDonough, my husband and Roddy's father." Rod and Martina spent that night telling them the whole story of how they found each other. Of course, the Denault's were delighted to welcome Rod to the family and ecstatic that Roddy now had his father. Rod, Uncle Jack and Shotgun soon became fast friends. After meeting Rod, Chloe Renfrew then completely understood why Martina had been so devoted to his "memory".

Within weeks of his move to California, Rod landed a job as a construction supervisor with Casa Verde Homes, a company that specialized in building earth friendly, solar powered houses. And within six months of kicking his addiction, Rod had regained most of his weight, muscle, and virility. To pacify Martina's aunt and uncle, the couple renewed their wedding vows with a beautifully orchestrated church ceremony. For his wedding gift to his bride, Rod gave Martina the keys to one of Casa Verde's custom built homes with all of the earth friendly bells and whistles, which was built over a creek in a woodsy enclave of Marin County that Casa Verde named Eco-logical Village. They did, however, keep their apartment in San Francisco to use as a "get away" destination for themselves and for visiting friends and family.

A year after their San Francisco wedding, Rod and Martina welcomed their baby daughter, whom they named Lani, after Martina's maternal great grandmother. Roddy was very proud of his big brother status.

Within three months of their meeting on that fateful day at Millborough Hospital, Travis McDonough and Nancy Farnsworth were married in a big church wedding and got right to the business of starting a family. Of course, Rod, Martina, and Roddy did return to Millborough just long enough to attend the wedding and reception, since Rod was the best man, Martina a bridesmaid, Roddy the ring bearer, and Jody the flower girl. Roddy and Jody stole the show.

Maggie and Jim McDonough sold their boat and took up permanent residence in their beloved stone house on Scenic Drive, and awaited the arrival of more grandchildren. They made frequent trips to California to spoil Roddy and Lani, and to prod their son and daughter-in-law into having more babies.

Oddly, the abandoned Georgian house that belonged to the Estate of Martino Fiasconi mysteriously burnt to the ground on the very day that Rod, Martina, and Roddy returned to California after attending Travis and Nancy's wedding. There was no official consensus as to the cause of the fire but it was agreed that the fire had started in Martina's old bedroom.

With Jody's playmate, Roddy, living so far away, Julie was able to talk Freebird into increasing the size of their family — it was an easy sell for Julie. They soon had another daughter, whom they named Wiyanna. And with his family now outgrowing their tiny house in Millborough, Freebird decided it was time he talked to Julie about the promise he had made to his parents. Within months of Wiyanna's birth, Freebird, Julie and the girls moved to a beautiful, new home on the Pequot Reservation in Connecticut, where Freebird took his place as a tribal healer alongside his father. A year after their move Freebird and Julie presented Hayward and Selma with another grandchild, this time a boy, whom they named Hayward Clay. Grandfather Hayward was fond of joking that Freebird turned out to be a "Blue Chip Stock: He keeps on paying dividends."

In nature, as the world turns round and round and the green of summer turns to the bright colored foliage of autumn, after which the dormancy of winter gives way to the great rebirth of spring; the earth is constantly replenished and renewed. With people, the passage of time causes the happenings of life to fade from the forefront of their respective awareness, while newer, more interesting happenings replace

331

the old. Life, too, follows its own seasons and seeks to renew and better itself by sloughing off that which is no longer suitable to hold onto.

And so it came to pass that the events which took place in the town of Millborough on July 18, 1975 also faded from the forefront of awareness. Nobody gave much thought to the deeds of Martino Fiasconi or even Carol Bennett anymore.

The End

ABOUT THE AUTHOR

ALBERTA L. MASON now lives in Central Florida and travels extensively. She attended Suffolk University, Boston, Massachusetts; San Francisco State University, San Francisco, California; and the University of Central Florida, Orlando, Florida; and has worked as a public relations copywriter in a California advertising agency and a reporter for a Florida newspaper. Ms. Mason has also been a community organizer and a consumer rights activist. She is currently at work on her next novel.

Visit Author's Websites at:

http://www.albertamason.info/

http://www.lulu.com/spotlight/albertamason